KININS—II
Biochemistry, Pathophysiology,
and Clinical Aspects

ADVANCES IN EXPERIMENTAL MEDICINE AND BIOLOGY

KININS—II
Biochemistry, Pathophysiology, and Clinical Aspects

Edited by

Setsuro Fujii
Institute for Protein Research
Osaka University
Osaka, Japan

Hiroshi Moriya
Science University of Tokyo
Tokyo, Japan

and

Tomoji Suzuki
Meiji College of Pharmacy
Tokyo, Japan

PLENUM PRESS • NEW YORK AND LONDON 1979

Library of Congress Cataloging in Publication Data

International Symposium on Kinins, Tokyo, 1978.
  Kinins II.

  (Advances in experimental medicine and biology; v. 120)
  Includes index.
  1. Kinins—Congresses. 2. Kallikrein—Congresses. I. Fujii, Setsuro, 1925-
II. Moriya, Hiroshi. III. Suzuki, Tomoji. IV. Title. V. Series.
QP552.K5I55 1978   615.7   79-9079
ISBN 0-306-40196-7 (part A)

Proceedings of the International Symposium on Kinins,
held in Tokyo, Japan, November 6–9, 1978.

© 1979 Plenum Press, New York
A Division of Plenum Publishing Corporation
227 West 17th Street, New York, N.Y. 10011

Preface

In this brief historical retrospect of kinin studies, we
recall the discovery of bradykinin by Professor M. Rocha e Silva
and the pioneer investigations on tissue kallikrein initiated by
Dr. E.K. Frey followed by the work of Professor H. Kraut and
Professor E. Werle who opened the way for the present flourishing
investigations of kinins. The elucidation of the structure of
bradykinin by Dr. F. Elliott in 1960 stimulated further research
of the vasoactive peptides. During the following years, the
physiological and pathological significance of kinins was explored
extensively, resulting in the rapid accumulation of information
regarding their potential importance. Tremendous progress in
our understanding of the involvement of the kallikrein-kinin system
in many physiological phenomena has been facilitated by the
friendly atmosphere among "kininologists" engendered at previous
international kinin symposia. During that time studies were
reported as to the role of kinins in functional vasodilation,
alteration of blood pressure and vascular permeability, shock,
inflammation, and pain production. Thus, through knowledge from
these basic studies, the action of kinins in morbidity is better
understood as are the counter measures for many diseases associated
with kinin formation.

Recent **discoveries** have focused on abnormally delayed blood
coagulation in the hereditary deficiency of high molecular weight
kininogen together with prekallikrein deficiency. Thus great **strides**
have been made in elucidating the interrelationships amongst the
blood coagulation, fibrinolysis, and vasopeptide kinin systems.
Moreover, apart from the aforementioned role of bradykinin as a
pharmacologically active substance, other important findings
involving the coordinated actions of prostaglandin and catecholamine
biosynthesis, particularly in the inflammatory process, have enhanced our appreciation of the complexity of the vasopeptide kinin
system.

The participation of more than 330 scientists from 16 countries
of the world in this International Symposium on Kinins-Kinin '78
Tokyo reflects accurately the interest and research activity in the

diverse and broad implications of the physiological and pathological functions of the kallikrein-kinin system. A total of 128 papers, including posters, were presented, attesting to the unquestioned success of the KININ '78 TOKYO Symposium. This volume in two sections contains the collective studies presented, studies of high scientific standard that provoked lively discussions. Also included in this volume are the two plenary lectures presented by Dr. K. Austen (USA) and Dr. Hamao Umezawa (JAPAN).

In the future, further closer exchange of information among investigators from varied bio-medical disciplines will contribute significantly to our understanding of the important roles played by the kallikrein-kinin and interrelated systems. Thus will the scope of the kinin studies be broadened thereby enhancing our appreciation of cell physiology as well as the possible clinical impact of the system.

On behalf of the Organizing Committee, the editors of this volume express their sincere gratitude for the support of the Ministry of Education, The Scientific Council of Japan, and the following academic societies in the various branches of medical science: The Japanese Biochemical Society, The Japanese Pharmacological Society, The Pharmaceutical Society of Japan, The Japan Hematological Society, Japanese College of Angiology, The Japanese Rheumatism Association, and the Japanese Society of Allergology. The editors also express their gratitude for the generous financial help provided by the Japan World Exposition Commemorative Fund and other Foundations and Corporations.

The editors deeply appreciate the dedicated assistance of Professor N. Back (USA) for helping facilitate the publication of this volume. Appreciation also is extended to Ms. Patricia Poczkalski of the State University of New York for her skillful transcription of the manuscripts to uniform type seen in this volume, and to Mr. Derrick Mancini, Editor at Plenum Press, and his associates for their cooperation in publishing attractively and speedily this volume. The editors express their indebtedness to Aaron I. Back for his meticulous proofreading of the manuscripts.

Setsuro Fujii
Hiroshi Moriya
Tomoji Suzuki

Contents

PHYSIOLOGICAL-PATHOLOGICAL SIGNIFICANCE OF KININS

CLINICAL SIGNIFICANCE OF KININS

PRESENTATION OF A FILM ON THE "CENTRAL EFFECTS OF BRADYKININ"

M. Rocha e Silva

Department of Pharmacology, Faculty of Medicine: USP,

Ribeirão Preto, São Paulo, Brazil

It was indeed the extraordinary kindness of the Japanese people in general, and most especially of Profs. Suzuki, Moriya, Katori, and all those mentioned in the Program, who made this Symposium a real feast of understanding, cordiality and exchange of information in the Kinin-field. It is a great pleasure to be present to this new Symposium on Kinins - Kinin 78 Tokyo. Soon we may start to stress the year with a subscript, because this year we had at least one more meeting in Paris, in July 1978 on Concepts of Kinin Research, organized by Profs. G. Haberland and U. Hamberg, and that filled a whole Saturday, immediately after the mammoth VII International Congress of Pharmacology.

Since its discovery in 1948, at the Instituto Biologico in São Paulo, Brazil, BRADYKININ and BRADYKININOGEN became important items of medical and biomedical literature, as peptide mediators of pain, in cardio-vascular phenomena, smooth muscle contraction, inflammation, regulation of blood pressure, and so forth. Their inbreeding with the enzymatic system in plasma: pre-kininogenin-kininogenin (or kininogenase = kallikrein system) expanded their field of application to a number of physio-pathological events, especially their implication in clotting events, shock, inflammatory reactions, and in the mechanism of regulation of blood pressure, coupled with the angiotensinogen-angiotensin system, as evidenced by the interaction of BPF or BPP peptide factor also originated from venoms as first studied in our laboratory by Dr. Sergio Ferreira.

All that has been of major concern in the many Symposia on Kinins, and we see that this one will not be an exception. If I am allowed to trace back the history of BRADYKININ, I have to stress that the first Symposium of this kind was the one held in Montreal in 1953, organized by von Euler and myself, on the

1

occasion of the International Congress of Physiology. For the publication of this Symposium, Prof. Gaddum assembled us and succeeded in publishing the Proceedings in 1955, in the form of a book in Edinburgh (E.& S. Livingstone), under the name of "Polypeptides which stimulate plain muscle". There, Bradykinin, Substance-P and Angiotensin were already discussed together, as done in this Symposium, though, in a very preliminary way. We should not forget that by that time Bradykinin was my own property, Substance-P von Euler's property, and Angiotensin Braun-Menendez' and Page's property. We had to manufacture the powders to send them as gifts to friends!

After that, came the Symposium organized by Schachter, at the Wellcome Foundation, in London, in 1959, under the name of "Polypeptides which affect smooth muscle and blood vessels", the Proceedings of which were published by Pergamon Press. It was at this Symposium that the first announcement of the sequence of Bradykinin was presented by Prof. Elliott, from Mill Hill, subsequently shown to lack one of the critical prolines in the bradykinin molecule. The group of Sandoz, in Basle, based on Elliott's results, succeeded in synthesizing the real nonapeptide, that I present in the first slide, and which is very well known to the distinguished group here present. The nonapeptide so synthesized, with the name of Bradykinin, corresponded in its physical, chemical and physiological activity to the substance isolated a few years earlier (Andrade and Rocha e Silva, 1956) and so the other names, such as plasma-kinin, became obsolete. This was the culmination of the intensive work done at the Biological Institute of São Paulo, by Prado, Andrade, Beraldo Diniz and myself, joined later on by Hamberg, on the study of the mechanism of release of bradykinin by the protease of <u>Bothrops jararaca</u> and by trypsin.

Through the work of the people at Sandoz, in Basle, it became possible to study thoroughly the nonapeptide BRS 640 generously supplied to all researchers, as Synthetic Bradykinin. Since then the number of investigators grew exponentially, as well as the number of Symposia: in New York, at the New York Academy of Sciences, in 1963; in Florence, in 1965, organized by the group of Sicuteri; in Ribeirão Preto, in 1966, at the occassion of the III International Congress of Pharmacology, held in São Paulo. Then, in quick succesion, in Fiesole in 1969 and 1970, when the Academia Kininensis Fiesolana was founded; in 1972, in San Francisco, then in Fiesole again, in 1975, when the Symposium received the name of KININ 75, still with the efficient collaboration of the group of Sicuteri; then in Rio de Janeiro, as Kinin 76, and now this extraordinary KININ 78, TOKYO.

After the synthesis of BK and derivatives such as kallidin (Lysyl-BK) and Methionyl-lysyl-BK, first by the group of Sandoz with Boissonnas and colleagues, and then the isolation and synthesis of kallidin (Lys-BK) by the group to which the researchers Moriya, Webster, Pierce and others belonged, the studies of the action of kinins gained an enormous impetus, especially in combination with

the investigations on the action of proteases that release them
from the precursor in plasma, namely BKg. The names of kininogenin
and kallikrein have both been considered as acceptable by the Biochemical Nomenclature Committee of the International Union of Biochemistry. Also the inhibitors of trypsin and kallikrein among
them trasylol or aprotinin, have been investigated in full detail.
Though there was some discussion on nomenclature by the main groups
working in the field, there is a kind of agreement, this agreement
being typical of the present stage of this kind of symposium, as
we read in the Mainichi Daily News, of Monday, November 6, 1978, in
which Prof. Moriya very nicely referred to us as "The Kinin Family".
This kind of Symposium is becoming now an Annual Classic, since Sicuteri started to call it Kinin-75. We called it Kinin-76 in Rio
de Janeiro, and now our Japanese Friends call it Kinin-78, Tokyo.
    Prof. Moriya asked me to present a film, reminiscent of the ol-
dest days of Bradykinin and Bradykininogen. This was supposed to
be a long 16 mm film presented in Europe, on the occasion of the
International Congress of Physiology, held in Copenhagen in 1950,
immediately after the first publication on the discovery of "Bradykinin, hypotensive and smooth muscle stimulating factor released
from plasma by snake venoms and by trypsin" in the Am. J. Physiology 156, 261 (1949) in collaboration with my colleagues Beraldo and
Rosenfeld. However the film is too long and inappropriate for a
pre-prandial period. Instead, I selected a Super-8 colored film,
showing the Central Effects of Bradykinin, when injected by the
intracerebroventricular route, showing the reactions of a bunch of
lively rabbits to pure bradykinin. To my advice, such central effects of Bradykinin are of the utmost timely importance and were
first described in our laboratory by Corrado, Čapek and myself,
joined immediately afterwards by the group of Drs. Graeff and Irene
Pelá using 1 µg of synthetic (Sandoz, BRS 640) bradykinin. The
film actually is a complete commentary to a paper published in the
Brit. J. Pharmacol. 37, 723 (1969), by F. G. Graeff, I. R. Pelá and
M. Rocha e Silva, under the title "Behavioural and somatic effects
of bradykinin injected into the cerebral ventricles of unanesthetized rabbits". The main effect to be shown in the film is an
early phase of extreme agitation, followed by a phase of quietness
where analgesia and tranquillization occur, followed by a prolonged
phase of catatonia. Analgesia and catatonia, were later on studied
in detail, in our laboratory, by S.A. Ribeiro and Rocha e Silva, and
published in the Brit. J. Pharmacol. 47, 517 (1973), under the title "Antinoceptive action of bradykinin and related kinins of larger molecular weights by the intraventricular route."Catatonia was
also studied by G. Ribeiro da Silva and myself, and published in
the Eur. J. Pharmacology 15, 180 (1971), under the title: "Catatonia induced in the rabbit by intracerebral injection of bradykinin
and morphine".
    Before presenting the film, I am showing you a few slides to call
attention to the problem, starting with some views about the origins

of bradykinin and some further central effects of the peptide on
thermal regulation, obtained recently by Dr. Irene R. Pelá and her
group, and which will be presented to the VII Latin American Congress of Pharmacology to be held next month in São Paulo, Brazil.
To my advice, such results put bradykinin in the same foot as sero-
tonin, catecholamines and prostaglandins as possible mediators of
thermo-regulation in mammals.

I hope that such a long story has not withdrawn your appetite
for the banquet that follows. Thank you. Arigató and Bon Appétit.

Chemistry of Kinins
and Related Peptides

THE NEW VASOACTIVE PEPTIDES IN AMPHIBIAN SKIN

V. Erspamer*, T. Yasuhara**, and T. Nakajima**

*Department of Medical Pharmacology, University of Rome
Rome, Italy
**Institute of Pharmaceutical Sciences, Hiroshima University, School of Medicine, Hiroshima, Japan.

Amphibian skin contains large amounts of many biological active substances of low molecular weight, such as steroids, pseudo-alkaloids, amines and/or polypeptides which reveal the potent action or toxicity for the other mammals.

Erspamer and his collegues have demonstrated the presence of many types of active polypeptides from the amphibian skin, including bradykinins, caeruleins, physalaemins, bombesins, etc., during the past 15 years (Erspamer et al., 1976, Bertaccini, 1976). From the outstanding research originating from his laboratory, we have also demonstrated the presence of some other polypeptides, such as ranatensin, xenopsin, thyrotropin releasing hormone and granuliberin-R, from the amphibian skin (Yasuhara and Nakajima, 1975, Nakajima, 1976, Nakajima and Yasuhara, 1977). As a result of cooperative work between both laboratories, chemical characterization of yet another vasoactive polypeptide has been elucidated.

The species of amphibians we examined in our laboratory, were Uperoleia, Litoria, Heleophryne and Crinia, in which the presence of active polypeptides has been pointed out by Erspamer et al. (1976). Uperoleia rugosa contains litorin-like and uperolein-like peptides. Heleophryne purcelli contains bradykinin-like peptides, and Crinia georgiana contains angiotensin-like peptides in the skin.

Isolation of the peptides in the skin of Uperoleia rugosa: Dried skin of 100g obtained from 1500 frogs were extracted with 80% methanol and the syrupy residue of the evaporated extract was

dissolved in 95% ethanol. The liquid was then passed through
aluminum columns which were eluted with decending concentrations
of ethanol, starting from 95% of the solvent.

The active principles were separated into 3 fractions, fraction
A, B, and C, and were eluted with 95%, 90%, and 60% ethanol respectively. The peptide in fraction A was subsequently purified with
droplet counter current chromatography with the solvent system of
n-butanol:acetic acid:water (4:1:5), with Sephadex LH-20, and with
Sephadex G-10 column chromatography, using ammonium formate in 50%
methanol or ammonium formate as the elution buffer.

Similarly, the peptide in fraction B was purified with Sephadex
LH-20 and Sephadex G-10 column chromatography. The peptide in
fractions A and B showed the property of becoming insoluble during
the purification procedure, and the insoluble materials formed in
the lyophilizate were of pure amino acid composition.

The active principle in fraction C mixture was separated
further in 2 active principles, C-I and -II by SP-Sephadex column
chromatography. These active principles were subsequently purified
with Sephadex G-25 and Sephadex LH-20 column chromatography.

The chemical characterization of the peptides in the skin of
Uperoleia rugosa. The amino acid composition of both peptides
obtained from fractions A and B, after usual acid hydrolysis, was
the same as that of litorin. The active principle in fraction B
was identified with litorin by co-chromatography of the standard.
The fragments of enzymatic digestion of the peptide with chymotrypsin
were also coincided chromatographically to those obtained from
the standard litorin.

The active principle in fraction A showed different RF values
(0.82) from those of Glu(OMe)^2-litorin (0.63) or litorin (0.51)
when chromatographed on thin layer Silica gel with the solvent
system of n-butanol:pyridine:acetic acid:water (4:1:1:1). When
the peptide was digested with chymotrypsin, the fragments produced
from the C-terminal region of the peptide were the same as those
from the litorin region, namely Ala-Val-Gly-His-Phe and methionine
amide. The intact peptide was digested with pyrrolidone carboxyl
peptidase, which was purified from Bacillus amyloliquefacience
(Tsuru et al., 1978), dansylated and successively digested with
a mixture of chymotrypsin and carboxypeptidase A. The dansyl
fragment was identical to dansyl glutamic acid γ-ethyl ester by
thin layer chromatography. The active principle in fraction A
was deduced to Glu(γ-OEt)^2-litorin as the result of these experiments (Fig. 1.).

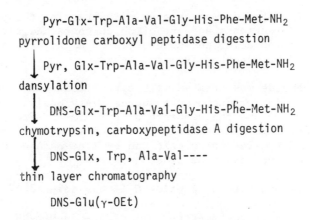

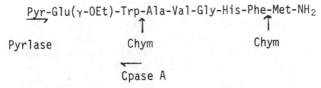

Figure 1.   Scheme of sequential degradation of $Glu(\gamma-OEt)^2-$
litorin.

The peptide in fraction C-I was identical to uperolein by co-
chromatography with uperolein on a thin layer of Silica gel, by
determination of the amino acid composition, and by the peptide
mapping analysis after the peptide was cleft with sodium in liquid
ammonia.

The peptide in fraction C-II was a new one, and composed of
one mole each of lysine, aspartic acid, threonine, glutamic acid,
proline, glycine, alanine, methionine, leucine, tyrosine and
phenylalanine, which was determined from its usual acid hydrolysate
by an amino acid analyser. This composition was similar to that of
physalaemin except additional threonine and lacking of 1 mole of
aspartic acid. The N-terminal amino acid could not be detected by
dansyl method.

When the peptide was cleft by Birch reduction, 1 mole of aspartic acid residue in the composition was lost by this procedure,
suggesting Asx-Pro bond in the sequence. The peptide cleft by
chymotrypsin digestion, produced the same C-terminal fragment,
$Gly-Leu-Met-NH_2$, which was identified by dansyl method and by
chromatography. This suggested that the C-terminal region of the
peptide was the same to physalaemin.

When the peptide was treated with trypsin, the peptide was cleft into 2 fragments and one of which contained threonine as an N-terminal amino acid, and no dansylated amino acid except ε-dansyl lysine could be detected from the other.

The peptide was treated with pyrrolidone carboxyl peptidase and the reaction products were successively analysed by dansyl-Edman procedure and the sequence of Pyr-Ala-Asx-Pro-Lys-Thr-Phe-Tyr- was obtained. Aspartic acid at position 3 was considered to be free acid by electrophoretic and by ionexchange chromatographic behaviors of the intact peptide.

The sequence of the peptide C-II was deduced as follows:

Pyr-Ala-Asp-Pro-Lys-Thr-Phe-Tyr-Gly-Leu-Met-NH$_2$

From the skin extract of Uperoleia rugosa, we have identified four kinds of active polypeptides. One of which was a new physalaemin type peptide. Two of which, uperolein and litorin, have already elucidated from this frog (Erspamer et al., 1974). On the estimation of naturally occurring of the last one, Glu(γ-OEt)^2-litorin, as well as Glu(γ-OMe)^2-litorin, which was recently characterized in the methanol extracts of the skin of Litoria aurea (Anastasi et al., 1978), it is not known whether these peptides pre-exist in the tissue or are the artifact produced during purification procedure. However, we cannot neglect the probability of the existence of the more unstable form of litorin, in other words, existence of the precursor of litorin bound its γ-carboxylic acid of glutamic acid residue at position 2 to some polysaccharides or other hydroxyl group of large molecular weight materials in the tissue.

Isolation and sequence analysis of bradykinin-like peptide in the skin of Heleophryne purcelli*   A very rare South-African frog, Heleophryne purcelli, contains bradykinin-like peptide in the skin. Active principle in the methanol extracts were eluted at 50% of ethanol from the aluminum column with the decending concentration from 95% ethanol. The 50% ethanol eluate was evaporated under the reduced pressure and lyophilized. The residue was dissolved in water and purified by SP-Sephadex column chromatography with stepwise elution of 0.15 N ammonium formate and 1.0 N ammonium formate as the eluent. The active principle was eluted at the front of 1.0 N of the buffer.

---

* submitted to EXPERIENTIA: Occurrence of Hyp^3-bradykinin in Methanol Extracts of the Skin of the Sourth-African Frog Heleophryne purcelli. Nakajima, T., Yasuhara, T., Erspamer, G.F., Erspamer, V., and Visser, J.

The peptide contained 1 mole of hydroxyproline instead of 1
mole of proline in the amino acid composition of bradykinin and
was considered to be hydroxyproline substituted analogue. The Rf
of its dansyl derivertive was slightly lower comparing to that of
bradykinin on a thin layer of Silica gel with the solvent system
of iso-propanol:Methyl acetate:28% ammonia (9:7:4).

Two of the chymotryptic fragments out of three were coincided
to Ser-Pro-Phe and arginine respectively. The fragment which did
not correspond to Arg-Pro-Pro-Gly-Phe of the digestive products
from bradykinin, contained arginine, proline, glycine, phenylalanine and hydroxyproline. Dansyl-Edman degradation for the
peptide resulted in the sequence of Hyp^3-bradykinin.

$$Arg-Pro-Hyp-Gly-Phe-Ser-Pro-Phe-Arg-Hyp^3-bradykinin$$

The occurrence of Hyp^3-bradykinin analogue has been reported
from the venom of Japanese hornet (Kishimura et al., 1976), and
this is the first case found in amphibian skin and as the free peptide. There is little known on the presence of hydroxyproline
containing peptides of small molecular size in animal kingdoms,
except the cleft products of collagen, gelatin or such hydroxyproline containing proteins, which exist in serum or urine of
mammals. The presence of Hyp^3-bradykinin and the analogous peptide
suggests the selective oxidation of the prolyl residue in the
third sequence of bradykinin with some proline hydroxylase.

Frog skin angiotensin, purification and chemical characterization*
Dry skin of approximately 17g obtained from 200 specimens of
Crinia georgiana, a very small Australian amphibian, was extracted
with methanol and chromatographed on an aluminum column in the
usual manner. Angiotensin-like material was eluted from the column
at 60% ethanol containing 3-4 mg equivalent to Asn^1-Val^5-angio-
tensin II (guinea pig ileum). One tenth of the aluminum eluate
was purified by SP-Sephadex column chromatography with the linear
concentration gradient elution from water to 0.5 N ammonium formate.
The major active principle was eluted at the concentration of
approximately 0.25 N of the buffer. The pure peptide of 0.35 μ
moles was obtained from 1/10 of the aluminum eluate.

The amino acid composition of the peptide was that of Ile^5-
angiotensin II plus each 1 mole of proline, alanine and glycine.
Aspartic acid was recovered and not asparagine when the peptide
was hydrolysed by amino peptidase M.

---

*submitted to EXPERIENTIA: Amino Acid Composition and Sequence of
Crinia Angiotensin. An Angiotensin II-like Endecapeptide from the
Skin of the Australian Frog Crinia georgiana. Erspamer, V.,
Melchioli, P., Nakajima, T., Yasuhara, T., and Endean, R.

When the peptide was split with trypsin, the newly formed N-terminal amino acid was isoleucine together with the original N-terminal alanine. On the other hand, when the peptide was split with chymotrypsin, the newly formed N-terminal was valine. These experiments suggested that the presence of Arg-Ile and Tyr-Val bonds in the sequence. Incubation products of the chymotrypsin digestion were dansylated and chromatographed, one of the dansyl-ated fragments was detected to Val-His-Pro-Phe from its amino acid composition and chromatographic behaviors comparing with the standard fragments.

The peptide was reduced with sodium in liquid ammonia, 1 mole each of alanine and histidine was lacked from the intact composi-tion which suggested the presence of Ala-Pro and His-Pro bonds in the sequence.

Dansyl-Edman procedure was performed and the sequence of Ala-Pro-Gly-Asp-Arg-Ile-Tyr-Val-His-Pro-Phe was obtained. This sequence obtained by the degradation, supported the other experimental results (Fig. 2).

This small Australian frog contains large amounts of free angiotensin II analogue in the skin. The content was at least 20 µg per one frog skin which is much higher than that of the other angiotensin produced from plasma in the other vertebrates. The skin angiotensin is quite notable. Tripeptide elongates at the N-terminal. Valine is replaced to isoleucine at the third position of angiotensin sequence, in which all of plasma angioten-sins ever elucidated in mammals, avians, reptiles, and teleosts are valine at this position. These structural features differed from plasma angiotensin produced by the renin in the kidney, and this finding suggests that the different renin-angiotensin system might exist in this frog skin.

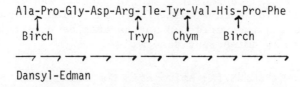

Figure 2. Scheme of sequential degradation of Crinia angiotensin

Amphibian skin is well known as a rich source of the biological active peptides and most of these peptides show the sequence homology or identity to mammalian hormones, transmitters or mediators. Angiotensin now entered this category. But some of these such as granuliberin-R, the potent mast cell degranulating peptide in the amphibian skin, have not yet been found in mammals. Similarly, physalaemin, xenopsin and others, prior to the establishment of their structures of substance P, neurotensin, etc., were considered to be unique and peculiar peptides in the lower vertebrates. Although none of these have been elucidated, their physiological significance in the amphibian skin may speculate that these peptides will serve as the local regulation of the vasculature, control of secretions, or water and electrolytes balance in the skin. Screening of the biological active peptides in the lower vertebrates and invertebrates based upon the other pharmacological techniques, may provide the new type of materials.

REFERENCES

Anastasi, A., Montecucchi, P., Angelucci, F., Erspamer, V. and
    Endean, R. 1978. Glu(OMe)^2-Litorin, The Second Bombesin-like
    Peptide Occurring in Methanol Extracts of the Skin of the
    Australian Frog Litoria aurea. submitted to Experientia.
Bertaccini, G. 1976. Active Polypeptides of Nonmammalian Origin.
    Pharmacol. Rev. 28: 127.
Erspamer, V., Negri, L., Erspamer, G.F. and Endean, R. 1975.
    Uperolein and Other Active Polypeptides in the Skin of the
    Australian Leptodactylid Frog Uperoleia and Taudactylus.
    Naunyn-Schmiedebergs Arch. Pharmakol. Exp. Pathol. 289: 41.
Erspamer, V., Erspamer, G.F. and Negri, F. 1976. Naturally
    Occurring Kinins. ed. by J.J. Pisano and K.F. Austen,
    Fogarty International Center Proceedings, No. 27: p. 153.
Kishimura, H., Yasuhara, T., Yoshida, H. and Nakajima, T. 1976.
    Vespakinin-M, a Novel Bradykinin Analogue Containing Hydro-
    xyproline in the Venom of Vespa mandarinia. Smith. Chem.
    Pharm. Bull. 24: 2896.
Nakajima, T. 1976. New Vasoactive Peptides of Nonmammalian
    Origin. ed. by J.J. Pisano and K.F. Austen, Fogarty Inter-
    national Center Proceedings, No. 27: p. 165.
Nakajima, T., and Yasuhara, T. 1977. A New Mast Cell Degranulating
    Peptide, Granuliberin-R, in the Frog (Rana rugosa) Skin.
    Chem. Pharm. Bull. 25: 2464.
Tsuru, D., Fujiwara, K. and Kado, K. 1978. Purification and
    Characterization of L-Pyrrolidone Carboxylate Peptidase from
    Bacillus amyloliquefaciens. J. Biochem. (Tokyo) 84: 467.
Yasuhara, T. and Nakajima, T. 1975. Occurrence of Pyr-His-Pro-
    NH$_2$ in the Frog Skin. Chem. Pharm. Bull. 23: 3301.

SPECIFIC ISOLATION OF BIOLOGICALLY-ACTIVE PEPTIDES BY MEANS OF

IMMOBILIZED ANHYDROTRYPSIN AND ANHYDROCHYMOTRYPSIN*

S. Ishii, H. Yokosawa, S. Shiba and K. Kasai

Department of Biochemistry, Faculty of Pharmaceutical

Sciences, Hokkaido University, Sapporo 060, Japan

ABSTRACT

Anhydrotrypsin, a derivative of bovine trypsin, immobilized on Sepharose tightly adsorbs various peptides containing L-arginine at the carboxyl termini, such as bradykinin and tuftsin. These peptides correspond to the specific products of the action of trypsin-like enzymes. Native trypsin immobilized on Sepharose does not show such strong affinity. Fragment 2, a peptide with 41 amino acid residues, which has been released together with brady-kinin from bovine high-molecular-weight kininogen by the action of plasma kallikrein, is also adsorbed on the immobilized anhydro-trypsin. When only the carboxyl-terminal arginine is removed with carboxy-peptidase B, however, the peptide loses its adsorptive ability. Immobilized anhydrochymotrypsin, on the other hand, exerts specific affinity for the peptides which correspond to the products of chymotrypsin. These results suggest that the anhydro-derivatives of serine-proteases in general may be of great use in the affinity chromatography of respective series of various naturally occurring peptides.

INTRODUCTION

Anhydrotrypsin, a catalytically inert derivative of bovine trypsin (EC 3.4.21.4) in which the active-site residue Ser-183

---

*This work was supported in part by a grant from the Ministry of Education, Science and Culture of Japan.

15

had been chemically converted to a dehydroalanine residue, was previously shown by us (Yokosawa and Ishii, 1977) to have much higher
affinity toward product-type ligands, containing an arginine residue
with free carboxyl group (e.g., K_d = 0.20 mM for Bz-L-arginine, at
pH 8.2 and 25°C), than that toward their cognate substrate-type
ligands with the carboxyl group substituted (e.g., K_d = 4.6 mM for
Bz-L-arginine amide, at pH 8.2 and 25°C). Native trypsin did not
show such distinctive behavior between these ligands (K_d = 5.9 and
3.3 mM, respectively, for Bz-L-arginine and its amide, at pH 8.2
and 25°C).

Anhydrotrypsin immobilized on Sepharose is expected, therefore,
to be useful as a biospecific affinity adsorbent for isolation of
the products generated by the action of various trypsin-like proteases. We have already reported some preliminary findings on the
promising properties of this affinity adsorbent (anhydrotrypsin-
Sepharose)(Yokosawa and Ishii, 1976). In this communication, we
report the further utility of anhydrotrypsin-Sepharose in isolation
of various biologically-active peptides and fractionation of tryptic
digest of some polypeptides.

It is also interesting to know whether the enhanced affinity
toward the product-type ligands is limited to the feature of anhydrotrypsin or is the general property of anhydro-derivatives of the
serine-proteases, in relation to the wider applicability of this
type of affinity chromatography for isolation and search of new
biologically-active peptides. Anhydrochymotrypsin was thus prepared from bovine chymotrypsin (EC 3.4.21.1) and examined in this
respect. The latter half of this paper deals with some basic
properties of anhydrochymotrypsin-Sepharose.

                        MATERIALS AND METHODS

Crystalline preparations of trypsin and α-chymotrypsin (bovine
pancreas) were purchased from Worthington Biochemical Co., Free-
hold. Anhydrotrypsin and anhydrochymotrypsin were prepared
according to the procedures of Yokosawa and Ishii (1977) and of
Ako et al., (1972), respectively. Immobilization of trypsin and
chemotrypsin, as well as their anhydro-derivatives, were carried
out by coupling these proteins to Sepharose 4B (Pharmacia Fine
Chemicals) according to the method of Axen and Ernback (1971)
with cyanogen bromide. Porcine pancreas carboxypeptidase B
purchased from Worthington was used after purification by the method
of Sokolovsky (1974).

Methionyl-lysyl-bradykinin, tuftsin, neurotensin, Ac-tryptophan
ethyl ester, Z=Gly-Phe, and Z-Glu-Phe were obtained from the
Protein Research Foundation, Osaka. Ig E peptide III was a product
of Peninsula Laboratories, San Carlos. Fibrinopeptide A was

prepared from bovine fibrinogen (Fraction I; Sigma Chemical Co.) by
the action of bovine topical thrombin (Parke-Davis) and the chromatographic separation on a column of Dowex 50-X2. Peptide C derived
from horseshoe crab coagulogen and Fragment 2 of bovine high-molecular-weight kininogen were kindly donated by Dr. S. Iwanaga, Osaka
University. Erabutoxin was a gift of Dr. N. Tamiya, Tohoku
University. Other peptides and amino acid derivatives were the
commercial products of various sources (Sigma Chemical Co., Mann
Research Lab., Nutritional Biochemical Co.).

Reduction and S-carboxymethylation of erabutoxin a, and tryptic
digestion of the reaction product were carried out as reported
(Sato and Tamiya, 1971). Neurotensin was digested as follows:
0.31 μmol of the peptide in 1 ml of 0.02 M borate buffer, pH 8.0,
containing 0.02 M $CaCl_2$ was incubated with 1 nmol of trypsin for
5.5 hr at 25°C.

Experiments of affinity chromatography, including frontal
analysis, were performed at 4°C throughout. Peptide concentrations
in the chromatographic effluents were determined by the fluorescamine
reaction for amino groups (Udenfriend et al., 1972), the ninhydrin
reaction for arginine residues (Conn and Davis, 1959), the fluorescence measurement for tryptophan residues (excitation at 290 nm and
emission at 370 nm), or Folin-Lowry's method for large peptides.
Amino acid compositions of peptides and immobilized proteins were
determined by analyzing their HCl-hydrolyzates on a Joel JLC-6AH
amino acid analyzer.

RESULTS AND DISCUSSION

Affinity Chromatography of Biologically-Active Peptides on Anhydrotrypsin-Sepharose

The affinity of anhydrotrypsin toward Bz-L-arginie has been
shown to be stronger in the medium of slightly acidic pH than in
that of slightly alkaline pH, such as pH 8 which is optimum for the
catalytic activity of native trypsin (K_d = 53 μM at pH 5.0; compare
with the value at pH 8.2 mentioned above), and the pK_a value for
the ionization form of anhydrotrypsin responsible for the interaction with this ligand has been estimated to be 7.60 ± 0.07
(Yokosawa and Ishii, 1977). In the following experiments, therefore, columns of anhydrotrypsin-Sepharose equilibrated with acetate
buffer, pH 5.0 were used throughout. (All amino acid residues are
of L-configuration unless otherwise indicated).

Six peptides, which differed from each other in molecular
size, electric charge and other properties but had carboxyl-
terminal arginine in common, were examined for the chromatographic

behavior on the anhydrotrypsin-Sepharose column. These were:
methionyl-lysyl-bradykinin, fibrinopeptide A, a phagocytosis-
stimulating tetrapeptide tuftsin (Thr-Lys-Pro-Arg), an inhibitory
pentapeptide of the Prausnitz-Kustner reaction Ig E peptide III
(Asp-Ser-Asp-Pro-Arg)(Hamburger, 1975), Peptide C derived from
horseshoe crab coagulogen (a peptide with 28 amino acid residues)
(Nakamura et al., 1976), and Fragment 2 of bovine high-molecular-
weight kininogen. All of them were adsorbed on the column at
pH 5.0 and desorbed with 5 mM HCl. A typical chromatogram with
Fragment 2 is shown in Fig. 1a. This peptide, one of the products
generated concomitantly with bradykinin from bovine high-molecualr-
weight kininogen by the action of plasma kallikrein, has been
reported by Oh-ishi et al (1977) to exhibit an inhibitory effect
on the activation reaction of Hageman factor. Its primary structure
consisting of 41 amino acid residues (11 His, 11 Gly, 7 Lys, 3 Asn,
2 Gln, 2 Leu, 1 Asp, 1 Ser, 1 Tyr, 1 Trp, 1 Arg) has been determined
by Han et al. (1975).

When the carboxyl-terminal arginine was released by the action
of carboxypeptidase B, Fragment 2 lost its adsorptive ability to
anhydrotrypsin-Sepharose (at pH 5.0) as shown in Fig. 1b, in spite
of the survival of 7 lysine residues within the peptide chain.

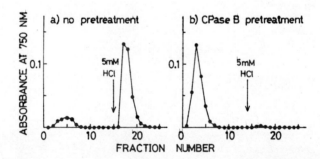

Figure 1. Affinity chromatography of a) bovine plasma Fragment 2
(18 nmol in 0.1 ml) and b) carboxypeptidase B-treated Fragment 2
(12 nmol in 0.3 ml) on a column (0.59 x 3.7 cm, 1 ml) of anhydrotrypsin-Sepharose (4.8 mg protein/ml wet gel). The column was
pre-equilibrated with 0.05 M acetate buffer, pH 5.0, containing
0.02 M CaCl$_2$. The indicated peptide in the same buffer was applied
and eluted stepwise with the same buffer and 5 mM HCl. The effluent
was collected in 1-ml fractions at the flow rate of about 5 ml per
hr. The peptide concentrations were determined by Folin-Lowry's
method. Each arrow indicates the replacement of the buffer with
5 mM HCl. The non-adsorbed fraction seen in the left figure may
be some contaminating peptide(s) in the preparation.

The essentiality of the presence of carboxyl-terminal L-arginine
for the adsorption was demonstrated also in the other peptides by
the similar experiments with carboxypeptidase B. We have already
reported that Bz-D-arginine, unlike its l-isomer, does not show any
substantial affinity to anhydrotrypsin-Sepharose (Yokosawa and
Ishii, 1976).

In the experiment shown in Fig. 2, methionyl-lysyl-bradykinin
was adsorbed on the column of anhydrotrypsin-Sepharose at pH 5.0,
and the eluent with a pH gradient decreasing to pH 2.7 was then
applied to the column. The peptide was eluted at pH 4.0. In the
same series of experiments, the lower pHs were required for the
elution of Peptide C (pH 3.2) and Fragment 2 (pH 2.7). The results
suggest that the structure of some moiety other than the carboxyl
terminus probably affects the interaction of these peptides with
anhydrotrypsin-Sepharose, and that anhydrotrypsin-Sepharose may be
usable even for the fractionation among various peptides containing
carboxyl-terminal arginine in common.

Fractionation of Tryptic Digests of Polypeptides
by Anhydrotrypsin-Sepharose

Figure 3 shows the chromatographic behavior of neurotensin, a
hypotensive tridecapeptide with leucine at the carboxyl-terminus,
and of its tryptic digest. Intact neurotensin passed through an
anhydrotrypsin-Sepharose column at pH 5.0. On the other hand,

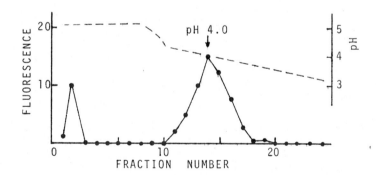

Figure 2. Affinity chromatography of methionyl-lysyl-bradykinin
(20 nmol) on anhydrotrypsin-Sepharose (1.75 ml). The chromatographic
conditions were the same as those described in the legend to Fig.
1, except that the elution with the acetate buffer, pH 5.0 was
followed by that with a pH gradient decreasing to pH 2.7, and 2.0
ml fractions of the effluent were collected. The peptide concentrations were determined by the fluorometry with ninhydrin (see
text).

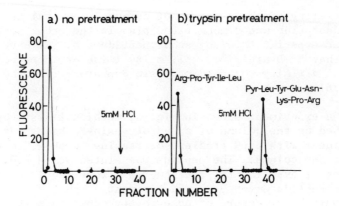

Figure 3. Affinity chromatography of a) neurotensin (88 nmol in
0.8 ml) and b) a tryptic digest of neurotensin (100 nmol in 1.0 ml)
on a column (0.74 x 14.7 cm, 6.3 ml) of anhydrotrypsin-Sepharose.
The chromatographic conditions were the same as those described in
the legend to Fig. 1, except that 3.0 ml fractions of the effluent
were collected. The peptide concentrations were measured by the
fluorometry with ninhydrin. Each arrow indicates the replacement
of the buffer with 5 mM HCl.

one of the peptides in the tryptic digest was adsorbed on the
column and desorbed with 5 mM HCl. Amino acid composition analysis
indicated that this is the amino-side octapeptide containing
arginine at its carboxyl terminus. Another peptide in the digest
also contained arginine but at the amino terminus. It passed
through the column at pH 5.0.

   Erabutoxin a is a neurotoxic protein of a sea-snake (Laticauda
semifasciata). Its primary structure consisting of 62 amino acid
residues (including 3 Arg and 4 Lys) has been elucidated by Sato
and Tamiya (1971). This protein was digested with trypsin after
the reductive cleavage of disulfide bridges and S-carboxymethylation, and the resulting peptide mixture was chromatographed on an
anhydrotrypsin-Sepharose column. Four peaks were depicted by the
fluorescamine reaction of amino groups, as illustrated in Fig. 4.
Among them, the first and the last peaks were detectable by the
ninhydrin fluorometry of guanidino groups. Amino acid analysis
indicated that the first peak contained a mixture of free arginine
released from residue No. 1 and the carboxyl-terminal peptide
(Nos. 52-62) which had neither arginine nor lysine. The second
and the third peaks corresponded to the peptide Nos. 16-27 and the
peptide Nos. 2-15, respectively, both of which had been produced by
the tryptic hydrolyses of lysyl bonds. The last peak contained two

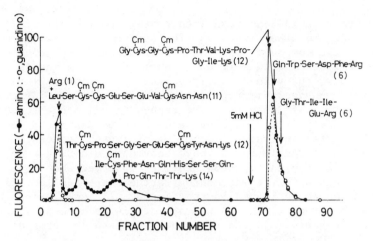

Figure 4. Affinity chromatography of a tryptic digest of reduced
and S-carboxymethylated erabutoxin a (100 nmol in 0.4 ml) on
anhydrotrypsin-Sepharose. The conditions were the same as those
described in the legend to Fig. 3, except that 1.5 ml fractions of
the effluent were collected. The peptide concentrations were
measured by the fluorometry with fluorescamine or with ninhydrin.
(——•——), fluorescence generated by the reaction with fluorescamine;
(- - o - -), fluorescence by the reaction with ninhydrin.

argine peptides (Nos. 28–33 and Nos. 34–39) and one lysine peptide
(Nos. 40–51). These peptides were adsorbed tightly on the column
at pH 5.0 and desorbed with 5 mM HCl. The affinity of the lysine
peptide, however, was considered to be less than that of the
arginine peptides, because the peak depicted by the fluorometry of
amino groups located slightly left-side compared with that by the
fluorometry of guanidino groups. In fact, when the elution of the
tightly adsorbed three peptides was carried out with gradually decreasing pH to 2.7, instead of the sudden change to 5 mM HCl, the
lysine peptide appeared first from the column separately from the
arginine peptides. We have previously reported the results of
comparative study between Bz-Gly-L-Arg and Bz-Gly-L-Lys, suggesting
the weaker interaction of the carboxyl-terminal lysine with anhydrotrypsin-Sepharose than that of the carboxyl-terminal arginine
(Yokosawa and Ishii, 1976).

Interaction of Anhydrochymotrypsin-Sepharose
with Various Ligands

The findings on the useful properties of anhydrotrypsin-
Sepharose as an affinity adsorbent gave an impetus to the study of

anhydrochymotrypsin-Sepharose with respect to its affinity toward product-type and other ligands. The product-type ligand in this case means the compound containing a tryptophan, tyrosine or phenylalanine residue with a free carboxyl group. As the first step of this study, the values of dissociation constant (K_d) of the immobilized anhydrochymotrypsin-ligand complexes were determined by quantitative affinity chromatography, in which the technique of frontal analysis was employed according to Kasai and Ishii (1978a, 1978b). For the analysis, a solution of ligand (concentration: $[A]_0$) was added continuously to an anhydrochymotrypsin-Sepharose column. Fig. 5 a shows typical elution profiles observed when Ac-L-tryptophan solutions of different concentrations were applied. $[A]_0$ of each solution is indicated in the figure. If the elution volume at which the front of the solute appears is defined as V, the relationship between $[A]_0$ and V can be expressed in terms of K_d as follows:

$$K_d = \frac{B_t}{V - V_0} - [A]_0, \tag{1}$$

where B_t is the total effective amount of immobilized anhydrochymotrypsin present in the column and V_0 is the void volume of the column. Equation 1 can be rearranged to:

$$\frac{1}{[A]_0 (V-V_0)} = \frac{K_d}{B_t} \cdot \frac{1}{[A]_0} + \frac{1}{B_t}. \tag{2}$$

Therefore, the plot of $1/[A]_0(V-V_0)$ versus $1/[A]_0$ (Fig. 5b) affords the values of K_d and B_t. A value of 14 µM was obtained, in this way, as K_d of anhydrochymotrypsin-Sepharose for Ac-L-tryptophan at pH 6.0 and 4°C.

Frontal analysis was performed also on a column of native chymotrypsin similarly immobilized on Sepharose. As the $V-V_0$ value was rather small even with the lowest concentration of Ac-L-tryptophan, the estimated value of K_d (0.4 mM) lacks high accuracy. The results suggest that chymotrypsin gained enhanced affinity toward the product-type ligands (Ac-L-tryptophan in this case) upon the dehydration at the serine residue in its active-site, as in the case of trypsin. In fact, the K_d value of anhydrochymotrypsin-Sepharose for Ac-L-tryptophan ethyl ester, one of the substrate-type ligands, was shown to be very large compared with that for Ac-L-tryptophan (300 µM versus 8.9 µM in 0.05 M acetate buffer containing 0.02 M $CaCl_2$, pH 4.0, at 4°C).

The pH dependence of K_d for Ac-L-tryptophan was examined (Fig. 6). K_d values decreased markedly from pH 8 to 7. Such pH dependence has been observed also with anhydrotrypsin-Sepharose.

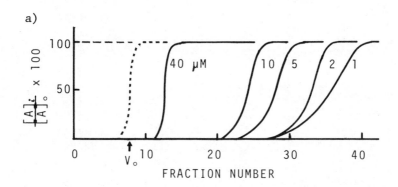

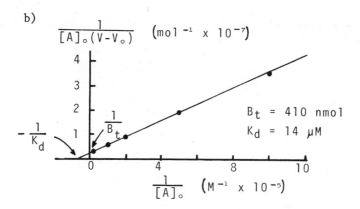

Figure 5.   a)   Elution profiles of Ac–L–tryptophan in frontal
analysis through a column (5 ml) of anhydrochymotrypsin–Sepharose
(3.3 mg protein/ml wet gel). The column was equilibrated with
0.05 M acetate buffer containing 0.02 M $CaCl_2$, pH 6.0, and one
of the Ac–L–tryptophan solutions (concentrations are indicated in
µM) in the same buffer was applied continuously. The effluent
was collected in 1 ml fractions at the flow rate of about 4 ml
per hr. A dotted line is the elution profile of 1 mM Ac–DL–
tryptophan.

        b) $1/[A]_o(V-V_o)$ versus $1/[A]_o$ plot of the data obtained
from the elution profiles shown above. V_o was estimated from the
profile with 1 mM Ac–DL–tryptophan.

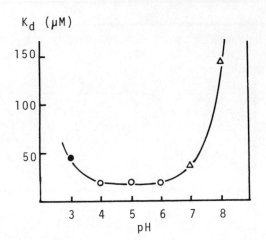

Figure 6. Effect of pH on K_d of anhydrochymotrypsin–Sepharose for Ac–L–tryptophan at 4°C. Δ, Tris buffer; o, acetate buffer; ●, formate buffer. Ionic strength, 0.27.

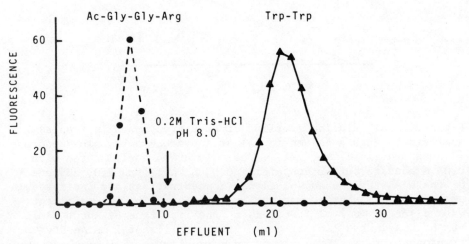

Figure 7. Chromatographic separation of Ac–Gly–Gly–Arg and Trp–Trp on a column of anhydrochymotrypsin–Sepharose (the same size and protein content as indicated in the legend to Fig. 5a). The first eluent, 0.05 M acetate buffer, pH 4.0, was replaced with 0.2 M Tris buffer, pH 8.0, as indicated in the figure. The peptide concentrations were determined by the fluorometry with ninhydrin (–o–) or by the fluorescence emitted from tryptophan residue (–Δ–) (see text).

The K_d values for various ligands estimated by the quantitative affinity chromatography are listed in Table I, where we can compare the data between optical isomers, between product-type and substrate-type ligands, and among different carboxyl-terminal and other residues. Fig. 7 illustrates an example of chromatographic separation of peptides on anhydrochymotrypsin-Sepharose. These results indicate that this affinity adsorbent may also be very useful in the fractionation of peptide mixtures and the search for new peptides which are functioning in various biological systems (e.g. chemotactic factors for neutrophils reported by Showell et al. (1976).

The appearance of enhanced affinity toward product-type ligands upon the chemical conversion of an active-site serine residue to a dehydroalanine residue is expected to be generally observable in the serine-proteases. The phenomenon is very important, we think, not only for the elucidation of the active-site charge-relay system in the serine-proteases, but also for the application of this type of affinity chromatography to wide varieties of naturally occurring peptides.

TABLE I

Dissociation Constants (K_d) of Anhydrochymotrypsin-
Sepharose for Various Ligands

	K_d (µM)		K_d (µM)
Ac-L-Trp	14	Ala-Trp	48
Ac-D-Trp	110	Val-Trp	48
Z-L-Trp	0.69	Leu-Trp	21
Z-D-Trp	16	Phe-Trp	26
Z-Tyr	7.8	Trp-Trp	6
Z-Phe	17	Trp-Phe	100
Z-Gly-Phe	120	Met-Phe	800
Z-Gly-Phe-NH$_2$	320	Gly-Tyr	600
Z-Ala-Phe	100	Ala-Tyr	440
Z-Val-Phe	33		
Z-Ile-Phe	55		
Z-Glu-Phe	270		

In 0.05 M acetate buffer containing 0.02 M CaCl$_2$, pH 6.0, 4°C.

REFERENCES

Ako, H., C.A. Ryan and R.J. Foster, 1972. The purification by affinity chromatography of a protease inhibitor binding species of anhydrochymotrypsin. Biochem. Biophys. Res. Commun. 46: 1639.

Axen, R. and S. Ernback, 1971. Chemical fixation of enzymes to cyanogen halide activated polysaccharide carriers, Eur. J. Biochem. 18: 351.

Conn, R.B., Jr. and R.B. Davis, 1959. Green fluorescence of guanidinium compounds with ninhydrin. Nature 183: 1053.

Hamburger, R.N., 1975. Peptide inhibition of the Prausnitz-Kustner reaction. Science 189: 389.

Han, Y.N., M. Komiya, S. Iwanaga and T. Suzuki, 1975. Studies on the primary structure of bovine high-molecular-weight kininogen. Amino acid sequence of a fragment ("Histidine-rich peptide") released by plasma kallikrein. J. Biochem. 77: 55.

Kasai, K. and S. Ishii, 1978a. Affinity chromatography of trypsin and related enzymes. V. Basic studies of quantitative affinity chromatography. J. Biochem. 84: 1051.

Kasai, K. and S. Ishii, 1978b. Studies on the interaction of immobilized trypsin and specific ligands by quantitative affinity chromatography. J. Biochem. 84: 1061.

Nakamura, S., T. Takagi, S. Iwanaga, M. Niwa and K. Takahashi, 1976. Amino acid sequence studies on the fragments produced from horseshoe crab coagulogen during gel formation: Homologies with primate fibrinopeptide B. Biochem. Biophys. Res. Commun. 72: 902.

Oh-ishi, S., K. Tanaka, M. Katori, Y.N. Han, H. Kato and S. Iwanaga, 1977. Further studies on biological activities of new peptide fragments derived from high molecular weight kininogen: An enhancement of the vascular permeability increase of the fragments by prostaglandin E_2. Life Sciences 20: 695.

Sato, S. and N. Tamiya, 1971. The amino acid sequences of erabutoxins, neurotoxic proteins of a sea-snake (Laticauda semifasciata) venom. Biochem. J. 122: 453.

Showell, H.J., R.J. Freer, S.H. Zigmond, E. Schiffmann, S. Aswanikumar, B. Corcoran and E.L. Becker, 1976. The structure-activity relations of synthetic peptides as chemotactic factors and inducers of lysosomal enzyme secretion for neutrophils. J. Exp. Med. 143: 1154.

Sokolovsky, M., Carboxypeptidase B, 1968. In: Methods in Enzymology, Vol. 34, eds. W.B. Jakoby and M. Wilchek (Academic Press, New York) p. 411.

Udenfriend, S., S. Stein, P. Bohoen, W. Dairman, W. Leimgruber and M. Weigele, 1972. Fluorescamine: A reagent for assay of amino acids, peptides, proteins, and primary amines in the picomole range. Science 178: 871.

Yokosawa, H. and S. Ishii, 1976. The effective use of immobilized
     anhydrotrypsin for the isolation of biologically active
     peptides containing L-arginine residues in C-termini.
     Biochem. Biophys. Res. Commun. 72: 1443.
Yokosawa, H. and S. Ishii. 1977. Anhydrotrypsin: New features in
     ligand interactions revealed by affinity chromatography and
     thionine replacement. J. Biochem. 81: 647.

COMPARATIVE STUDY ON DISTRIBUTION OF BOMBESIN-, NEUROTENSIN- AND

α-ENDORPHIN-LIKE IMMUNOREACTIVITIES IN CANINE TISSUES

N. Yanaihara, H. Sato, A. Inoue, N. Sakura, M. Sakagami,
T. Mochizuki, H. Nakamura and C. Yanaihara

Laboratory of Bioorganic Chemistry, Shizuoka College
of Pharmacy, Shizuoka, Japan 422

Bombesin and neurotensin, which have recently been found in
both brain and intestine tissues, were originally isolated from frog
skin (Anastasi et al., 1971) and from bovine hypothalamus (Carraway
and Leeman, 1973 and 1975), respectively. Both the peptides have
been reported to show a wide spectrum of actions in mammals. Neurotensin possesses pharmacological actions which are similar to those
of the mammalian plasma kinins. Bombesin is also known to possess
a variety of actions on isolated smooth muscle preparations and
cardiovascular system (Melchiorri, 1978). It has recently reported
that bombesin and neurotensin show potent action on thermoregulation
(Brown et al., 1977).
On the other hand, endorphins have been well-characterized as
endogenous opiate-like peptides which were isolated from ACTH containing pituitary extracts (Bradbury et al., 1976). By combination
of immunocytochemistry and radioimmunoassay, Bloom et al. (1977)
have indicated that endorphin-like immunoreactivity is found exclusively in the intermediate lobe of the pituitary. α-Endorphin having the hexadecapeptide sequence (β-LPH 61-76) is the shortest
peptide among α-, β- and γ-endorphins (Ling et al., 1976). Although
the sequence of enkephalin, another opiate-like peptide, is embodied
in the endorphin molecule, recent studies have suggested the completely different localizations between endorphins and enkephalin
(Rossier et al., 1977).
We have recently completed the syntheses of bombesin, neurotensin and their analogues (Yanaihara et al., 1978). Synthesis of
α-endorphin was also achieved (Sakura and Yanaihara, 1978). The
present paper describes the distributions of bombesin-, neurotensin-
and α-endorphin-like immunoreactivities in canine tissues which were
measured by radioimmunoassays specific for the respective hormones

developed by using the above-mentioned highly purified synthetic
polypeptides. Concentrations of the immunoreactivities of these
three peptide hormones in rat pituitary and pineal body were also
compared.

METHODS

Synthetic peptides: Bombesin, neurotensin, α-endorphin and
their related peptides were synthesized by the conventional method
for peptide synthesis. The chain elongation was conducted mainly
by the azide fragment condensation. Purity of the synthetic peptides was assessed in the usual analytical methods. Ranatensin C
(Yoshida et al., 1974) having amino acid sequence very similar to
that of bombesin was also synthesized in order to compare its
immunoreactivity with that of bombesin. Table I shows the amino
acid sequences of the synthetic peptides used in this study.

Extraction of tissue: The procedure of extraction was similar to that described previously (Yanaihara et al., 1976). Freezed
canine or rat tissue was minced and heated with about 10-fold
weight of boiling water for 10 min. After acidification with
acetic acid on cooling followed by centrifugation, the supernatant
was evaporated and lyophilized. Each of the lyophilized materials
was dissolved in 1 M acetic acid and the solution was submitted
to gel filtration on Sephadex G-25 using 1 M acetic acid as eluent.
Fractions containing the materials of molecular weight over approximately 500 were collected, lyophilized and used for radioimmunoassay determination.

Radioimmunoassay: Radioimmunoassay systems for the three respective active peptides, i.e. bombesin, neurotensin and α-endorphin,
have been developed using the synthetic peptides prepared in this
study. The assay systems are summarized in Table II.

The anti-bombesin serum GP-3303 was obtained from one of the
guinea pigs received N^{α}-glycyl-[Gln^1]-bombesin-BSA conjugate,
which had been prepared by coupling N^{α}-glycyl-[Gln^1]-bombesin with
BSA in the presence of water-soluble carbodiimide. The anti-
neurotensin sera GP-3501 and R-3502 were produced in one of the
guinea pigs and one of the rabbits immunized with neurotensin-
BSA conjugate which had been prepared by coupling the peptide
with BSA by means of glutaraldehyde. The anti-α-endorphin serum
was raised in one of the rabbits received glutaraldehyde-coupled
α-endorphin-BSA conjugate.

Radioiodination was performed by the chloramine T or lactoper-
oxidase method. Since bombesin does not contain tyrosine residue,
N^{α}-tyrosyl-[Gln^1]-bombesin was used as substrate for radioiodination. The reaction proceeded for 20 seconds and the resulting

TABLE I. AMINO ACID SEQUENCES OF SYNTHETIC PEPTIDES

Bombesin	: pGlu-Gln-Arg-Leu-Gly-Asn-Gln-Trp-Ala-Val-Gly-His-Leu-Met-NH$_2$
H-Tyr-[Gln^1]-Bombesin	: H-Tyr-Gln-Gln-Arg-Leu-Gln-Asn-Gln-Trp-Ala-Val-Gly-His-Leu-Met-NH$_2$
H-Gly-[Gln^1]-Bombesin	: H-Gly-Gln-Gln-Arg-Leu-Gln-Asn-Gln-Trp-Ala-Val-Gly-His-Leu-Met-NH$_2$
Ranatensin	: pGlu-Thr-Pro-Gln-Trp-Ala-Val-Gly-His-Phe-Met-NH$_2$
Neurotensin	: pGlu-Leu-Tyr-Glu-Asn-Lys-Pro-Arg-Arg-Pro-Tyr-Ile-Leu-OH
α-Endorphin	: H-Tyr-Gly-Gly-Phe-Met-Thr-Ser-Glu-Lys-Ser-Gln-Thr-Pro-Leu-Val-Thr-OH

TABLE II.   RADIOIMMUNOASSAY SYSTEMS FOR BOMBESIN, NEUROTENSIN
AND α-ENDORPHIN

	Bombesin	Neurotensin	α-Endorphin
Tracer	^{125}I-Tyr-[Gln^1]-Bombesin (Lactoperoxidase)	^{125}I-Neurotensin (Chloramine T)	^{125}I-α-Endorphin (Chloramin T)
Antiserum	GP3303 (x14000 final)	GP3501 (x3500 final) R3502 (x2800 final)	R3402 (x14000 final)
Antigen	H-Gly-[Gln^1]-Bombesin-BSA	Neurotensin-BSA	α-Endorphin-BSA
B.F-Separation	Dextran-Charcoal	Dextran-Charcoal	Double Antibody

radioiodinated material was purified by gel filtration on Sephadex
G-25.

RESULTS AND DISCUSSION

Antigenic determinants: Crossreactivities of bombesin and
its analogues in the system using antiserum GP-3303 were examined.
N^{α}-tyrosyl-[Gln^1]-bombesin and N^{α}-glycyl-[gln^1]-bombesin showed
crossreactions identical with that of synthetic bombesin itself.
Fig. 1 shows the dose-response curves of bombesin-related peptides.
In addition, bombesin(6-14) also showed nearly 100% activity,
indicating that this antiserum is C-terminal specific. Elimination
of asparaginyl-glutamine residues in positions 6 and 7 resulted in
a marked decrease in the reactivity. Crossreactivity of bombesin
(8-14) was less than 0.01%. Ranatensin C in which the C-terminal
octapeptide is analogous to that of bombesin showed approximately
2.5% crossreactivity in this system.

We have obtained two kinds of antisera against neurotensin
having entirely different specificities. It was found that antiserum GP-3501 is N-terminal specific, while R-3502 is C-terminal
specific. In the radioimmunoassay with antiserum GP-3501, the N-
terminal neurotensin fragments having the 1-9 and 1-8 sequences
crossreacted 21% and 16% respectively, whereas the C-terminal fragment neurotensin (6-13) did not crossreact. On the other hand, with
antiserum R-3502, the C-terminal hexapeptide showed 75% crossreaction, while the N-terminal nonapetide did not crossreact. Any of
neurotensin C-terminal analogues which were substituted with D-Leu,
Phe or Val residue in position 12 or 13 did not crossreact in the
system using either of the antisera.

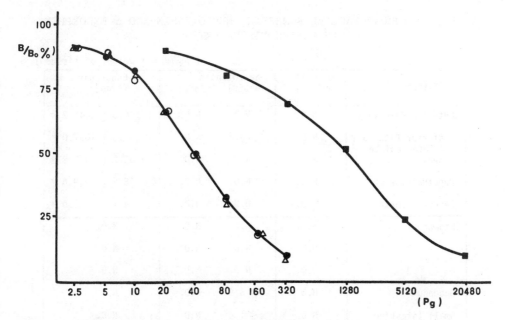

Fig. 1.   Dose-response curves of bombesin-related peptides.   The
radioimmunoassay system used is described in Table II. ($\bullet$) Synthe-
tic bombesin, ($\circ$) N^{α}-tyrosyl-[Gln^1]-bombesin, ($\triangle$) N^{α}-glycyl-
[Gln^1]-bombesin and ($\blacksquare$) synthetic ranatensin C.

In the case of α-endorphin radioimmunoassay developed in this
study, crossreactivities of β- and γ-endorphins were 6 and 17%
respectively.   Neither enkephalin, ACTH, β-MSH, bombesin nor neurotensin crossreacted.   This antiserum R-3402 was found to be C-terminal specific by examination of the crossreactivities of various
synthetic α-endorphin fragments.   The C-terminal fragment β-LPH
(65-76) showed 55% crossreaction, while the C-terminal heptapeptide
β-LPH (70-76) did not crossreact in the concentration employed.

Distribution: Using the radioimmunoassay systems for the
three respective active peptides, canine brain and gut tissue
extracts were assayed.   The results are summarized in Table III.
Interestingly, bombesin-like immunoreactivity was not detectable
in the crude extracts from both gut and brain tissues.   In the case
of neurotensin, only the N-terminal specific antiserum GP-3501 was
crossreacted with the extracts from the small intestine, ileum and
posterior pituitary with the intermediate lobe, while the C-terminal
specific antiserum R-3502 did not crossreact with any of the
extracts.   The highest concentration of immunoreactive neurotensin

TABLE 3.   IMMUNOREACTIVE BOMBESIN, NEUROTENSIN AND α-ENDORPHIN
IN CANINE TISSUE EXTRACTS

(pg/mg wet weight of tissue)

Tissue	Bombesin (GP3303)	Neurotensin (GP3501)	(R3502)	α-Endorphin (R3402)
Anterior Pituitary	N.D.	N.D.	N.D.	35506.3 ± 2041.2 *
Posterior Pituitary & Intermediate	N.D.	24.6	N.D.	28039.8 ± 1057.0 *
Pineal	N.D.	N.D.	N.D.	1153.2 ± 368.9 *
Hypothalamus	N.D.	N.D.	N.D.	98.5 ± 29.6 *
Cerebral Cortex	N.D.	N.D.	N.D.	6.5 ± 2.0 *
Stomach 1	N.D.	N.D.	N.D.	N.D.
2	N.D.	N.D.	N.D.	N.D.
3	N.D.	N.D.	N.D.	N.D.
Duodenum	N.D.	≤ 3.8	N.D.	N.D.
Small Intestine 1	N.D.	≤ 1.8	N.D.	N.D.
2	N.D.	1.3	N.D.	N.D.
3	N.D.	3.0 ± 2.1**	N.D.	N.D.
4	N.D.	4.5 ± 0.9**	N.D.	N.D.
Cecum	N.D.	N.D.	N.D.	N.D.
Colon	N.D.	N.D.	N.D.	N.D.

*   n = 5
** n = 3

was found in the ileum extract, as reported in the cases of human
(Polak et al., 1977) and rat (Uhl and Snyder, 1976; Kobayashi et
al., 1977). Localization of immunoreactive neurotensin in dog
intestinal mucosa has also been described (Orci et al., 1976).
High concentration of immunoreactive α-endorphin was found in the
pituitary extract as expected. On the other hand, any of the
reactivity was not detected in the gut extracts. All of bombesin-,
neurotensin- and α-endorphin-like immunoreactivities were detected
in the extracts from the rat pituitary and pineal body as shown
in Table IV. The presence of immunoreactive bombesin in human and
rat tissue extracts has already been reported (Polak et al., 1976;
Brown et al., 1977). The present result clearly indicated that
the failure to detect bombesin immunoreactivity in the extracts
from canine or monkey tissues may be due to some species differences

Table IV.   IMMUNOREACTIVE BOMBESIN, NEUROTENSIN AND
             α-ENDORPHIN IN RAT PITUITARY AND PINEAL EXTRACTS

| Tissue (n=2) | (pg/mg wet weight of tissue) | | |
	Bombesin (GP3303)	Neurotensin (GP3501)	α-Endorphin (R3402)
Pituitary (whole)	105.8	46.0	44866
Pineal body	217.5	521.4	240000

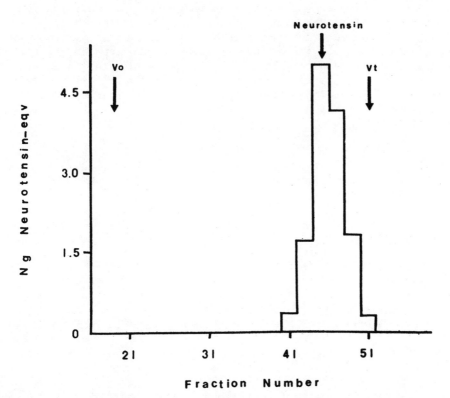

Fig. 2. Elution profile of immunoreactive neurotensin in canine
ileum extract from Sephadex G-50 (fine). Column: 1.5 x 85 cm,
eluent: 3M acetic acid and fraction: 3 ml each.

in the C-terminal portion of the molecule, or species differences
in existence of the immunoreactivity. Similar observation was
reported with the case of cholecystokinin between porcine and
canine or monkey (Straus and Yalow, 1978). Dose-response curves
of the rat pituitary extracts are parallel to that of the standard
synthetic bombesin. This indicates that bombesin immunoreactivity
in the rat pituitary extract is indistinguishable from the immunoreactivity of bombesin extracted from the frog skin.

Fig. 2 shows the gel filtration pattern of canine ileum extract
on Sephadex G-50 in which neurotensin immunoreactivity of each
fraction was determined by the N-terminal specific antiserum GP-3501.
The immunoreactivities appeared as a single peak in the elution
volume where the standard neurotensin was eluted. Any detectable
big form of neurotensin immunoreactivity was not found in the fractions. When the C-terminal specific antiserum R-3502 was used,
neurotensin immunoreactivities in the fractions were undetectable.
The result may indicate possible species differences in the carboxy-
terminal sequence of the neurotensin molecule. In addition, our
antiserum specific for synthetic frog skin bombesin also failed
to detect bombesin immunoreactivity in the extracts from canine
and monkey tissues. Since the antigenic determinant of the present
bombesin radioimmunoassay is located within the 6-14 sequence,
some substitution(s) that greatly affects immunological recognition
may occur at least in the C-terminal portion of the bombesin
molecule of canine and monkey origins.

REFERENCES

Anastasi, A., V. Erspamer and M. Bucci, 1971, Isolation and structure
    of bombesin and alytensin, two analogous active peptides from the
    skin of the European amphibians, Bombina and Alytes, Experientia
    27,166.
Bloom, F., E. Battenberg, J. Rossier, N. Ling, J. Leppalusto, T.M.
    Vargo and R. Guillemin, 1977, Endorphins are localised in the
    intermediate and anterior lobes of the pituitary gland, not in the
    neurohypophysis, Life Sciences, 20,43.
Bradburg, A.F., D.G. Smyth and C.R. Snell, 1975, Biosynthesis of
    β-MSH and ACTH, in: Peptides: Chemistry, Structure and Biology,
    eds. R. Walter and J. Meienhofer (Ann Arbor Sci. Inc., Michigan)
    p.609.
Brown, M.R., J.R. Rivier and W.W. Vale, 1977, Bombesin: potent effects
    of thermoregulation in the rat, Science, 196,998.
Carraway, R., and S.E. Leeman, 1973, The isolation of a new hypothala-
    mic peptide, neurotensin, from bovine hypothalamic, J.Biol.Chem.,
    248,6854.
Carraway, R., and S.E. Leeman, 1975, The amino acid sequence of a

hypothalamic peptide, neurotensin, J.Biol.Chem., 250,1907.

Kobayashi, R.M., M.R. Brown and W. Vale, 1977, Regional distribution of neurotensin and somatostatin in rat brain, Brain Research, 126,584.

Ling, N., R. Burgus and R. Guilemin, 1976, Isolation, primary structure and synthesis of α-endorphin and γ-endorphin, two peptides of hypothalamic-hypophysial origin with morphinomimatic activity, Proc.Natl.Acad.Sci., 73,3942.

Melchiorri, P., 1978, Bombesin and bombesin-like peptides of amphibian skin, in: Gut Hormones, ed. S.R. Bloom (Churchill Livingstone, Edinburgh) p.534.

Orci, L., O. Baetens, C. Rufener, M. Brown, W. Vale and R. Guillemin, 1976, Evidence for immunoreactive neurotensin in dog intestinal mucosa, Life Sciences, 19,559.

Polak, J.M., S. Hobbs, S.R. Bloom, E. Solcia and A.G.E. Pearse, 1976, Distribution of a bombesin-like peptide in human gastrointestinal tract, Lancet,1.,1109.

Polak, J.M., S.N. Sullivan, S.R, Bloom, A.M.J. Buchan, P. Facer, M.R. Brown and A.G.E. Pearse, 1977, Specific localisation of neurotensin to the N cell in human intestine by radioimmunoassay and immunocytochemistry, Nature, 270,183.

Rossier, J., T.M. Vargo, S. Minick, N. Ling, F.E. Bloom and R. Guillemin,1977, Regional dissociation of β-endorphin and enkephalin contents in rat brain and pituitary, Proc.Natl.Acad.Sci.USA, 74, 5162.

Sakura, N., and N. Yanaihara, 1978, Syntheses of some β-LPH-related peptides, in: Peptide Chemistry 1977, ed. T. Shiba (Protein Research Foundation Press, Osaka) p.183.

Straus, E., and R.S. Yalow, 1978, Species specificity of cholecystokinin in gut and several mammalian species, Proc.Natl.Acad.Sci. USA, 75,486.

Uhl, G.R. and S.H. Snyder, 1976, Regional and subcellular distribution of brain neurotensin, Life Sciences, 19,1827.

Yanaihara, C., H. Sato, M. Hirohashi, M. Sakagami, K. Yamamoto, T. Hashimoto, N. Yanaihara, K. Abe and T. Kaneko, 1976, Substance P radioimmunoassay using N^{α}-tyrosyl-substance P and demonstration of the presence of substance P-like immunoreactivities in human blood and porcine tissue extracts, Endocrinol.Japon.,23,457.

Yanaihara, C., A. Inoue, T. Mochizuki, N. Sakura, H. Sato and N. Yanaihara, 1978, Synthesis of bombesin-related peptides and their use for bombesin-specific radioimmunoassay, in: Peptide Chemistry 1978, ed. N. Izumiya (Protein Research Foundation Press, Osaka) in press.

Yoshida, H., T. Nakajima, K. Sakurai and Y. Fujita, 1974, Studies on high speed liquid chromatography on porous polymer and the separation of peptides. Isolation of biologically active peptides from the skin of Rana catesbeiana, in: Peptide Chemistry 1973, ed. H. Kotake(Protein Research Foundation Press, Osaka) p.115.

PREPARATION OF INTRINSICALLY-LABELLED KININS

Alfred Chung, James W. Ryan, and Pierre Berryer

Department of Medicine, University of Miami School
of Medicine, Miami, Florida 33101, U.S.A.

And Ronald Block, Papanicolaou Cancer Research Institue,
Miami, Florida 33136, U.S.A.

ABSTRACT

As part of a program to prepare bradykinin (H-Arg-Pro-Pro-
Gly-Phe-Ser-Pro-Phe-Arg-OH) labelled at high specific radioactivities, we have synthesized three analogs for dehalogenation in
tritium gas: [4-Br-Phe^5]-bradykinin (BK), [4-Br-Phe^8]-BK and
[4-Br-Phe^{5,8}]-BK. The analogs were synthesized by the Merrifield
solid-phase method and were purified by molecular sieve and partition chromatography. The analogs themselves possess biological
activity (as assayed for effects on mean arterial blood pressure
and isolated rat uterus). [4-Br-Phe^8]-BK was 1.5 to 3 times as
active as bradykinin. [4-Br-Phe^{5,8}]-BK was approx. 22% as active
as BK and [4-Br-Phe^5]-BK was approx. 18% as active. [4-Br-Phe^5]-BK
was submitted to catalytic dehalogenation with 10% Pd/C and 5%
Rh/CaCO$_3$ in H$_2$O and DMF (1:1) plus 10 Ci of ^{3}H$_2$. [4-^{3}H-Phe^5]-BK
was obtained at 6.7 Ci/mmole in an overall yield of 15%. [4-^{3}H-
Phe^8]-BK was prepared similarly to yield an intrinsically-labelled
peptide with a specific radioactivity of 21 Ci/mmole.

INTRODUCTION

Bradykinin (H-Arg-Pro-Pro-Gly-Phe-Ser-Pro-Phe-Arg-OH) is a
vasoactive substance thought to play a role in a variety of pathophysiologic events, including function vasodilation, systemic blood
pressure control, and the shock phase of acute hemorrhagic pancreatitis (for review, see Eisen, 1970). However, relatively little is
known of the means by which the biological activity of bradykinin
is terminated. Its biologic half-life in blood or plasma is short
(<15 sec), and its clearance rates in various vascular beds imply

far shorter half-lives (<1 sec in the pulmonary vascular bed, cf. Ryan and Ryan, 1977). Angiotensin converting enzyme (also known as kininase II) can degrade bradykinin to yield inactive metabolites, but the inactivation of bradykinin proceeds in vivo, even under conditions in which angiotensin converting enzyme is inhibited (e.g., after treatment with the specific inhibitors, SQ 14,225 and SQ 20,881 [BPP_{9a}]; e.g., see Ryan, U.S. et al., this volume).

The present study was begun as part of a program to help clarify the characteristics of other enzymes which inactivate bradykinin. Specifically, we set out to prepare a series of halogenated analogs of bradykinin, which, on catalytic dehalogenation in $^3H_2$ gas, would yield bradykinin intrinsically-labelled at high specific radioactivity. For these purposes, we prepared 4-Br-L-phenylalanine and substituted this residue to yield the three analogs, [4-Br-Phe[5]]-bradykinin (BK), [4-Br-Phe[8]]-BK and [4-Br-Phe[5,8]]-BK. Catalytic dehalogenation of these analogs to yield the respective [^3H]-Phe-bradykinins will allow us to monitor the actions of both endo- and exopeptidase enzymes (the latter including the dipeptidyl carboxypeptidase, angiotensin converting enzyme), when bradykinin is infused or perfused through organs at physiologic concentrations. This report describes the synthesis of the derivatized pehnylalanine, synthesis of the bradykinin analogs, and the procedures developed for radio-labelling. During the course of these studies, it was found that [4-Br-Phe[8]]-BK is more active than bradykinin itself.

MATERIALS AND METHODS

4-Br-L-phenylalanine was prepared from 4-amino-L-phenylalanine by the Sandemeyer reaction, and was protected with t-butyloxcarbo-nylazide, according to Scheme I. Properties of 4-Br-L-phenylalanine and derivatives are shown in Table I. Protected amino acids were obtained from Peninsula Laboratories, Inc.

Boc Arginine-Resin

According to the method of Gisin (1973), 4 g of resin (chloro-methylated Bio-Beads SX1, 0.75 meq/g) were treated in purified DMF at 50°C with dry cesium salt of Aoc-arginate(Tos) (prepared from 1.60 g of Aoc-Tosyl-L-arginine and 1 equivalent of CsOH in aqueous ethanol). The degree of amino acid substitution was determined by dry weight to be 0.25 meq/g.

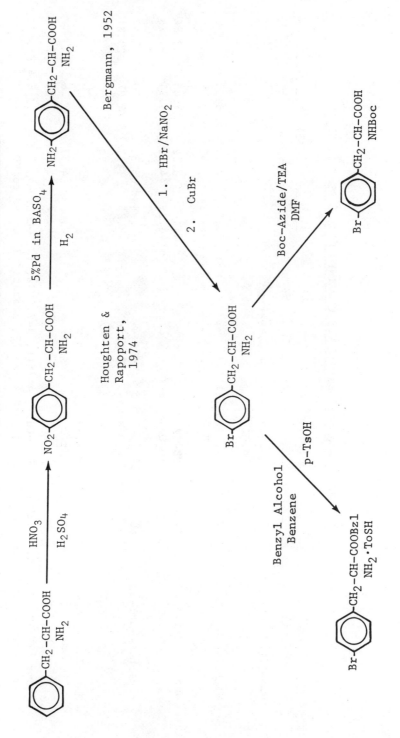

Scheme I

THE SYNTHESIS OF 4-BROMO-L-PHENYLALANINE AND ITS DERIVATIVES

Table I

PROPERTIES OF L-PHENYLALANINE DERIVATIVES OBTAINED FROM L-PHENALNINE

Compound	% Yield	m.p., °C	$[\alpha]^{25}_D$	Analysis			
				C	H	N	Br
H-Phe-(4-NO$_2$)-OH*	74	242-243 (H$_2$O)	+10.39**				
H-Phe(4-NH$_2$)-OH	89	249.5-250(d) (H$_2$O)		Cal. 59.94 Fd. 59.34	6.71 7.44	15.55 15.34	
H-Phe(4-Br)-OH	66	228-229 (H$_2$O)		44.09 44.29	4.12 4.13	5.66 5.74	32.86 32.74
Boc-Phe(4-Br)-OH	80	114.5-115.5 (Et$_2$O/Hex)	+24.4 (1% in EtOAc)	47.98 48.85	5.31 5.27	4.30 4.07	23.47 23.21
H-Phe(4-Br)-OBzl TsOH		181-182 (Et$_2$O)		54.50 54.37	4.77 4.77	2.76 2.94	

* nmr [TFA-d] 3.71(d, J=7.0 Hz, 2H, -CH$_2$-, 4.78(t, J=7.0 Hz, 1H, -CHCOO-), 7.63(d, J=8.4 Hz, 2H, aromatic H, ortho to -CH$_2$-), 8.23(d, J=8.4 Hz, 2H, aromatic H, ortho to NO$_2$).

** (0.98 in 1.0 N HCl).

The Peptide-Forming Step

Solid phase peptide synthesis was carried out in an upright vessel clamped to a power shaker. Peptide synthesis was carried out by the solid phase method (Stewart and Young, 1969). For incorporation of proline[7] and 4-bromophenylalanine[8], the dipeptide Boc-Pro-Phe(4-Br)-OH was used, which was prepared by coupling Boc-Pro-ONSu to H-Phe(4-Br)-OH.

The couplings were mediated with N,N'-dicyclohexyl-carbodiimide in the presence of 1-hydroxybenzotriazole (Koenig and Geiger, 1970). One cycle of the synthesis consisted of: (a) methylene chloride three times for 6 min; (b) 25% trifluoroacetic acid-methylene chloride containing 0.4 ml of 2-mercaptoethanol per 100 ml, 1.5 min; (c) 25% trifluoroacetic acid-methylene chloride containing 0.4 ml per 100 ml of 2-mercaptoethanol, 30 min; (d) methylene chloride six times for 6 min; (e) 10% triethylamine in methlene chloride, 2 min; (f) 10% triethylamine in methylene chloride, 10 min; (g) methylene chloride, six times for 6 min; (h) Boc-amino acid (2.5 equivalents), 5 min; (i) DCC-HOBt, 2 h; (j) methylene chloride, three times for 3 min; (k) DMF, three times for 3 min; (1) absolute ethanol, three times for 3 min; (m) methylene chloride, three times for 6 min.

Ninhydrin assay (Kaiser et al., 1970) of small samples of peptide resin intermediates before and after each coupling reaction served to test for completion of each acylation step.

Isolation Step

The peptides were deprotected and cleaved from the resin by anhydrous HF (Sakakibara, 1971), in the presence of anisole at 0°C for 60 min. After evaporation of the HF, the reaction mixture was washed thoroughly three times with ethyl acetate. The peptide was extracted from the resin with three 20 ml portions of 1% acetic acid. The aqueous extracts were combined and dried by lyophilization.

The crude peptides were purified by a series of column chromatography systems: (a) gel filtration on Sephadex G-25, elution with 1% acetic acid; (b) partition chromatography on Sephadex G-25 with n-butanol-acetic acid-H_2O (4:1:5); (c) chromatography on Sephadex LH-20, elution with 6% n-butanol in water. The peptides appeared as a single spot on four TLC systems and on electrophoresis at pH 1.9 and pH 5. The peptides were visualized with ninhydrin, O-tolidine/Cl_2 reagents and Sakaguchi spray (Irreverre, 1965).

RESULTS AND DISCUSSION

Synthesis

Our interests in preparing ^{3}H-labelled bradykinin by catalytic dehalogenation arose from the study of Morgat et al., 1970), who iodinated angiotensin II (H-Asp-Arg-Val-Tyr-Ile-His-Pro-Phe-OH) with ^{125}I and then dehalogenated the product in ^{3}H$_2$ to yield [^{3}H-Tyr^4]-angiotensin II at an apparent specific radioactivity near theoretical. However, bradykinin does not contain an amino acid residue that would allow iodination of the intact polypeptide. Furthermore, in the case of angiotensin II, iodination of the final peptide may not be specific, as both tyrosine and histidine may be iodinated. Similarly, histidine could be oxidized under the conditions used by Morgat et al.

Therefore, we chose to prepare a well-characterized halogenated phenylalanine, 4-Br-L-phenylalanine (Table I) for use in de novo synthesis of the relevant bradykinin analogs. To our knowledge, 4-Br-L-Phenylalanine has not been prepared previously by the Sandemeyer reaction. Dornow and Winter (1951) prepared 4-Br-D,L-phenylalanine by alkylation of α,4-dibromo toluene with diethyl formamidomalonate. Schwyzer and Surbeck-Wegmann (1960) resolved the corresponding D,L-methyl ester with dibenzoyl-L-tartaric acid. Others (e.g., Vine et al., 1973) have used enzymic resolution techniques. More recently, Brundish and Wade (1976) prepared Br-phenylalanine by exposure of L-phenylalanine to bromine gas. However, to obtain 4-Br-L-phenylalanine, it was necessary to resolve six ring-isomers by extensive ion exchange chromatography. We prepared 4-Br-L-phenylalanine directly from 4-NH$_2$-L-phenylalanine. The final step is straightforward and efficient, and can be generalized for use with all halogens. In addition to Br, we have used Cl and I. However, the final reaction assumes access to the corresponding NH$_2$-phenylalanine.

Incorporation of the corresponding N$^\alpha$-Boc-4-Br-L-phenylalanine into the final peptide presented no unusual problems: [4-Br-Phe^5]-BK and [4-Br-Phe^{5,8}]-BK were synthesized by the Merrifield technique at respective yields of 94%, 61%, and 78%.

Labelling

The dehalogenation in ^{3}H$_2$ gas was performed by two commercial firms. The Phe^5-BK derivative was obtained at 6.7 Ci/mmole and [4-^{3}H]Phe^8-BK was obtained at 21 Ci/mmole (theoretical 27 Ci/mmole) (Table III). We do not know whether the differences are owing to relative accessibilities of the phenylalanines to the catalysts, to the quality of ^{3}H$_2$ gas used by the different firms, or to use of different catalysts.

Table II

CHARACTERIZATION OF PHE(4-Br)-BRADYKININ ANALOGS

Peptide	TLC R_{Arg}				Electrophoresis E_{Arg}		Amino Acid Analysis					
	A	B	C	D	pH 1.9	pH 5.0	Arg	Pro	Gly	Phe	Phe(4-Br)	Ser
Phe(4-Br)[8]-BK	1.98	6.20	0.72	4.03	0.47	0.64	2.07	3.06	1.00	0.99	1.06	0.95
Phe(4-Br)[5,8]-BK	1.98	6.20	0.80	4.62	0.50	0.67	2.05	3.00	1.03		1.96	0.96
Phe(4-Br)[5]-BK	1.98	6.20	0.71	4.00	0.43	0.61	2.07	3.07	1.00	0.98	1.03	0.96

TLC buffer systems: A n-Butanol-pyridine-acetic acid-water (15:10:3:12)
                     B Chloroform-methanol-ammonium hydroxide (60:45:20)
                     C n-Butanol-acetic acid-ethyl acetate-water (1:1:1:1)
                     D Ethyl acetate-pyridine-acetic acid-water (5:5:1:3)

Electrophoresis pH 1.9 Formic acid-aceti acid-water (14:10:75)
           buffers: pH 5.0 Diethylene glycol-acetic acid-pyridine-water (100:6:8.5:885.5)

Table III

METHODS OF LABELLING

Precursor	Catalyst	Labelled Peptide	Specific Radioactivity
Phe(4-Br)^5-Bradykinin	10% Pd/C-5% Rh/CaCO$_3$	[4-^{3}H]Phe^5-Bradykinin	6.7 Ci/mmole
Phe(4-Br)^8-Bradykinin	10% Pd/CaCO$_3$	[4-^{3}H]Phe^8-Bradykinin	21 Ci/mmole

Table IV

COMPARISON OF BIOLOGIC ACTIVITIES OF 4-BROMO-L-PHENYLA-
LANINE ANALOGS OF BRADYKININ WITH THOSE OF BRADYKININ

(% of Bradykinin)

Analogs	Rat Uterus (Isolated)	Guinea Pig Ileum (Isolated)	Rat Blood Pressure	
			Intravenous	Intra Aortic
Bradykinin	100	100	100	100
[4-Br-Phe^5]-BK	17.5	55.5	22	44.5
[4-Br-Phe^8]-BK	143	153	360	337
[4-Br-Phe^{5,8}]-BK	21.8	35.6	113	50

(For assay techniques, see Robler et al., 1973)

Specificity of Labelling

Non-specific labelling did not appear to be a problem in either tritiation: Analyses of acid hydrolysates showed that phenylalanine possessed 98% of the ^{3}H label. None of the other amino acids showed definite evidence of labelling. However, since phenylalanine did not contain 100% of the label, we cannot rule out the presence of small amounts of slowly exchangeable ^{3}H. Hydrolysis of [4-^{3}H]Phe^5-BK with either chymotrypsin or human urinary angiotensin converting enzyme yielded Arg-Pro-Pro-Gly(^{3}H)Phe as the limit product. Similarly, ^{3}H-Phe^8-BK was hydrolyzed by converting enzyme to yield (^{3}H)Phe-Arg and by chymotrypsin to yield Ser-Pro-(^{3}H)Phe. Thus, the specificity of labelling and the efficiency of ^{3}H incorporation are fully adequate to permit future metabolic studies to proceed (See Ryan, U.S. et al., this volume).

Biological Activities of the Precursors

One finding was unexpected: Depending on the assay tissue, [4-Br-Phe^8]-BK was found to be 1.4 to 3.6-times more active than bradykinin. [4-Br-Phe^5]-BK was clearly less active than bradykinin (Table IV). These results, taken with those presented elsewhere (Chung et al., 1978) appear to indicate that the interaction of bradykinin with its receptors (and probably with its metabolic enzymes) can be critically affected by the nature of substituents on the phenylalanine rings. If one takes the relative potencies of a given analog on mean arterial blood pressure when injected intravenously, versus when injected into the ascending aorta as a measure of metabolic degradation, the [4-Br-Phe^{5,8}]-BK is clearly resistant to degradation and [4-Br-Phe^5]-BK is more vulnerable. [4-Br-Phe^8]-BK appears to be metabolized, presumably by enzymes of the lungs, at a rate like that for bradykinin itself. Thus, the superactivity of [4-Br-Phe^8]-BK is unlikely to be due to resistance to metabolic degradation. Possibly the bromo-atom has favorable effects on the conformation of bradykinin or on the relative affinity of the analog to the receptor. However, neither of these two possibilities is readily tested.

ACKNOWLEDGEMENTS

This work was supported in part by the U.S. Public Health Service (HL22087 and HL22896), the John A. Harford Foundation, Inc., and the Council for Tobacco Research-U.S.A, Inc.

REFERENCES

Bergman, E.P., 1952, p-Amino- and p-fluoro-β-phenylalanine, J. Amer. Chem. Soc., 74, 4947.

Brundish, D. and R. Wade, 1976, Tritiated peptides, Part 3, Synthesis of [4-^{3}H-Phe^7]-β-corticotrophin-(1-24)-tetracosapeptide, J. Chem. Soc., Perkin I, 2186.

Chung, A., J.W. Ryan, P. Berryer and A. Day, 1978, Influence of phenylalanine residues on the activity of bradykinin, 176th Nat. Meet. Amer. Chem. Soc., Miami Beach, Sept. 9-15, 1978.

Dornow, A. and G. Winter, 1951, Some chloromycetin-like N-dichloroacetyl derivatives of the "phenylalaninol" series, Chem. Ber., 84, 307.

Eisen, V., Formation and functions of kinins, 1970, in: The Immunochemistry and Biochemistry of Connective Tissue and Its Disease States, Rheumatology, Vol. 3, (Karger Basel), p. 103.

Gisin, B.F., 1973, The preparation of Merrifield-resins through total esterification with cesium salts, Helv. Chim. Acta, 56, 1476.

Houghten, R.A. and H. Rapoport, 1974, Synthesis of pure p-chlorophenyl-L-alanine from L-phenylalanine, J. Med. Chem., 17, 556.

Irreverre, F., 1965, A modified Sakaguchi spray, Biochim. Biophys. Acta, 111, 551.

Kaiser, E., R.L. Colescott, C.D. Bossinger and P.I. Cook, 1970, Color test for detection of free terminal amino groups in the solid-phase synthesis of peptides, Anal. Biochem, 34, 595.

Koenig, W. and R. Geiger, 1970, New method for the synthesis of peptides: Activation of the carboxyl group with dicyclohexylcarbodiimide by using 1-hydroxybenzoltriazoles as additives, Chem. Ber., 103, 788.

Roblero, J., J.W. Ryan and J.M. Stewart, 1973, Assay of kinins by their effects on blood pressure, Res. Commun. Chem. Path. Pharmac., 6, 207.

Ryan, J.W. and U.S. Ryan, 1977, Pulmonary endothelial cells, Fed. Proc., 36, 2683.

Ryan, U.S., J.W. Ryan, D. Habliston and G. Pena, Endothelial cells and components of the kallikrein-kinin system, this volume.

Sakakibara, S., The use of hydrogen fluoride in peptide chemistry, 1971, in: Chemistry and Biochemistry of Amino Acids, ed. C.B. Weinstein (Marcel Dekker, New York), p. 51.

Schwyzer, R. and E. Surbeck-Wegmann, 1960, Resolution of D,L-p-bromophenylalanine, Helv. Chim. Acta, 63, 1073.

Stewart, J.M. and J.D. Young, 1969, Solid Phase Peptide Synthesis, (W.H. Freeman Co., San Francisco).

Vine, W.H., D.A. Brueckner, P. Needleman, and G.R. Marshall, 1973, Synthesis, biological activity and ^{19}F nuclear magnetic resonance spectra of angiotensin II analogs containing fluorine, Biochemistry, 12, 1630.

KININOGENASE ACTIVITY AND KININ-LIKE SUBSTANCE IN THE

VENOMOUS SPICULES AND SPINES OF LEPIDOPTERAN LARVAE

F. Kawamoto and N. Kumada

Department of Medical Zoology, Nagoya University

School of Medicine, Showa, Nagoya 466 Japan

Of the medically important caterpillars of Lepidopteran insects (moths and butterflies) in Japan, some species of the genus Euproctis (tussock moth) and three kinds of slug moths, Parasa consocia, Parasa sinica, Cnidocampa flavescens, are known to be the most harmful.   Recently, the pioneer work was performed by de Jong and Bleumink (1-2) concerning the spicule venom of the brown tail moth, E. chrysorrhoea, and they found the presence of enzymic activities of protease, esterase and phospholipase A_2 in its extract.   However, there is little knowledge about the nature of the venoms involved in the venomous spicules and spines of the above insects.

We studied the venomous hairs by electron microscopy, and their venoms were investigated biochemically and pharmacologically. Parts of our findings have been reported previously (3-5).

Euproctis spicule

A single caterpillar of the oriental tussock moth, E. subflava (Fig. 1a) has millions of venomous spicules with a length of about 150 μm on each subdorsal tubercle (Fig. 1b).   It penetrates into the skin with the pointed proximal end after detached from its socket in the cap-shaped papilla (Fig. 1c).   As shown in Fig. 1d, we found that the electron-dense and osmiophilic materials secreted from spicule-formative cells enter the spicule cavity passing through holes on the spicule and socket.   It was considered that the electron-dense materials were the main toxic substances involved in the spicule.

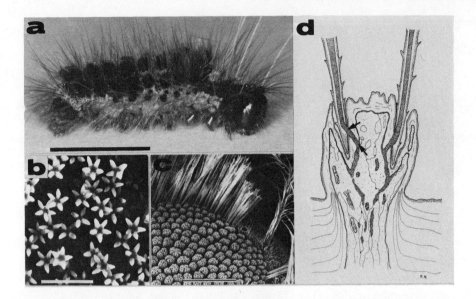

Fig. 1.   (a) E. subflava caterpillar.   (b) Top portion of
spicules located on the subdorsal tubercles.   (c) Spicules and
sockets in the papillae.   (d) A schematic presentation of a
papilla and two spicules.   Arrows show holes on spicule and
socket.   Bars represent 1 cm (a), 10 μm (b) and 50 μm (c).

The crude venom was extracted with PBS (pH 7.2) from the
spicule.   A high molecular (HM) fraction of the venom was
separated from a lower molecular (LM) one by a single hollow fiber
concentrator (SHFC, cut-off molecular weight of 15,000).   Then,
HM was further fractionated with a Sephadex G-100 column.   Among
the four fractions (HM-I~IV) obtained, HM-II~III were proved to
contain potent proteolytic (casein as substarate) and esterolytic
(TAME as substrate) activities (Fig. 2a).   After an incubation
with heated plasma of guinea pig as substrate, kininogenase
activity was also found in the same fraction (Fig. 2).   This
seems to be the first finding on the presence of a kininogenase
in arthropod venoms.

Pain-producing substances in the venomous hairs of the slug moth caterpillars

Dermatitis caused by spines and spicules of slug moth larvae (Fig. 3, a-b) is characterized by accompanying severe pain with erythema or edema. Crude venoms from these hairs also involved severe pain-producing activity. After the separation of the crude venoms into HM and LM fractions with SHFC, the presence of the pain-producing activity in each of these fractions was

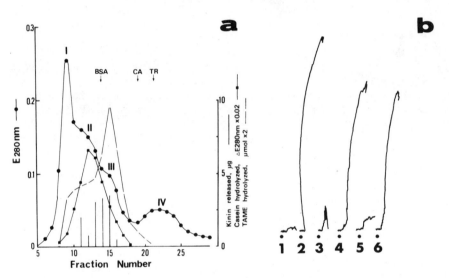

Fig. 2a. Chromatography of HM fraction obtained from the spicule venom on a Sephadex G-100 column (0.9 x 28 cm) equilibrated with 0.05M phosphate buffer (pH 7.2). Enzymic activities were expressed in the amounts of substrates hydrolyzed by 0.1 ml of each fraction in 30 min at 37°C. BSA, bovine serum albumin; CA, casein; TR, trypsin.

Fig. 2b. Contraction by released kinin and inactivation of kinin by chymotrypsin. Guinea pig ileum was used in a 20 ml bath. The reaction mixture containing 0.5 ml of heated plasma and 0.1 ml of pooled HM-III was incubated for 15 min at 37°C. After heating, the mixture was treated with 100 μg of chymotrypsin (CH) or trypsin (TR) for 15 min at 37°C, and the remaining kinin was assayed. 1, Control plasma added with 0.1 ml of PBS, 0.3 ml; 2, Bradykinin (BK), 1 μg; 3, BK+CH; 4, Kinin released by venom, 0.15 ml; 5, Kinin+CH, 0.45 ml; 6, Kinin+TR, 0.15 ml.

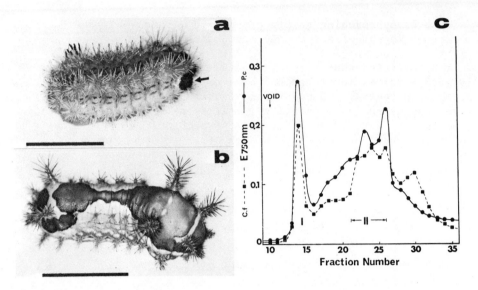

Fig. 3.   (a) P. consocia caterpillar.   Arrow shows the cluster
of spicules morphologically similar to the Euproctis spicule.
(b) C. flavescens caterpillar.   Bars represent 1 cm in (a-b).
(c) Gel-filtration of LM fractions from P. consocia (P.c) and
C. flavescens (C.f) spines in a Sephadex G-50 column (1.6 x 38 cm)
equilibrated with 0.05M phosphate buffer (pH 7.2).

assayed by the skin scratch method in man; strong activity was
detected in HMs of Parasa spines and spicules.   LMs of
P. consocia and C. flavescens also showed this activity, however,
it differed from that of HMs in its rapid action and shorter
duration, and it was not so stable as HMs.   It appeared that the
activity in LMs might be diminished or lost during the extraction
and storage of the crude venoms with PBS.

    Experiments with fractions obtained on Sephadex G-100 and
G-50 column chromatographies, respectively for HM and LM,
demonstrated that the second peak of HM (HM-II) and the first peak
of LM (LM-I, Fig. 3c) had activities to produce pain and to
contract smooth muscle of the isolated guinea pig ileum.   The
contraction induced by HM-II differed from that by histamine,
bradykinin and LM-I in that the former showed marked tachyphylaxis.
Enzymic activity (protease, esterase, kininogenase) or a possible
involvement of kininogen in HM-II has not been observed so far.

LM-I was revealed to be a protein or polypeptide with a molecular weight of several thousands, lacking the absorbancy at 280 nm. Since LM-I also had a permeability-increasing activity, it was suggested that it might be related to a kinin-like substance or peptide found in the venoms of bees, hornets, ants, etc (6). However, we consider that methods of extraction and storage must be improved for the final characterization of LM-I.

ACKNOWLEDGEMENTS

We are grateful to Prof. T. Shigei, Department of Pharmacology, Nagoya University School of Medicine, for his valuable suggestions and advice during this study.

REFERENCES

1. de Jong, M.C.J.M. and E. Bleumink (1977): Investigative studies of the dermatitis caused by the larvae of the Brown-tail moth, Euproctis chrysorrhoea Linn. (Lepidoptera, Lymantriidae) III. Chemical analysis of skin reactive substances. Arch. Derm. Res., 259, 247-262.

2. de Jong, M.C.J.M. and E. Bleumink (1977): Investigative studies of the dermatitis caused by the larvae of the Brown-tail moth, Euproctis chrysorrhoea Linn. (Lepidoptera, Lymantriidae) IV. Further characterization of skin reactive substances. Arch. Derm. Res., 259, 263-281.

3. Kawamoto, F., C. Suto and N. Kumada (1978): Studies on the venomous spicules and spines of moth caterpillars I. Fine structure and development of the venomous spicules of the Euproctis caterpillars. Jap. J. Med. Sci. Biol., 31, 291-299.

4. Kawamoto, F. (1978): Studies on the venomous spicules and spines of moth caterpillars II. Pharmacological and biochemical properties of the spicule venom of the Oriental tussock moth caterpillar, Euproctis subflava. Jap. J. Sanit. Zool., 29, 175-183.

5. Kawamoto, F. (1978): Studies on the venomous spicules and spines of moth caterpillars III. Scanning electron microscopic examination of spines and spicules of the slug moth caterpillar, Parasa consocia, and some properties of pain-producing substances in their venoms. Jap. J. Sanit. Zool., 29, 185-196.

6. Pisano, J.J. (1968): Vasoactive peptides in venoms. Fed. Proc., 27, 58-62.

Assays of Components of the
Kallikrein-Kinin System

AN APPROACH TO THE CHEMICAL QUANTITATION OF KININS FOR THE ASSAY

OF KININOGENASES

B.T. Khouw

Research Centre, Canada Packers, Ltd.,

Toronto, Ontario, M6N 1K4, Canada

ABSTRACT

A method was developed for the rapid isolation and identification of kallidin produced by hog pancreatic kallikrein on a partially purified bovine plasma kininogen preparation. By means of a reversed phase chromatography on a C_{18}-silica gel column, kallidin was rapidly concentrated from the reaction mixture, and subsequently resolved on a thin-layer plate of silica gel 60. Fluorescamine was used to locate the kinin. Efforts to elute the kinin from the TLC plates for quantitation were not successful.

INTRODUCTION

Presently two types of assay methods for kininogenases are used. One type is based on the determination of the kinin activity in a biological system, such as hypotensive activity, increased blood flow or contractive activity on smooth muscle preparations. This type of assay requires an external standard whose unit (KU or FU) has been arbitrarily assigned. The other type of assay is based on the esterase activity of the enzymes in N-substituted arginine esters such as BAEE or TAME. Although an external standard is not required, these esters are susceptible to hydrolysis by other proteases, and specific inhibitors to eliminate or differentiate these proteases are not always available. Furthermore, the esterase activity obtained may not necessarily reflect the kinin-yielding activity of the kininogenases on the naturally occurring substrate (Mares-Guia, et al., 1975).

Despite the sensitivity exhibited by these types of assay systems, their specificity is questionable. On the other hand, a chemical assay based on the measurement of the reaction product, kinin, produced from a kininogen by a kininogenase would offer a distinct advantage in specificity. However, like all specific chemical assay systems, a preliminary isolation of the type of kinin produced is necessary. This is often difficult to achieve in a relatively simple and rapid manner, particularly when the quantity involved is small (ng). In order to circumvent this, advantage has been taken to use the resolving power of a non-polar bonded phase to quickly separate the kinin or other peptides produced from an acidified reaction mixture, and to further resolve the product in a simple system consisting of thin-layer chromatography. The preliminary results at such an attempt are presented.

MATERIALS AND METHODS

A highly purified hog pancreatic kallikrein, 1100 FU/mg, was produced in Canada Packers Research Centre. Soybean trypsin inhibitor (SBTI), 5x crystallized, was a product of Nutritional Biochemicals. Hog trypsin, crystallized, was purchased from Miles Biochemicals. Bradykinin (BK) and kallidin (KD) were obtained from Beckman, the purity and the quantity of which were checked by means of their amino acid contents. Octadecyltrichlorosilane was supplied by Aldrich Chemicals. Fluorescamine was a product of Hoffmann-La Roche. BDH Chemicals supplied the trifluoroacetic acid (TFA) and the pre-coated TLC plates (5x20 cm) of silica gel 60 without fluorescent indicator. All other chemicals and solvents were of reagent grade and used as such without further purification.

A partially purified bovine plasma kininogen was prepared from heated (60°C, 30 minutes) citrated plasma by DEAE-A-50 and Sephadex G-150 chromatography (Komiya, et al., 1974). On extensive digestion with hog pancreatic kallikrein in the presence of SBTI and EDTA, the kininogen preparation showed a specific activity of 2.13 ug KD equivalent/mg protein as measured in the guinea pig ileum assay (Webster and Prado, 1970). Protein was determined by means of biuret reagent (Gornall, et al., 1949).

Preparation of C_{18}-Silica Gel. 15 g dry silica gel (SilicAR, CC-7, 200-325 mesh, Mallinckrodt), was refluxed for 2 hours with 160 ml 10% octadecyltrichlorosilane in chloroform. After cooling, the silanized gel was repeatedly washed with chloroform, methanol, and finally sucked dry in air. For use, 1 g of silanized gel was packed in a 3 ml disposable plastic syringe (0.9x6 cm) fitted with a porous teflon or polyethylene disc. The gel column, about 1.8 ml, was washed with 8 ml methanol, followed by 8 ml 1% TFA, and was then ready for use.

Assay System for Hog Pancreatic Kallikrein. The reaction
mixture consisted of 0.1 ml 0.1M phosphate buffer containing 0.01M
EDTA at pH 8.0, 0.1 ml SBTI (1 mg/ml), 0.1 ml enzyme (200 ug/ml),
0.1 ml kininogen (50 mg/ml) and water to 1.0 ml. Prior to kininogen
addition, the enzyme was allowed to incubate with the inhibitor for
10 minutes. The reaction was carried out at 38°C for 2 minutes,
and 0.2 ml ice cold 30% TFA was used to terminate the reaction.
After 30 minutes at 0°C, the mixture was centrifuged at top speed
in a clinical centrifuge, and the hazy supernatant was used for
kinin isolation and identification as described below.

Kinin Isolation and Identification. An aliquot (0.2 - 0.5 ml)
of the reaction supernatant was applied to the packed and conditioned
(in 1% TFA) silanized gel. The gel column was subsequently washed
with 2 ml 1% TFA, and the retained kinin was eluted with 4 ml 80%
methanol containing 1% TFA. The flow rate of the gel column was
maintained at about 1 ml/min with the aid of an infusion pump
(Harvard Apparatus). The acidic eluate was then neutralized with
2 g moist freshly regenerated Dowex 1-X1 (OH⁻), 50-100 mesh, and
the anion exchange resin was washed with 80% methanol. The resin-
treated solution (pH 5-6), was evaporated to dryness under reduced
pressure at 40°C, and the residue was subsequently taken up in 5-10 ul
methanol for spotting on a TLC plate. The TLC solvent used was 1-
butanol:acetic acid:pyridine:water (BAPW) in a ratio of 30:6:20:24.
Following the TLC run, the plate was air-dried, stained with fluorescamine (Mendez and Lai, 1975), and visualized under UV light to
locate the kinin spot. A standard bradykinin or kallidin (100-200 ng)
each, was concurrently run. Alternatively, the sample was prestained
prior to the TLC run. This was carried out by adding 10 ul 1% triethylamine in acetone to 5-10 ul sample in methanol or water, followed by
20 ul fluorescamine 0.3 mg/ml in acetone. After 10-15 minutes, the
reaction mixture was evaporated to dryness under reduced pressure
and the residue was taken up in 5-10 ul methanol which was then
used for spotting on TLC plate and developed in BAPW. Following
the TLC run, and drying of the plate, the fluorescent spot was
visualized under UV light.

All glassware used was treated with silicone (Siliclad, Clay
Adams). When fluorescent measurements were attempted, a Turner
fluorometer (model No. 111) was used, equipped with No. 7-60 (360 nm)
primary, and No. 8 (485 nm) secondary filter.

RESULTS AND DISCUSSION

When different amounts of bradykinin and kallidin were
chromatographed on a TLC plate, and stained with fluorescamine,
quantities as low as 30 ng of the kinins fluoresced clearly under

UV light. When the free kinin was reacted with fluorescamine in
solutions, the fluorescence intensity was linearly related to the
amount of the kinin and a quantity as low as 4 ng was readily
measurable. Since the measurements of fluorescence attempted in
this study were not at the optimal excitation (390 nm) and emission
(480 nm), wavelength of fluorescamine, a lower kinin detection level
is certainly anticipated. Thus fluorescamine could be adequately
used to detect and quantify the kinins as represented by bradykinin
and kallidin. The limit of detection was certainly within the
scope of the kinin generated during the course of an enzyme reaction
as monitored in a guinea pig ileum assay.

Since the fluorescamine reaction is a general one for peptides
or amino acids bearing free amino groups (Udenfriend, et al., 1972),
it was therefore necessary to isolate the kinin prior to reacting it
with this reagent. To this end the method described above was used
to initially and rapidly isolate the kinin from a reaction mixture.
As much as 0.5 ug of free kallidin, when applied in 1% TFA, was
effectively retained by 1 g dry silanized gel (1.8 ml bed volume)
conditioned in the same acid. Increasing the solvent polarity by
means of 80% methanol (4 column volumes) applied to the non-polar
gel resulted in an effective elution of the retained kinin. In
order to further resolve the kinin as a distinct spot following TLC
it was found necessary to treat briefly the acidic eluate obtained
from the silanized gel with anion exchanger, Dowex 1-X1 (OH⁻), which
brought the eluate to about pH 5-6.

Based on such simple and relatively rapid isolation and elution
operation in a non-polar bonded phase (or reversed-phase chromatography), peptides including kinin generated from a kininogenase
reaction were readily separated and resolved on a TLC plate of
silica gel. Figure 1A illustrates the thin-layer chromatogram of
processing reaction aliquots made from an undigested reaction mixture
(a), the products of kininogen treated with hog pancreatic kallikrein (c) or with hog crystalline trypsin (b) together with the
corresponding standard kallidin and bradykinin spots (d). No bradykinin spot was noted from the pattern of tryptic digest. This was
also confirmed by a negative response registered in a guinea pig
ileum assay. The trypsin used contained about 0.3% chymotrypsin
which would act as a kininase. Thus the fluorescent peptide spots
were possibly representing fractions of degraded kinin. On the
other hand, a fluorescent spot corresponding to kallidin was brightly
registered from the kallikrein digest. However, two other very
faintly fluorescent spots were observed but their identity was not
determined.

As an alternative method for resolving these digestion mixtures,
the peptides were prestained with fluorescamine prior to TLC, as
illustrated in Figure 1B. Again the results were essentially similar

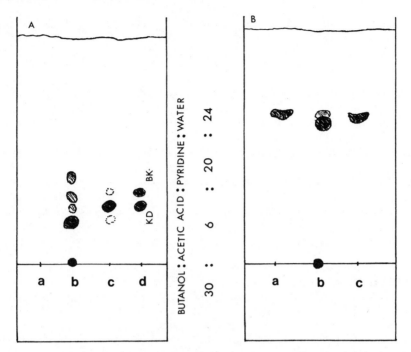

Figure 1A. Thin-layer chromatogram of kinins and peptides on silica gel 60. (a) Undigested kininogen, (b) trypsin digest, (c) kallikrein digest and (d) standard kallidin, KD, and bradykinin, BK.

1B. Same as 1A, but samples were prestained with fluorescamine prior to TLC. (a) Standard kallidin, (b) trypsin digest and (c) kallikrein digest.

to the unstained TLC run, but a far cleaner (non-fluorescent) background was noted in the prestained chromatogram. Furthermore, the mobility of the stained kinins was greatly increased, because of increased polarity originating from the fluorescamine. However, the TLC based on prestained samples showed diffused fluorescence, and also the resolution as indicated by the number of spots was less defined compared to the chromatographic run made with the non-stained sample. This was illustrated by the reduction in the number of spots obtained by prestaining the tryptic digest.

Attempts thus far to quantitate the fluorescent intensity of kinins by eluting the TLC spots were not successful. This failure thus precluded the development of a quantitative assay method for kinins. There were numerous factors contributing to the difficulty of eluting and quantifying the kinins from the TLC plate. One such factor was associated with the highly charged properties of both the silica gel and the kinins; perhaps TLC based on cellulose or on alumina gel medium would circumvent this. No doubt the use of paper electrophoresis would also facilitate not only kinin resolution and elution, but also the sensitivity of kinin detection. Another important factor was the purity of the solvents used during the isolation as well as during the TLC run, since the fluorescamine reaction was highly sensitive, and many impurities present in these solvents were also reactive; extraneous fluorescence could thus complicate the measurements of fluorescence generated from minute quantities of kinins.

To summarize, despite the failure to develop a quantitative assay method for kininogenases based on a chemical kinin estimation, a system for rapidly isolating the kinin on a non-polar bonded phase was developed. It is hoped that future efforts will enable us to conveniently and reliably quantitate the isolated kinins, and the activity of the enzyme will thus be more clearly defined in terms of its reactive product.

ACKNOWLEDGEMENT

The excellent assistance of Miss Laurie Michal is greatly appreciated.

REFERENCES

Gornall, A.G., C.J. Bardawill and M.M. David, 1949, Determination of serum proteins by means of biuret reaction, J. Biol. Chem., 177: 751.
Mares-Guia, M., et al., A comparative study of urinary kallikrein isolated from man and the rat, 1975 In: Chemistry and Biology of the Kallikrein-Kinin System in Health and Disease, eds., J.J. Pisano and K.F. Austen (Fogarty Internat. Center Proc. No. 27, U.S. Gov. Printing Office, Washington) p. 97.
Mendez, E. and C.Y. Lai, 1975, Reaction of peptides with fluorescamine on paper after chromatography or electrophoresis, Analyt. Biochem. 65: 281.
Komiya, M., H. Kato and T. Suzuki, 1974, Bovine plasma kininogen. III. Structural comparison of high molecular weight and low molecular weight kininogens. J. Biochem. (Tokyo), 76: 833.

Udenfriend, S., et al., 1972, Applications of fluorescamine, a new reagent for assay of amino acids, peptides, proteins and other primary amines in the picomole range. Science, $\underline{178}$: 871.

Webster, M.E. and E.S. Prado, Glandular kallikreins from horse and human urine and from hog pancreas, 1970, In: Methods in Enzymology, Vol. 14, Eds., G.E. Perlmann and L. Lorand (Academic Press, New York) p. 681.

DETERMINATION OF PREKALLIKREIN IN PLASMA BY MEANS OF A CHROMOGENIC TRIPEPTIDE SUBSTRATE FOR PLASMA KALLIKREIN

P. Friberger, E. Eriksson, S. Gustavsson, & G. Claeson

AB Kabi, Peptide Research

Mölndal, Sweden

ABSTRACT

A method for plasma prekallikrein determination utilizing a chromogenic tripeptide substrate is presented. The method has a good reproducibility and can easily be automized. Several parameters have been optimized. By using mixtures of deficient plasmas and pooled normal plasma or purified factors it was proved that prekallikrein was the factor determined and that more than 10% (of normal plasma concentration) of FXII and HMW kininogen were essential for the activation of prekallikrein in our method. Further experiments showed that the method was fairly selective and was not influenced by inhibitors present in normal plasma. The later finding was attributed to the high dilution of plasma made possible by using a potent activator and a sensitive substrate.

INTRODUCTION

In the Hageman factor mediated activation of the coagulation-, fibrinolytic- and kinin systems in blood, prekallikrein (prekininogenase, Fletcher factor) is an important link (Fig. 1). These initial reactions mainly take place on negatively charged surfaces (10, 11, 13, 15) and high molecular weight (HMW) kininogen (Fitzgerald factor) is essential for the efficiency of this activation (6, 10, 11, 13).

Mainly the inhibitor of C 1 esterase activity (C 1 INH) but also α_2-macroglobulin (α_2-M) and antithrombin (AT III) in combination with heparin control these reactions in vivo (4, 14).

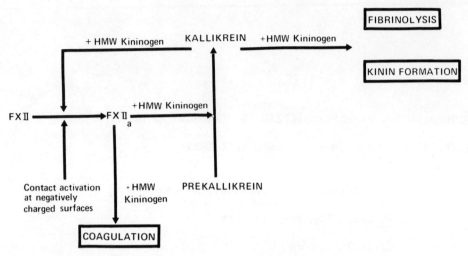

Fig 1. A schematic sketch on the initial phase of the activation
of the coagulation-, fibrinolytic-, and kinin systems in blood.

The amount of prekallikrein in human plasma can after activation be
determined as an active enzyme by using a suitable chromogenic
substrate. Such methods have been reported by several research
groups (1, 5, 7, 9, 12). We have made a series of experiments to
optimize the method and to study factors that may influence the
assay of plasma prekallikrein.

MATERIALS AND METHODS

Normal human plasmas: Citrated pooled plasma from 25 healthy donors
was kept at -25°C for less than 3 months. Lyophilized normal human
plasma from Ortho Diagnostics (Raritan, N.J.) was also used.
Activators: Cephotest ^{R} from Nyco (Oslo, Norway), Activated Thrombofax Reagent^R from Ortho Diagnostics and Dextran sulphate sodium salt,
MW ~ 500 000 from Pharmacia Fine Chemicals (Uppsala, Sweden).
Buffers: 0.05 mol/l Tris buffer with pH adjusted with hydrochloric
acid and I adjusted with sodium chloride.
Substrates: S-2302 (H-D-Pro-Phe-Arg-pNA), S-2222 and S-2251 (Plasmakallikrein, FXa and plasmin substrates) from Kabi Diagnostica (Stockholm, Sweden). S-2249 (Bz-Pro-Phe-Arg-pNA) was synthesized in our
laboratory.
Deficient plasmas: FXIII-, Fitzgerald- and Fletcher factor deficient
plasmas were obtained from George King Bio-Medical Inc. (Overland
Park, Kansas). FXI deficient plasma (lyophilized) was kindly supplied
from Ortho Diagnostics.

Purified human plasma prekallikrein: was kindly supplied from
Dr D Schroeder, Cutter Laboratories (Berkeley, California).
Purified human plasma kallikrein: prepared according to Gallimore
et al (9) was obtained from Dr M Gallimore (Oslo, Norway).
Purified bovine HMW kininogen: was kindly supplied from Dr S Iwanaga
(Osaka, Japan).
Sodium flufenamate: Flufenamic acid from Troponwerke (Köln, FRG) was
dissolved in an equivalent amount of sodium hydroxide solution.
Equipment: A Hitachi 101 Spectrophotometer connected over an Optilab
Multianolog lin-log converter to a Tohshin linear recorder was used.
Plastic disposable tubes were used for the plasma samples.

Determination of Purified Plasma Kallikrein Activity.

The plasma kallikrein preparation was diluted 1+40 with distilled
water (other solvents: saline, 0.5% Carbowax 6000 were also tested
and gave the same results and stability). The substrate S-2302 was
used at a concentration of $2 \cdot 10^{-3}$ mol/l.

Tris buffer pH 7.8, I 0.05	µl	700
thermostate at 37°C (5-6 min)		x
Enzyme	µl	100
Substrate	µl	200
mix and read ΔA/min at 405 nm (37°C)		

Determination of Prekallikrein after Cephotest Activation.

The plasma was kept frozen (-25°) or during the analysis (< 8 hr) at
room temperature (not on ice) in order to avoid "cold promoted activation". 50 µl of test plasma was diluted with 600 µl of the 0.05
mol/l Tris buffer pH 7.8, I 0.05. The activator was prepared by diluting Cephotest with 9 parts of 0.05 mol/l Tris buffer pH 7.8, I 0.05.
This solution was stable for one working day at room temperature. The
substrate (S-2302) was used at a concentration of $6 \cdot 10^{-3}$ mol/l.

Activator	µl	800
thermostate at 37°C (5-6 min)		x
Diluted plasma sample or standard	µl	100
mix and incubate at 37°C for	sec	120
Substrate (37°C)	µl	100
mix and read ΔA/min at 405 nm (37°C)		x
or		
incubate for exactly	sec	60
Acetic acid, 50%	µl	100
mix and read A405 against a sample blank		x

Standards (25, 50, 75, 100, and 125% of normal) were made by diluting
500 µl of plasma with 2.10 ml of buffer and then 100, 200, 300, 400,
and 500 µl were further diluted to 1 ml.

Determination of Prekallikrein after Activation with Dextran sulphate.

Dextran sulphate was dissolved and diluted to a concentration of
25 mg/l. A Tris buffer pH 7.8, I 0.15 was used. The substrates were
used at a concentration of $1.5 \cdot 10^{-3}$ mol/l. In order to be able to
use the same amount of plasma as in the method above 150 µl of
saline was added to 500 µl of plasma.

Dextran sulphate solution	µl	100
Diluted plasma sample or standard	µl	100
incubate at 0°C	min	7
Tris buffer	µl	1500
thermostate at 37°C (5-6 min)		
Activated plasma from the incubate (0°C)	µl	20
Substrate (37°C)	µl	500
mix and read ΔA/min at 405 nm (37°C)		

Standards (25, 50, 75, and 100%) were made by diluting the normal
plasma 1+3, 1+1, 3+1, and 1+0 with saline. Method according to
Kluft (12).

RESULTS

All data presented are mean values of double determinations, if not
otherwise stated.

Optimation for the Determination of Purified Plasma Kallikrein.

It was found that a 0.05 mol/l Tris-HCl buffer with a pH from 7.6
to 8.3 was optimal for kallikrein determination (Fig 2 a). The ionic
strength could be changed from 0.05 to 0.25 with NaCl without affecting
the activity (Fig 2 b). Tris buffer pH 7.8, I 0.15 was used for further
experiments. By using seven different substrate concentrations with
four determinations on each concentration, we found in a Lineweaver-
Burk plot a $K_m = 1.8 \cdot 10^{-4}$ mol/l. Therefore a final substrate concentration of $4 \cdot 10^{-4}$ mol/l would be reasonable for the determination of
kallikrein activity in a purified system using an initial rate method.

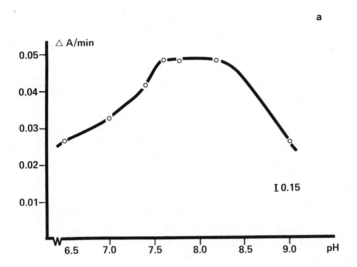

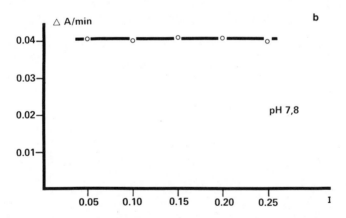

Fig 2. Optimation of pH and I of the Tris buffer used in the determination of plasma kallikrein. a) pH was varied using a constant I (0.15) and b) I was varied using a constant pH (7.8).

Prekallikrein Determination after Cephotest Activation

When kaolin or ellagic acid were used as contact activators, we did not succeed in obtaining a fast and total activation. Therefore we tried Cephotest which contains ellagic acid and phospholipid. During our work with a preliminary method (5), we found that an ionic strength of 0.05 mol/l gave a maximal rate of activation. We also found a better reproducibility and higher rate of activation, when the Cephotest was prediluted 1:10. When the activation time was varied, using different amounts of plasma, it was found that 2 min was the ideal incubation time (Fig 3 a). By using shorter time, the highest dilutions will not be completely activated but by using longer time, there will be some inhibition when less diluted plasma is used.

By using different amounts or different dilutions of Cephotest, we found that 800 μl of Cephotest diluted 1:10 with buffer would be an optimal activator (Fig 3 b). When four different batches of Cephotest were used, no difference between batches was found. Activated Thrombofax Reagent was also used under the conditions that were found optimal for Cephotest and gave then equivalent results.

Using different amounts of substrate with Cephotest activated plasma and with help of the Lineweaver-Burk plot (two series of determinations) the $K_m = 2.1 \cdot 10^{-4}$ mol/l and $V_{max} = 6.8 \cdot 10^{-6}$ mol/min per PEU (plasma equivalent unit = activity in 1 ml of normal plasma). The K_m was in good agreement with that obtained with purified plasma kallikrein (see above).

The standard curves are shown in Fig 4 a (initial rate method) and 4 b (end point method). Freshly taken plasma from a few single individuals gave 0-10% higher activity than after freezing and thawing of the same plasma.

The reproducibility of the method is good. Within one series of determinations (n=10) the coefficient of variation (C.V.) was 2.2% and between days C.V. = 3.7% (n=11).

Experiments with Deficient Plasmas and Purified Factors

FXII deficient plasma gave almost no activity. When a purified FXII was added to the deficient plasma, it was found that 2 μg of this preparation gave >70% of the activity that could be generated in normal plasma (Fig 5 a). When more of the FXII preparation was added, some inhibition, however, occurred, probably because of inhibitors (Benzamidine and aprotinin) added to stabilize the preparation.

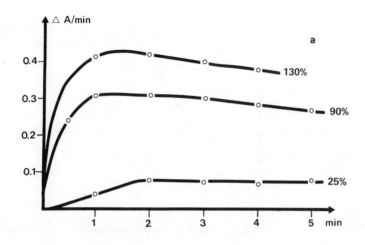

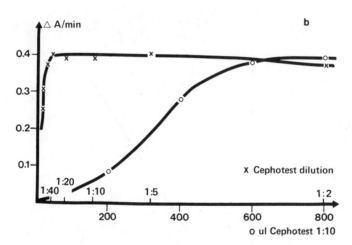

Fig 3. a)   Optimation of incubation time using 800 µl of 10%
            Cephotest in buffer with different plasma dilutions
            (100% see method).

       b)   Different dilutions (x) and different amounts of a 10%
            Cephotest solution (o).

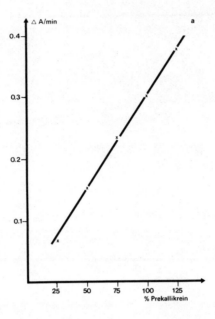

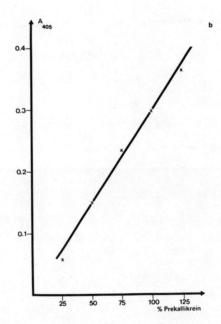

Fig 4.   Standard curves using the initial rate (a) and the acetic
         acid stopped (b) methods. Three different series of
         determinations are used.

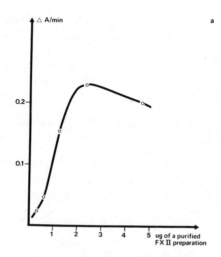

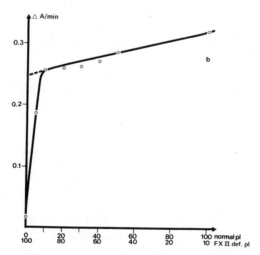

Fig 5. To FXII deficient plasma was added purified FXII (a)
and to normal plasma (b).

When normal plasma was added to the FXII deficient plasma, full
activity was obtained when only 10% of normal plasma was used
(Fig 5 b). The prekallikrein concentration in the FXII deficient
plasma was about 85% of that found in normal plasma.

The other factor needed for prekallikrein activation, HMW kininogen
(Fitzgerald Factor) was tested by using deficient plasma. When a
purified HMW kininogen preparation was added to the Fitzgerald
plasma or to the same plasma with an extra addition of purified
prekallikrein, it was found that 2 µg of this kininogen preparation
gave full activity (Fig 6 a).

When normal plasma was added to the Fitzgerald plasma containing
extra prekallikrein, full activity was obtained when only 10-20%
of normal plasma was used (Fig 6 b).

FXI deficient plasma gave the same activity as normal plasma (both
lyophilized). This shows that FXI is not needed for prekallikrein
activation. The lyophilized normal plasma gave about 80% of the
activity found in fresh frozen normal plasma.

When finally a purified prekallikrein preparation was added to
Fletcher plasma (prekallikrein deficient), the increase of activity
was linearly proportional to the amount of added prekallikrein
(Fig 7 a). Corresponding results were obtained by using a mixture
of Fletcher plasma and normal plasma (Fig 7 b).

Various Experiments

The activation of later coagulation and fibrinolytic factors was
checked by using the FXa sensitive substrate S-2222 (13) and the
plasmin sensitive substrate S-2251 (14) respectively. No significant
activity was found (<10% of what can be activated in plasma).

In order to neutralize the possible effect of the Cl 1NH, sodium
flufenamate may be added to the sample (12). By adding 50 µl of
the flufenamate solutions (0.01, 0.1, and 1 mg/ml) to the 125%
standard sample and incubate it for 10 min with Cephotest, a 6%
higher activity was obtained in each case compared with a control
without flufenamate. When a 2 min incubation time was used, we
found a 5% lower activity in all experiments where flufenamate was
used.

When dextran sulphate was used as an activator for plasma prekallikrein, we obtained the results shown in Fig 8 with the two substrates
H-D-Phe-Pro-Arg-pNA (S-2302) and Bz-Phe-Pro-Arg-pNA (S-2249, Chromozy
PK). This method gives about half the activity obtained with
Cephotest (c.f. Fig 4 a) because of the larger volume (2 ml compared
to 1 ml) used in this method. The minor difference can be explained
by the lower substrate concentration in the dextran sulphate method.

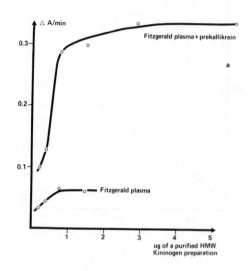

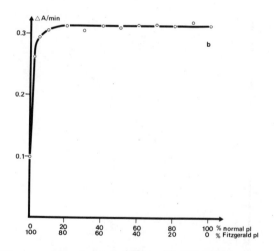

Fig 6.   To a Fitzgerald plasma (with extra prekallikrein added)
was added purified HMW kininogen (a) and normal plasma (b).

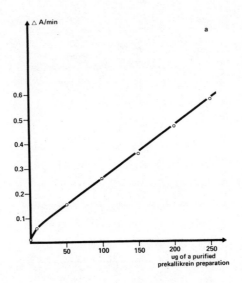

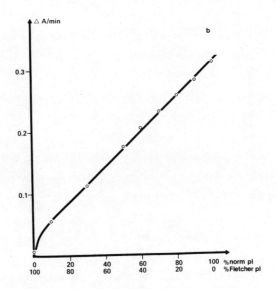

Fig 7. To a Fletcher plasma was added purified prekallikrein (a)
and normal plasma (b).

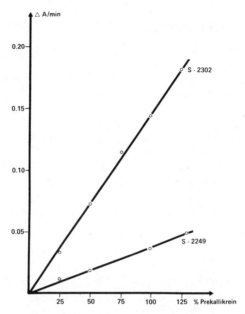

Fig 8. Standard Curves for the method using dextran sulphate as activator. Two different substrates S-2302 and S-2249 (equivalent to chromozym PK) were used.

The activity of purified kallikrein and Cephotest activated plasma on 21 different chromogenic tripeptide substrates (-Phe-Arg-pNA and -Leu-Arg-pNA), using S-2302 as 100, showed a good correlation, r=0.98.

DISCUSSION

In order to avoid inhibition by plasma inhibitors, prekallikrein has generally been activated at low temperatures by using kaolin as an activator. Kaolin is, among other reasons, not suitable in spectrophotometric methods because it makes the sample opaque. Ellagic acid and dextran sulphate are more suitable activators. As ellagic acid was difficult to dissolve and our results with this activator were poor, we decided to use the commercially available preparation Cephotest. Its potency allowed a rapid activation of plasma prekallikrein at high plasma dilutions. When the activator was prediluted, it gave more reproducible results than the same amount undiluted. The larger errors when using undiluted Cephotest probably depends on insufficient activation but by using larger amounts of undiluted activator a significant opaquenes was observed.

The optimized method described above was then checked by using deficient plasmas. Our data show that both FXII and HMW kininogen are needed for the activation of prekallikrein. About 10% of these factors are sufficient for a fast activation (Fig 5, 6). A low level of prekallikrein can thus be checked by adding 10-20% of normal plasma to the sample. This also explains our difficulties to get a sufficient rate of activation when the plasma was diluted to $\leqslant 20\%$ of normal (see method). Our findings about factors needed for prekallikrein activation are in accordance with the accepted model of the phase of contact activation. The low concentration of prekallikrein in Fitzgerald plasma has also been reported earlier (6).

The extra activity (5-10%) found in Fletcher plasma when purified prekallikrein or normal plasma was added could naturally not have been observed when normal plasma dilutions (Fig 4, 7) were used. This effect may be explained by presence of minor amounts of pre-kallikrein in the Fletcher plasma or possibly by the activation of other enzymes. However, in this diluted system without Ca^{2+}, no activation (<10%) of the coagulation (FXa) or the fibrinolytic (plasmin) system was observed. This is important because the sub-strate is readily split by those two enzymes but not by activated FXII or XI (according to E. Davie, personal communications).

For comparison, a method using dextran sulphate was used. Similar activities were obtained by the two methods.

By comparing data from purified human plasma kallikrein with Cephotest activated human normal plasma, we found equivalent substrate specificity and Michaelis constant. These data prove that the method is fairly selective.

The diluted system also proved to be effective in avoiding the inhibition by C 1 1NH. This was shown in the experiments with flu-fenamic acid but also by comparing the kallikrein activity in dilution of normal plasma (Fig 4) with the activity in mixed normal and deficient plasma (Fig 8).

We have concluded that the method presented, measures plasma pre-kallikrein selectively, it is easy to perform, it is highly repro-ducible and it can easily be automized.

Severe deficiency in FXII, HMW kininogen and kallikrein inhibitors may be detected and even quantified by using similar methods.

It has been shown that the plasma prekallikrein concentration in the blood from healthy volunteers is within a rather narrow range; ± 10% (S.D.) (9, 12). Decreased levels have been reported in liver cirrhosis and DIC (3). Much data about the clinical significance of the prekallikrein level, is, however, still lacking.

REFERENCES

1. Amundsen, E. and Svendsen, L.: A new method for plasma kalli-krein utilizing a synthetic chromogenic substrate. In: New methods for the analysis of coagulation using chromogenic substrates. Ed. I. Witt, Walter de Gruyter. p. 211, 1977.
2. Aurell, L., Friberger, P., Karlsson, G. and Claeson, G.: A new sensitive and highly specific chromogenic peptide substrate for factor Xa. Thromb. Res. II: 595-609, 1977.
3. Bang, N.U. and Mattler, L.E.: Serine Protease Specificity for Peptide Chromogenic Substrates. Thromb. Haemost. 38: 776-92, 1977.
4. Burrowes, C.E., Habal, F.M. and Movat, H.Z.: The inhibition of human plasma kallikrein by antithrombia III. Thromb. Res. 7: 175-83, 1975.
5. Claeson, G., Friberger, P., Knös, M., and Eriksson, E.: Methods for determination of prekallikrein in plasma, glandular kallikrein and urokinase. Haemostasis 7: 76-78, 1978.
6. Donaldson, V.H., Glueck, H.I., Miller, M.A., Movat, H.Z. and Habal, F.: Kininogen deficiency in Fitzgerald trait: role of high molecular weight kininogen in clotting and fibrinolysis. J. Lab. Clin. Med. 87: 327-37, 1976.
7. Egberg, N. and Bergström, K.: Studies on assays for plasma pre-kallikrein and for the monitoring of cumarol therapy. Haemo-stasis 7: 85-91, 1978.
8. Friberger, P., Knös, M., Gustafsson, S., Aurell, L. and Claeson, G.: A new specific substrate for the determination of plasmin activity. In: Chromogenic Substrates. Ed. V.V. Kakkar. Churchill Livingstone. In press.
9. Gallimore, T.M., Fareid, E. and Stormorken, H.: The purification of a human plasma kallikrein with weak plasminogen activator activity. Thromb. Res. 12: 409-20, 1978.
10. Griffin, J.H.: Role of surface-dependent activation of Hageman factor (Blood coagulation Factor XII). Proc. Natl. Acad. Sci. 75: 1998-2002, 1978.
11. Kaplan, A.P., Meier, H.L. and Mandle, R.: The Hageman factor dependent pathway of coagulation, fibrinolysis and kinin generation. Seminars in Thrombosis and Haemostasis 3: 1-26, 1976.
12. Kluft, C.: Blood Fibrinolysis. Preactivators and activators in human plasma. Thesis. Dutch Efficiency Bureau-Pijnacker. p. 104, 1978.

13. Meier, H.L., Scott, C.F., Mandle, R., Webster, M.E., Pierce, J.V., Colman, R.W., and Kaplan, A.P.: Requirements for contact activation of human Hageman factor. Ann. N.Y. Acad. Sci. 283: 93-103, 1977.

14. Schreiber, A.D.: Plasma inhibitors of the Hageman factor dependent pathways. Seminars in Thrombosis and Haemostasis 3: 43-51, 1976.

15. Wiggins, R.C., Bouma, B.N., Cochrane, C.G. and Griffin, J.H.: Role of high-molecular-weight kininogen in surface binding and activation of coagulation Factor XI and prekallikrein. Proc. Natl. Acad. Sci. 74: 4634-40, 1977.

METHODS FOR THE DETERMINATION OF GLANDULAR KALLIKREIN BY MEANS OF A CHROMOGENIC TRIPEPTIDE SUBSTRATE

Egil Amundsen[x], J. Putter[+], P. Friberger[o], M. Knos[o], M. Larsbraten[x] and G. Claeson[o].
[x]Institute for Surgical Research, Rikshospitalet, Oslo, Norway; [+]Bayer AG, Institute for Pharmacokinetics, Wuppertal, FRG; [o]AB KABI, Peptide Research, Molndal, Sweden.

ABSTRACT

A chromogenic peptide substrate H-D-Val-Leu-Arg-pNA (S-2266) has been used for the determination of glandular kallikrein derived from pancreas, urine and saliva. The conditions used have been optimized. The methods developed are simple and shown to have good reproducibility.

INTRODUCTION

The first assay using a tripeptide chromogenic substrate for estimation of plasmakallikrein and prekallikrein was presented at the Reston Conference in 1974 (Amundsen et al. 1974). The amino acid sequence in this substrate was Pro-Phe-Arg, i.e. the three C-terminal amino acids in bradykinin. It was a great surprise to us that glandular kallikrein, even in very high concentrations, did not split this substrate.

In the present communication a new assay for glandular kallikreins utilizing a tripeptide chromogenic substrate is presented. The amino acid sequence in this substrate has no obvious relation to the sequence of amino acids around the cleavage points in low molecular weight kininogen. The sequence was discovered by screening of a number of different peptide substrates with a purified glandular kallikrein preparation. Special procedures for determination of glandular kallikrein in urine and saliva are given.

MATERIALS AND METHODS

Pancreas kallikrein[R] of porcine origin, KZC 1/75, 1180 KU/mg
(Bayer, Leverkusen, GFR) with a purity of 85%, containing no known
inhibitor or enzyme impurities.
Urokinase of reagent quality, 10000 Ploug U/vial (Leo, Copenhagen,
Denmark)
Aprotinin, Trasylol[R] (Bayer)
Chromogenic substrate, S-2266, H-D-Val-Leu-Arg-pNA (AB KABI
Diagnostica, Stockholm, Sweden).
Tris-HCl buffers, Tris, reagent grade (Merch, Darmstadt, GFR)
Sterile water was used as solvent for the reagents.
Human urine was collected from four apparently healthy persons.
Human saliva was collected from three apparently healthy persons.
The spectrophotometer (Hitachi 101) was connected over a lin-log
converter (Multianalog 311) to a linear recorder (Tohshin) for the
initial rate methods. A Zeiss PM 23 spectrophotometer was used for
the end point determinations.
50% acetic acid (p.a., Merck) was otherwise used to stop the
reaction. (The colour was stable for at least four hours).
Semimicro cuvettes (Helma) were used for sample volumes of about
1 ml.

Determination of Pancreas Kallikrein Activity

The procedure is described in Table I. The pH and I (adjusted
with NaCl) of the buffer (0.05 mol/1 Tris) were optimized by varying
one parameter at the time. The kinetic constants in the optimal
buffer were obtained by varying the amount of substrate and by
using the Lineweaver-Burk plot.

Determination of Kallikrein in Urine

For practical reasons some changes in the former method were
made. Because of the low activity of kallikrein in urine an end-
point method was used. To check for interfering enzymes, Trasylol
was added to the buffer used in the blank. The risk of turbidity
and pH instability was counteracted by using a 0.2 mol/1 Tris-HCl
buffer with pH 8.2. The procedure is described in Table II.
Experiments adding the reagents in different combinations were
performed using this method. Purified urokinase, a serine protease
in urine, was also studied in combination with Trasylol.

Determination of Kallikrein in Saliva

Saliva generates a higher kallikrein activity than urine.
Therefore, approximately the same method as for purified pancreas
kallikrein was used. (Table III). The saliva was first diluted
with equal parts of sterile water and the precipitate was centrifuged down. The supernatant was used as a source of kallikrein.

A blank determination with Trasylol was made and subtracted from the results to correct for enzyme activities not inhibited by Trasylol.

Table I.   Procedure for the determination of glandular kallikrein (pancreatic)

	Reagents/ Procedure	Volume (µl)
1	Buffer pH 9.0 I 0.05 (37°) Enzyme dilution (59 KU/ml)	2250 50
	Mix well in a cuvette	X
2	S-2266, 2 mmol/l	200
	Mix well and record the increase of absorbance at 405 nm (ΔA/min ~ 0.08)	

Table II.   Procedure for the determination of kallikrein in urine

	Reagents/ Procedure	Volume (µl)
1	Buffer pH 8.2 I 0.1 (37°) Urine	500 400
	Mix well in a test tube or cuvette	X
2	S-2266, 1 mmol/l	100
	Mix well and incubate for 30 min at 37°C	X
3	HAc, 50%	100
	Mix well and read the absorbance (A) at 405 nm against a blank using the same reagents but with Trasylol (10 KIU/ml) in the buffer	X

Table III. Procedure for the determination of kallikrein
            in saliva.

	Reagents/ Procedure	Volume (µl)
1	Buffer pH 9.0 I 0.05 (37°) Saliva diluted 1:1	800 100
	Mix well in a cuvette	X
2	S-2266, 4 mmol/l	200
	Mix well and record the increase of absorbance at 405 nm	X
3	Blank: use Trasylol (10 KU/ml) in the buffer	X

Table IV. Absorbances resulting from kallikrein determinations
          as described for urine with and without addition of
          kallikrein (K) (0.1 KU), Trasylol (T), urine (U) and
          substrate (S) to 0.2 mol/l Tris buffer (B); all
          additives dissolved in the same buffer; additions
          indicated in ml.

No.	B	K	T	U	S	A
1	1.0	-	-	-	-	0.052
2	0.9	-	-	-	0.1	0.055
3	0.8	0.1	-	-	0.1	0.264
4	0.6	-	-	0.4	-	0.212
5	0.5	-	-	0.4	0.1	0.307
6	0.4	-	0.1	0.4	0.1	0.227
7	0.4	0.1	-	0.4	0.1	0.511
8	0.3	0.1	0.1	0.4	0.1	0.231

RESULTS

The enzymatic activities of the pancreas kallikrein preparations, urine and saliva were stable for several hours at room temperature (25°) and for at least one working day in a refrigerator (5°). The substrate solution was stable for several months in a refrigerator. All results are mean values of double or triple determinations when not otherwise stated.

Determination of Pancreas Kallikrein Activity

The standard curve for purified pancreas kallikrein was linear to at least 1 KU/ml in the cuvette (Fig.1). The optimal ranges of the buffer pH and I were wide (Fig.2 a,b). The pH 9.0 and I 0.05 were chosen for the method. The kinetic constants K_m = 2.2 x 10^{-5} mol/1 and V_{max} = 8 nmol/min per KU were obtained (Fig.3a). The rate obtained by using the method described in Table I was only about 10% below the V_{max} value. The coefficient of variation (C.V. = 100 x $\frac{S.D.}{mean}$) within one series of determinations was less than 3% (n = 10).

Determination of Kallikrein in Urine

A linear relation was found between the amount of urine and the amount of pNA formed up to approximately 400 µl of urine. Above this volume of urine, the amount of Trasylol in the blank has to be increased to 20-50 KIU/ml and some inhibition was also observed. When purified pancreas kallikrein was used in this method instead of urine, the standard curve was approximately linear from 0.003 KU up to 0.10 KU of kallikrein (Fig.4). The activity was almost the same as that calculated from the method for purified pancreatic kallikrein. No significant increase in activity was found when Carbowax 6000 was added to the highly diluted enzymes in order to avoid absorption e.g. to the cuvette walls. This curve (Fig.4) or the activity figure in nkat/1 (=146 x A) was used for the standardization of the kallikrein activity in urine.

In Table IV the contribution of the different reagents to the absorbance is shown. When the purified pancreatic kallikrein was added to urine in the method, no inhibition was found. Some experiments with other urines showed however, a small inhibition (0-15%) of the activity.

All enzymatic activity of added kallikrein to urine was inhibited by Trasylol (Table IV). When 40 Ploug U of urokinase was added to the urine this activity was not at all inhibited by Trasylol. This amount of urokinase cleaved the substrate with a rate that was only about 15% of that caused by the kallikrein in urine.

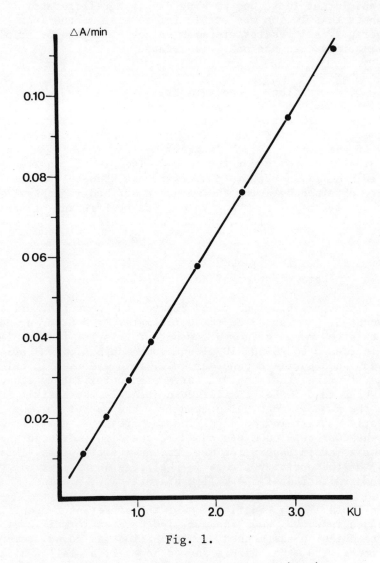

Fig. 1.

Standard curve for purified pancreas kallikrein.
Method see Table I. Kallikrein activity (ΔA/min) is
plotted against the total amount of enzyme added.

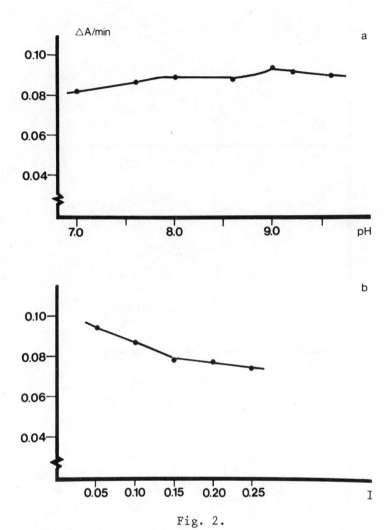

Fig. 2.

Optimation of the pH (a) and the ionic strength (b) of
the buffer used for the determination of pancreas
kallikrein. When the pH was optimized I was 0.05 and
when the I was optimized pH was 9.0.

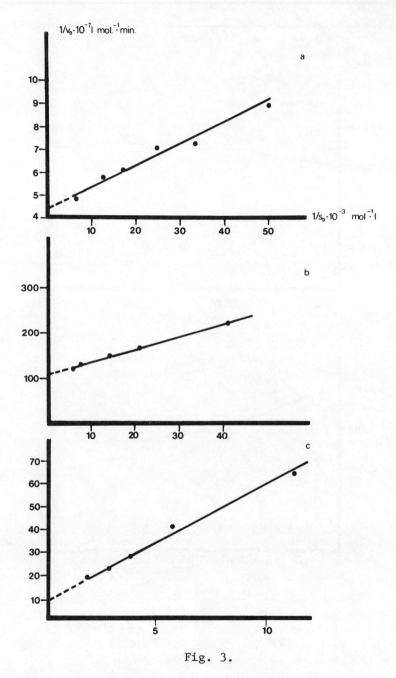

Fig. 3.

Lineweaver–Burk plots using (a) purified pancreatic kallikrein (b) urine and (c) saliva using the sub-strate S-2266.

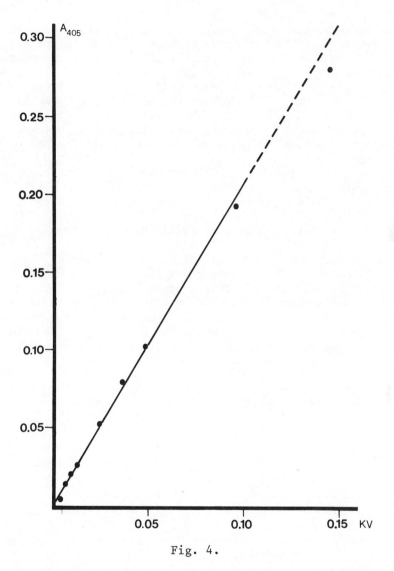

Fig. 4.

Standard curve for the urine kallikrein method (Table II)
using the purified pancreatic kallikrein as a standard
instead of urine. Absorbance (A) after 30 min plotted
against the total amount of kallikrein added.

The K_m for the kallikrein excreted in urine was 3.0×10^{-5} mol/l (Fig.3b). This value is similar to that of purified pancreas kallikrein.

In one laboratory the results from the determination of kallikrein activity in the urine of four individuals are shown in Table V. In another laboratory the 24 hr urine from 12 apparently healthy persons in the ages from 25-60 years, the total kallikrein activity was 11.0 ± 7.3 nkat (mean $\pm$ SD). After freezing and thawing the activity was 9.9 ± 7.7 nkat ($\varepsilon = 10500$ for pNA). One urine investigated lost successively 15% of its activity during storage for 14 days at $+4^\circ$C. The morning urine sampled from one person at 4 different occasions within 5 months were within a range of $\pm 25\%$ of the mean.
The C.V. for the method was within one series of determinations on the same urine sample less than 1% (n=10).

Determination of Kallikrein in Saliva

The kallikrein activity in saliva was considerably higher than that in urine. The enzymatic activity upon the substrate was however not totally inhibited by Trasylol but about 15% remained. The buffer optima for pH and ionic strength were approximately the same as those for the purified pancreatic kallikrein. The standard curve for pooled saliva is shown in Fig.5. The K_m value for the kallikrein-like activity in saliva using the substrate S-2266 was 5×10^{-4} mol/l (Fig.3c). This figure was considerably higher than for the other two enzymes.
The C.V. for the method was within one series of determinations on the same saliva about 3% (n=10).

Table V. Measured absorbances after determination of enzymatic activity in the 24 hr urine (U) of four persons without and with added Trasylol (T);calculation of the kallikrein content per ml and the kallikrein excretion per day.

Person	Volume (ml)	A U	A U + T	ΔA	Kallikrein calculated KE/ml	Kallikrein calculated KE/day
A	1260	0.307	0.227	0.080	0.099	124
B	840	0.454	0.398	0.056	0.069	58
C	1180	0.780	0.577	0.203	0.250	296
D	1230	0.311	0.213	0.098	0.120	148

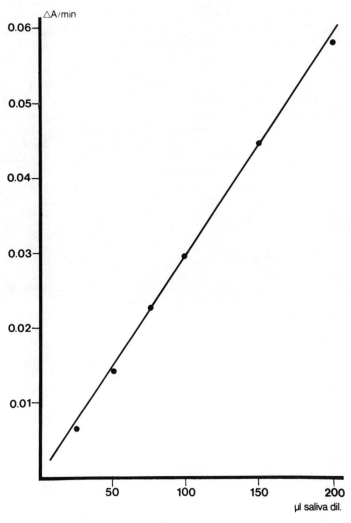

Fig. 5.

Standard curve for saliva kallikrein (Table III).
Activity plotted against the amount of saliva
dilution used.

DISCUSSION

When different substrates of the tri-peptide-pNA type were screened
against the three different kallikreins used here they proved to
have the same substrate specificity requirements,(G. Claeson et al.
1978).It was also shown that 1×10^{-11} mol of a purified pancreatic
kallikrein (KZC Bayer) in 2.5 ml (total volume) of an optimal
buffer gives $\Delta A/min = 0.09$ using the chromogenic substrate S-2266.
This sensitivity is of the same order of magnitude as that of other
serine proteases (thrombin, Factor Xa and plasmin) and their pep-
tide-pNA substrates,(G. Claeson et al. to be published).The S-2266
is more selective than BAPNA or BAEE but is less selective than
the above mentioned substrates for other serine proteases. By using
specific inhibitors the methods can, however, be made fairly selective for glandular kallikreins. The determination of kallikrein
with S-2266 is not quite as sensitive as the BAEE method comparing
the change of absorbance per minute. However, by using a 30 minute
incubation time the method described above for urinary kallikrein
is in practice more sensitive than the usual BAEE methods,
(J.J.Pisano, 1975).

The methods described are simple and reproducible. The conditions for the determination of kallikrein have been optimized, but
for practical reasons the pH, ionic strength and amount of buffer
substance were somewhat changed in the method for kallikrein determination in urine.

There are two well-known serine proteases in urine viz. urokinase and kallikrein. Trasylol added to the blank inhibits the
kallikrein activity whereas urokinase is unaffected. The influence
of increased levels (normal level 1 Ploug U/ml) of urokinase can
thus be determined. Bacterial amidase activities which are generally not inhibited by low concentrations of Trasylol would be excluded
at the same time.

It has been shown by Geiger et al. (personal communications)
that the activity of different urines from apparently healthy
persons on the pNA substrate used here was very well correlated to
the activity upon a peptide ethyl ester substrate as well as upon
the dog blood pressure.

The maximal amount of urine recommended in the method was
400 ul. This amount is needed because the kallikrein activity in
urine is normally low (corresponding to about 0.05 KU per test).
The method was adopted for this level down to an activity of about
0.003 KU. If the kallikrein activity in urine is higher than that
corresponding to 0.10 KU, less urine (e.g.200 ul) should be used
in the method The small inhibitory effect in some urine samples
may be caused by high salt concentrations in these urines

(c.f. Fig.2b). This phenomenon was however not further investigated
in this study. The kallikrein activity has been given in ĸU using
the purified pancreatic kallikrein as a standard. This seems practical but it can of course also be expressed in change in absorbance per 30 min or preferably nkat/l.

The kallikrein-like activity in saliva is much higher than
that in urine. The K_m for the salivary kallikrein deviated from
that of the purified pancreatic enzyme but the buffer pH and ionic
strength optima were the same.

Glandular kallikrein activity has previously been difficult
to determine. The assay presented here provides a good tool for
such determinations. The pNA released by the enzymatic action on
the substrate could also be used as an accurate unit for expression
of glandular kallikrein activity.

REFERENCES

Amundsen, E., Svendsen, L., Vennerød, A.M. and Laake, K., 1974,
    Determination of plasma kallikrein with a new chromogenic
    tripeptide derivative, in:Chemistry and Biology of the
    Kallikrein-kinin system in Health and Disease, eds. J.J.Pisano
    and K.F. Austen, Fogarty International Center Proceedings No.27,
    U.S. Government Printing Office, Washington D.C., p.215.
Claeson, G., Amundsen, E. et al., To be published, Chromogenic
    peptide substrates for kallikrein.
Claeson, G., Friberger, P., Knös, M. and Ericsson, E., 1978,
    Methods for determination of prekallikrein in plasma, glandular
    kallikrein and urokinase, Haemostasis 7, p.76.
Geiger, R., Personal communications.
Pisano, J.J., 1975, Chemistry and biology of the kallikrein-kinin
    system, in: Proteases and Biological Control, eds. E. Reich,
    D.B. Rifkin and E. Shaw, Cold Spring Harbor Laboratory, p.199.

A DIRECT RADIOIMMUNOASSAY FOR HUMAN URINARY KALLIKREIN

Narendra B. Oza and James W. Ryan

Department of Medicine, University of Miami School of
Medicine, Miami, Florida 33101, U.S.A.

ABSTRACT

A protein-binding radioimmunoassay (RIA) has been developed
for human urinary kallikrein (HUK). HUK was purified to apparent
homogeneity and rabbit anti-human urinary kallikrein serum was
prepared. Radio-iodination of HUK was performed in 20 µg batches
with 1 mCi of ^{125}I-Bolton-Hunter reagent in 0.1 M sodium borate
buffer, pH 8.5, at 0°C. The 30 min reaction was terminated by
adding 0.5 ml of 0.2 M glycine. Radiolabelled HUK was purified on
a Sephacryl S-200 column (1 x 50 cm) in 0.05 M Tris·HCl plus 0.2%
gelatin, pH 7.4 (RIA buffer). ^{125}I-HUK emerged as a single, uniform peak at V_e/V_o of 1.3. The RIA reaction mixture contained
15,000 cpm of ^{125}I-HUK, 0.1 ml of diluted anti-kallikrein serum,
0.1 ml unlabelled kallikrein (1-100 ng) or the unknown sample and
RIA buffer to a total of 0.5 ml. The reaction mixture was incubated at 22°C for 18 hr, and 100 µl of goat-anti-rabbit IgG serum
was added to each tube. The tubes were incubated 18 hr at 4°C,
centrifuged 4,000 rpm for 30 min and, after decantation, the
precipitate was counted for ^{125}I. The RIA reported here is
sufficiently sensitive to detect 1 ng of kallikrein and should
offer a useful technique to determine alterations of the kallikrein-kinin system in response to stimuli; both physiologic and
pathologic.

INTRODUCTION

Many investigators have found alterations in the excretion of
kallikrein (EC 3.4.28.8) in urine with the induction of renovas-
cular hypertension and mineralocorticoid hypertension. Dietary

97

NaCl and H_2O also affect excretion rates (e.g. Keiser et al., 1976; Mills et al., 1976). However, the physiological and/or pathological roles of the renal or urinary kallikrein-kinin system are not known. In addition, there is a controversy (cf. Mills et al. and Keiser et al., loc. cit.) on the levels of kallikrein in urine during high and low intake of dietary sodium. It seems that part of the controversy may have arisen from differences in the analytical methods which were employed to determine kallikrein activity.

Kallikreins of both the plasma and glandular types show a high degree of specificity for the native substrate kininogen. A similar degree of specificity is difficult to obtain with a variety of synthetic substrates; notably, those of N-α-substituted L-arginine esters. Thus, measurement of kallikrein activity by functional assay is subject to possible interference by trypsin-like enzymes other than kallikrein to variable levels of endogenous substrate and to endogenous inhibitors of kallikrein.

Component binding radioimmunoassays have made it possible to gain an appreciation of biologically inactive, yet immunoreactive, macromolecules which compose part of the renin-angiotensin system (e.g. Malling and Poulsen, 1977). We have isolated human urinary kallikrein and prepared antibodies against it (Oza and Ryan, 1978). The antibodies were used to develop a direct radioimmunoassay.

MATERIALS AND METHODS

[125]I-Labelling of Kallikrein

Human urinary kallikrein was isolated by anion-exchange, affinity (Trasylol-Sepharose) and molecular sieve (Sephacryl S-200) chromatography as described in a previous communication (Oza and Ryan, 1978).

Pure kallikrein was radiolabelled in 16-80 µg batches with 1-2 mCi of the Bolton-Hunter reagents, according to the published procedure (Bolton and Hunter, 1973). The iodination reaction was carried out for 30 min and terminated by the addition of 0.5 ml of 0.2 M glycine in 0.1 M sodium borate buffer, pH 8.5. The reaction mixture, approx. 0.6 ml, was passed through a 1 x 50 cm column of Sephacryl S-200 (Pharmacia Fine Chemicals, Piscatawy, NJ, U.S.A.). The column was equilibrated in 0.05 M Tris·HCl, pH 7.4, containing 0.1% (w/v) gelatin (RIA buffer) and was calibrated (for its void volume) with 1 mg of Blue Dextran 2000 (Pharmacia Fine Chemicals). The effluent was collected in 1 ml fractions and counted for radioactivity. In addition, each fraction was analyzed for immunoreactivity with the anti-kallikrein serum. Selected fractions were also analyzed for their catalytic activity, using Pro-Phe-Arg-[^{3}H]-benzylamide as a substrate (see Chung et al., this volume).

Rabbit Anti-(Human Urinary Kallikrein) Serum

The antiserum was that described in a previous paper (Oza and Ryan, loc. cit). A sample of a high titer antiserum was pretreated to inactivate kallikrein inhibitors normally present in blood. The inhibitors were inactivated by acidification and heat denaturation as described in an earlier report (Oza, 1977). Following the denaturation treatment, the antiserum was centrifuged at 4,000 rpm for 30 min. The supernatant was employed, in appropriate dilutions, in the radioimmunoassay. Nonspecific binding was determined by using non-immune rabbit serum pretreated in an identical manner. This serum was also used as a source of carrier IgG.

Radioimmunoassay

Unlabelled kallikrein (0.5-100 ng, for preparation of a standard curve) or 50-100 µl of human urine (unknown) were pipetted into polyethylene tubes. Thereafter, 0.1 ml of a 1:200 dilution of non-immune serum (carrier IgG), 0.1 ml of suitably diluted anti-kallikrein serum and approx. 15,000 cpm of ^{125}I-kallikrein were added to each tube. The total volume was brought to 0.5 ml by the addition of RIA buffer. The assay tubes were incubated at 25°C for 18 hr and 0.1 ml of a 1:5 dilution of second antibody (goat anti-rabbit IgG serum purchased from Miles Laboratories, Inc., Elkhart, IN, U.S.A.) was added to all tubes. The tubes were then incubated at 4°C for 18 hr and centrifuged at 4,000 rpm for 30 min. At this stage, the ^{125}I-kallikrein-anti-kallikrein-double antibody complex was sedimented as a fine ring of white precipitate. The supernatant was decanted, and the precipitate was counted for radioactivity. The initial binding obtained with the incubation of ^{125}I-kallikrein and anti-kallikrein serum (about 30%) was regarded as 100%. The displacements obtained with the addition of different amounts of unlabelled kallikrein were expressed as a percentage of initial binding. Nonspecific binding was determined by substituting non-immune serum instead of the anti-kallikrein serum. Duplicate determinations were made and the unknown samples were interpolated from a standard plot of percent of initial binding versus the amount of added kallikrein.

RESULTS AND DISCUSSION

Purification of ^{125}I-kallikrein on Sephacryl S-200 is shown in Fig. 1. The homogeneity of the enzyme was unchanged following radiolabelling as is evident from the symmetrical peak. The V_e/V_o ratio for the native enzyme was 1.5, and that for ^{125}I-kallikrein was 1.3. Fractions 16 through 22 were found to contain immunoreactive and functional ^{125}I-kallikrein. The labelled kallikrein can hydrolyze Pro-Phe-Arg-[^{3}H]benzylamide (Chung et al., this volume). Therefore, these fractions were combined and stored

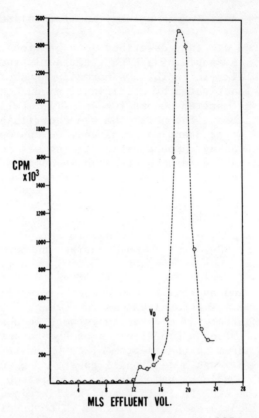

Fig. 1. Gel filtration of kallikrein, after ^{125}I-labelling, on a
1 cm x 50 cm column of Sephacryl S-200 eluted with the RIA buffer.
One ml fractions were collected, counted for radioactivity and
analyzed for ability to bind with anti-kallikrein. In this
experiment, fractions 16-22 were pooled for use in the radioimmunoassay.

at 4°C. Appropriate samples of the material were used directly in
the radioimmunoassay.

The percentage of binding obtained with a series of dilutions
(ranging from 1:10 to 1:100) of anti-kallikrein serum is shown in
Fig. 2. It was evident that approx. 30% binding was obtainable
when the anti-kallikrein was diluted 1:60. Therefore, in subsequent experiments, anti-kallikrein was employed in a 1:60 dilution.
Nonspecific binding was consistently less than 2%, irrespective of

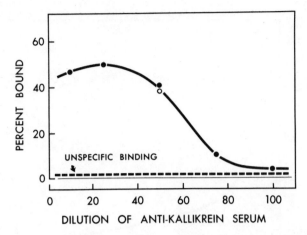

Fig. 2.   Antiserum titration curve.   The tubes contained 100 µl of
antiserum in dilutions given in the figure and approx. 15,000 cpm
of ^{125}I-kallikrein in a final volume of 0.6 ml.   The percentage of
binding was determined in duplicates (open and closed circles).
Unspecific binding (broken line) was determined by substituting
normal rabbit serum instead of the anti-kallikrein serum.

the dilution of non-immune serum, and, therefore, no corrections
were necessary.

In Fig. 3 is shown a standard curve of the radioimmunoassay
for the direct measurement of human urinary kallikrein.   Each point
on the curve represents an average and its standard error of the
mean from five different experiments.   It is evident that the assay
is sufficiently sensitive to measure 0.5 ng of urinary kallikrein.
As a routine we used human urine in 50-100 µl samples.   In six
normal subjects, the kallikrein concentration was found to be
204 ± 30.4 ng/ml (avg. ± SEM: n = 6).   On the basis of esterase
and kinin-forming activity, we had obtained an average of approx.
110 ng/ml (Oza and Ryan, 1978; see also Chung et al., this volume).
Therefore, it is conceivable that our radioimmunoassay measures
inactive (prekallikrein or inhibitor-bound kallikrein) as well as
active forms of kallikrein.   As discussed elsewhere (Ryan, J.W., et
al., this volume), the functional assays may accumulate errors
owing to competition between substrates, e.g. Pro-Phe-Arg-[^{3}H]-
benzylamine vs. urokininogen.

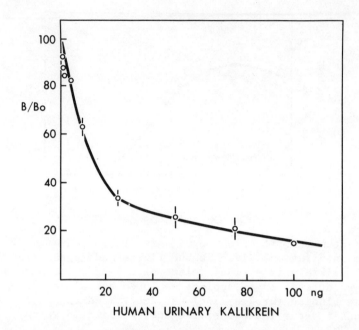

Fig. 3. Standard curve of percentage of initial binding (B/B_0)
versus the amount of added unlabelled human urinary kallikrein.
The first point of displacement in the standard curve was obtained
with 0.5 ng of kallikrein.

In conclusion, the radioimmunoassay of human urinary kallikrein should eliminate or decrease the artifacts due to trypsin-
like enzymes other than kallikrein and should improve understanding
of active and inactive forms of kallikrein.

ACKNOWLEDGEMENTS

This work was supported in part by grants from the U.S. Public
Health Service (HL22087), from the American Heart Association
(Palm Beach County Chapter, Inc.), and from the John A. Hartford
Foundation, Inc.

REFERENCES

Bolton, A.E. and W.M. Hunter, 1973, The labelling of proteins to high specific radioactivities by conjugation to a ^{125}I-containing acylating agent, Biochem. J., 133, 529.

Chung, A., J.W. Ryan, G.A. Pena and N.B. Oza (this volume), A simple radioassay for human urinary kallikrein.

Keiser, H.R., R.G. Geller, H.S. Margolius and J.J. Pisano, 1976, Urinary kallikrein in hypertensive animal models, Fed. Proc., 35, 199.

Malling, C. and K. Poulsen, 1977, A direct radioimmunoassay for plasma renin in mice and its evaluation, Biochim. Biophys. Acta, 491, 532.

Mills, I.H., N.A.A. MacFarlane, P.E. Ward and L.F.O. Obika, 1976, The renal kallikrein-kinin system in the regulation of salt and water excretion, Fed. Proc., 35, 181.

Oza, N.B., 1977, A direct assay for urinary kallikrein, Biochem. J., 167, 305.

Oza, N.B. and J. W. Ryan, 1978, A simple high-yield procedure for isolation of human urinary kallikrein, Biochem. J., 171, 285.

Ryan, J.W., N.B. Oza, L.C. Martin and G.A. Pena (this volume), Components of the kallikrein-kinin system in urine.

ESTIMATION OF URINARY KININOGENASE ACTIVITY USING BOVINE SERUM

LOW MOLECULAR WEIGHT KININOGEN

Keishi Abe, Hisao Kato*, Yataka Sakurai, Toru Itoh,
Keitaro Saito, Toshiaki Haruyama, Yoichi Otsuka and
Kaoru Yoshinaga

Department of Internal Medicine, Tohoku University
School of Medicine and *Protein Research Institute
Osaka University. 1-1, Seiryocho, Sendai 980, Japan

ABSTRACT

Estimation of urinary kininogenase activity by radioimmunoassay
of generated kinin was studied. Bovine serum low molecular weight
kininogen was proved not to cross-react with kallidin antibody and
also bradykinin antibody. This kininogen was used as substrate
measuring urinary kininogenase activity. Separation of released
kinin from the kininogen was not required in the present method.
Urinary kallikrein activity was found to be significantly decreased
in essential hypertension, in chronic glomerulonephritis and in
patients who had received renal transplantation. On the contrary,
an increase in urinary kallikrein was found in primary aldosteronism
and in Bartter's syndrome. The present method was very useful for
measuring kininogenase activity.

INTRODUCTION

There is evidence that urinary kallikrein is originated in
the kidney and its excretion rate reflects the biosynthesis of
renal kallikrein or its release (Nustad 1970). Therefore, the
urinary excretion of kallikrein is measured as an indicator of
renal biosynthesis of this substance.

Measurement of urinary kallikrein is more specific when it is
assayed by its kininogenase activity than when assayed by esterolytic
activity. Recently, Carretero and his coworkers (1976) developed
an estimation method of urinary kininogenase activity by means

of radioimmunoassay of generated kinin. In their method, partially purified dog plasma kininogen was used as a substrate, but this substrate was found to cross-react with the antibody against kallidin. Therefore, isolation of generated kinin from the kininogen was necessary to remove the interference of the substrate in the kinin assay. In the present study, a direct estimation of urinary kininogenase activity was studied using bovine serum low molecular weight kininogen as the substrate. Using this simplified method, urinary excretion of kallikrein was measured in healthy subjects and in patients with various diseases.

MATERIALS AND METHODS

Measurement of urinary kininogenase activity

Bovine serum low molecular weight kininogen prepared according to Suzuki's procedure (Suzuki et al. 1965) was used in this method. The urine sample (0.05~0.1 ml) was incubated with 4 µg of bovine serum low molecular weight kininogen dissolved in 0.4 ml of 0.1 M phosphate buffer, pH 8.4, containing 0.1% neomycin, 3 mM 8 hydroxy-quinoline and 30 mM disodium ethylenediaminetetraacetic acid at 37°C for 20 minutes. After the incubation, the mixture was diluted 5-fold with cold water and heated at 80°C for 15 minutes to stop the enzymatic reaction, and the generated kinin was measured radio-immunologically using the kallidin antibody. The kinin present in the urine before incubation was also measured, the urinary kallikrein activity was calculated by subtracting the preincubation kinin value from that obtained postincubation. In the present study, kallikrein activity was expressed as total kinin generated during the incubation of 20 minutes.

Kinin was measured by Carretero's method (1976). The incubation system consisted of ^{125}I-8-tyrosine-bradykinin, 3000 cpm (specific radiological activity, 800~1000 mci/µM, Daiichi Radio-isotope Corp), 0.01~0.02 ml of urine and 0.1 ml of antiserum (1: 16,000) adjusted to a final volume of 0.8 ml with 0.1 M Tris buffer, pH 7.4, containing 0.2% of gelatin and 0.1% of neomycin. The mixture was incubated for 24 hours at 4°C and free kinin was separated with dextran-coated charcoal. After counting radio-activity, kinin content was calculated. The recovery rate of added kallidin (50~500 pg) was 97 ± 4% (mean ± SE, n=15). The metabolic fragments produced by incubating bradykinin, kallidin and methionyl-lysyl-bradykinin with chymotrypsin showed 0.5% cross-reaction with the kallidin antiserum. In the present studies, plastic tubes were used in all procedures.

Measurement of urinary TAME esterase activity.

TAME esterolytic activity was measured by the method modified by Matsuda and coworkers (1976). Urine sample, 8 ml, was dialysed against running tap water for 16 hrs at 4°C and then concentrated to 1/2~1/3 volume with polyethylene glycol at 4°C. The esterolytic activity was determined as follows: The concentrated urine, 0.1 ml, was incubated with 5 mM of p-tosyl-arginine-methyl-ester (TAME) dissolved in 0.1 M phosphate buffer, pH 8.0, at 37°C for 30 minutes, and 0.2 ml of 10% HC10 solution was added to terminate the reaction. To oxidize methanol formed by the enzymatic reaction, 0.2 ml of 0.1% $KMnO_4$ solution was added, and then 0.1 ml of 0.1% $NH_2OH \cdot HCl$ solution and 3.0 ml of 0.2% acetylacetone in 0.5 M ammonium malate solution, pH 6.0 were added. After the mixture was kept in a water bath at 56°C for 20 minutes, the fluorescence was measured at 410 nm excitation and at 510 nm emission. Esterolytic activity was expressed in terms of esterase unit which is defined as the amount of kallikrein hydrolyzing 1 μM of TAME per minutes per ml.

Urine collection

Twenty-four hour urine was collected in a bottle kept in a refrigerator from 84 normal subjects, 55 patients with essential hypertension, 9 patients with primary aldosteronism, 9 patients with Bartter's syndrome, 40 patients with chronic glomerulonephritis and 16 patients received with kidney transplantation and was then stored at -20°C until assay.

RESULTS

Measurement of kininogenase activity

The problem of cross reaction of antibody against kallidin with bovine serum low molecular weight kininogen was examined. As shown in Figure 1, bradykinin had higher affinity than kallidin. Bovine serum low molecular weight kininogen (0.01~1000 ng) had no cross reaction with the kallidin antibody. In the present experiment, cross reaction of this kininogen with antiserum against bradykinin (Johnston et al. 1976) was also examined. As shown in Figure 2, no cross reaction was proved. Thus, bovine serum low molecular weight kininogen could be used to measure the urinary kininogenase activity directly.

Time course of the kinin generation was studied. Figure 3 shows the time course of the kinin generation when 0.05 ml of urines obtained from 2 subjects were incubated with each 4 μg of bovine low molecular weight kininogen at 37°C. A linear correlation was found between the amounts of the generated kinin and

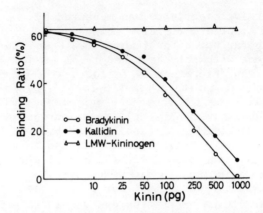

Figure 1.   Inhibition curves of kallidin, bradykinin and
bovine serum low molecular weight kininogen on
the reaction of antibody against kallidin and
^{125}I-8-tyrosine-bradykinin.

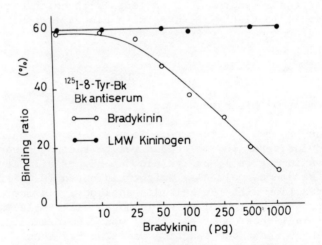

Figure 2.   Inhibition curves of bradykinin and bovine
serum low molecular weight kininogen on the
reaction of antibody against bradykinin and
^{125}-I-8-tyrosine-bradykinin.

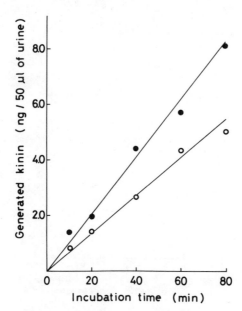

Figure 3.   Time course of kinin generation in each
            0.05 ml of urine from 2 subjects.

the incubation time in all samples.   From this result, the incubation time was fixed at 20 minutes.

To investigate the relationship between enzyme concentration
and the amounts of generated kinin, 0.025, 0.05, 0.075, 0.1 and
0.15 ml of urines were incubated with each 4 µg of bovine serum
low molecular weight kininogen at 37°C for 20 minutes.   As shown
in Figure 4, a linear correlation was found between the amounts
of the generated kinin and the urine volumes in 2 subjects.   From
this result, 0.05 to 0.1 ml of urine was used in the present
method.

The relationship between the amounts of generated kinin and
the substrate concentration was also investigated.   Urine specimens,
0.05 ml, obtained from 2 normal subjects were incubated with 0.25,
0.5, 1.0, 2.0, 4.0, 6.0, 8.0 and 10 µg of bovine serum low molecular
weight kininogen at 37°C for 20 minutes, respectively.   The increment of added bovene serum low molecualr weight kininogen enhanced
the amounts of the generated kinin, and the kinin generation
reached a plateau at the substrate concentration of more than 1.0
µg of the kininogen.   Therefore, 4 µg of bovine serum low molecular
weight kininogen was used in the present method (Figure 5).

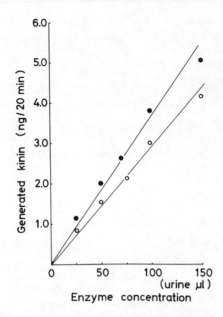

Figure 4. Relationships between the amounts of generated
           kinin and enzyme concentration in urine specimens
           from 2 subjects.

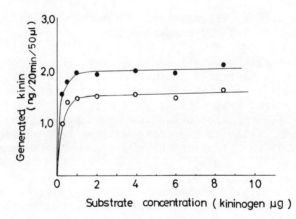

Figure 5. Relationship between the amounts of generated
           kinin and substrate concentration in urine
           specimens from 2 normal subjects.

Relationship between urinary kallikrein determined by kininogenase activity and that by TAME esterolytic activity.

Urinary excretion of kallikrein measured by kininogenase activity using kinin radioimmunoassay was compared with that by TAME esterolytic activity. Figure 6 shows the relationship between urinary kallikrein excretion rates determined by both methods in 31 healthy subjects. There was a significant correlation.

Urinary kallikrein excretion in normal subjects and in patients with various diseases.

Urinary kallikrein excretion was measured by the present method in normal subjects and in patients with various diseases (Fig. 7). The estimated values were 34.5 ± 4.0 µg/day in 84 healthy subjects and 18.3 ± 2.8 µg/day in 55 patients with essential hypertension. Urinary kallikrein excretion was significantly lower in essential hypertension than in healthy subjects ($p<0.05$). A significant decrease in urinary kallikrein output was also found in chronic glomerulonephritis and in patients who received the kidney transplantation as compared with that in healthy subjects. The excretion rates were 14.9 ± 3.3 µg/day in 21 patients without renal failure ($p<0.005$) contrast with 4.8 ± 1.7 µg/day in 19 patients with renal failure ($p<0.001$) in chronic glomerulonephritis and 9.8 ± 3.9 µg/day in 12 normotensive patients ($p<0.001$ contrast with 3.4 ± 2.0 µg/day in 4 hypertensive patients ($p<0.005$) who received the kidney transplantation. On the contrary, significant increase in urinary kallikrein output was found in primary aldosteronism and in Bartter's syndrome. The excretion rates were 80.8 ± 10.0 µg/day in 10 patients with primary aldosteronism ($p<0.05$) and 181.6 ± 45.2 µg/day in 9 patients with Bartter's syndrome ($p<0.01$).

DISCUSSION

According to recent paper by Carretero and his coworkers (1978) regarding urinary kallikrein in hypertensive rats developed by Dahl and his coworkers (1962), it is convinced that urinary kininogenase activity indicates only active kallikrein, whereas a direct radioimmunoassay of kallikrein measures total kallikrein which includes active and inactive kallikrein. Thus, they consider that measurement of kallikrein by the kininogenase method is preferable, since the possible effects of this enzyme in the kidney are not direct but mediated through the release of kinin.

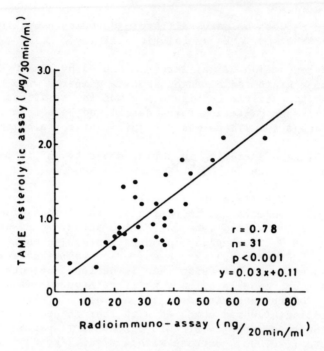

Figure 6. Relationship between urinary kallikrein activity
determined by kininogenase activity using kinin
radioimmunoassay and that by TAME esterolytic activity
in 31 healthy subjects.

In the original report in the estimation of urinary kininogenase activity by kinin radioimmunoassay, Carretero and coworkers
(1976) described that antibody against kallidin had cross reaction
with bradykinin (153%), methionyl-lysyl-bradykinin (83%) and
partially purified dog plasma kininogen (83%). Therefore, it was
necessary to avoid interference of substrate prior to the radioimmunoassay of generated kinin. In their method, ethanol precipitation and QAE-sephadex-A50 chromatography were used to separate
generated kinin from the substrate. In the present study, it was
confirmed that 1000 ng of bovine serum low molecular weight kininogen had no cross reaction with antibody against kallidin and
antibody against bradykinin. Thus, the application of this
kininogen in the system made it possible to skip the complicated
isolation procedure of released kinin from the substrate. When
urine, 0.05 ml was incubated with various amounts of bovine serum
low molecular weight kininogen, the kinin generation reached a
plateau at the substrate concentration of more than 1.0 µg. Therefore, 4 µg of the kininogen was used in the present method.

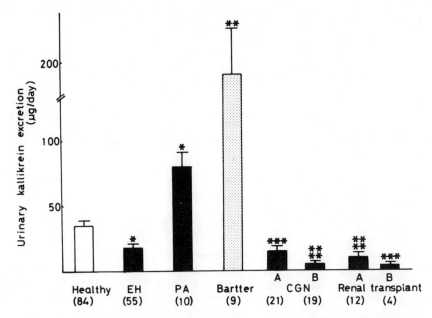

Figure 7. Urinary kallikrein excretion in normal subjects and
in patients with various diseases. Abbreviations:
EH; essential hypertension, PA; primary aldosteronism,
CGN; chronic glomerulonephritis.

The present method was very useful for the determination of
kininogenase activity and may contribute to studies on the pathophysiological roles of renal kallikrein-kinin system in various
diseases. The estimated values of urinary kallikrein excretion
in essential hypertension and in primary aldosteronism by the
present method was in good accordance with the data reported
previously by Margolius and his coworkers (1971) using TAME
esterolytic activity. In 1976, Lechi reported an increase in
urinary kallikrein excretion in a patient with Bartter's syndrome.
Recently, Haluska and his coworkers (1977) reported similar data
in 2 children with Bartter's syndrome. In the present study, 5
out of 9 patients with Bartter's syndrome had extremely high
values of urinary kallikrein output, while the remaining 4 had
normal values.

In chronic glomerulonephritis, there was a significant
correlation between urinary kallikrein excretion and mean blood
pressure (r= -0.589). This result suggests that reduced renal
kallikrein generation may be involved in the pathogenesis of
hypertension in this disease. A marked decrease in urinary kallikrein output was found in renal transplant patients with normal

renal function. It is not clear whether this lowered activity of renal kallikrein-kinin system in this disease is due to the denervation of the transplanted kidney.

ACKNOWLEDGEMENTS

We thank Dr. O.A. Carretero of Henry Ford Hospital, Detroit for the supply of kallidin antiserum and Dr. C.I. Johnston of Manash University, Melbourne for the supply of bradykinin antiserum.

REFERENCES

Carretero, O.A., N.B. Oza, A. Piwonska, T. Ocholik and A.G. Scicli, 1976. Measurement of urinary kallikrein activity by kinin radioimmunoassay. Biochem. Pharmacol. 25: 2265.

Carretero, O.A., V.M. Amin, T. Ocholik, A.G. Scicli and J. Koch, 1978. Urinary kallikrein in rats bred for their susceptibility and resistance to the hypertensive effect of salt. Circ. Res. 42: 727.

Dahl, L.K., M. Heine and L. Tassinary, 1962. Effects of chronic excess salt ingestion: Evidence that genetic factors play an important role in susceptibility to experimental hypertension J. Exp. Med. 115: 1173.

Halushka, P.U., H. Wohltmann, P.J. Privitera, G. Hurwitz and H.S. Margolius, 1977. Bartter's syndrome: Urinary prostaglandin E-like material and kallikrein; Indomethacin effects. Ann. Int. Med. 87: 281.

Johnston, C.I., P.G. Mathews and E. Dax, 1976. Renin-angiotensin and kallikrein-kinin systems in sodium homeostasis and hypertension. Clin. Sci. Mol. Med. 51: Suppl. 3, 283.

Lechi, A., G. Covi, C. Lechi, F. Mantero and L.A. Scuro, 1976. Urinary kallikrein excretion in Bartter's syndrome. J. Clin. Endocinol. Metab. 43: 1175.

Margolius, H.S., R. Geller and J.J. Pisano, 1971. Altered urinary kallikrein excretion in human hypertension. Lancet 2: 1063.

Matsuda, Y., H. Moriya, C. Moriwaki, Y. Fujimoto and M. Mastuda, 1976. Fluorometric method for assay of kallikrein-like arginine esterases. J. Biochem. 79: 1197.

Nustak, K., 1970. The relationship between kidney and urinary kininogenase. Brit. J. Pharmac. 39: 73.

Suzuki, T., Y. Mizushima, T. Sato and S. Iwanaga, 1965. Purification of bovine bradykinin. J. Biochem. 57: 14.

A SIMPLE RADIOASSAY FOR HUMAN URINARY KALLIKREIN

Alfred Chung, James W. Ryan, Guillermo Pena and
Narendra B. Oza

Department of Medicine, University of Miami School
of Medicine, Miami, Florida 33101, USA

ABSTRACT

We have developed a sensitive, highly selective assay for
human urinary kallikrein (HUK) that uses Pro-Phe-Arg-[^{3}H]benzyl-
amide as substrate. The substrate was prepared from Pro-Phe-Arg-
3-iodo-benzylamide by dehalogenation in ^{3}H$_2$ gas. HUK is measured
by its ability to release [^{3}H]benzylamine. The pH optimum is 9.5.
Urokinase, plasmin and thrombin do not interfere. The assay can
measure as little as 5 ng of HUK in a 15 min incubation at 37° C.
Typically, we use 50 µl of dialyzed urine for HUK assays. Reactions
are terminated by adding 0.1 M NaOH, and reaction product is
separated from substrate by partitioning with an equal volume of
toluene. A sample of the toluene phase is submitted for liquid
scintillation counting. As judged by separations obtained on
molecular sieve chromatography (Sephacryl), only one urinary enzyme
possesses the ability to hydrolyze our substrate. The enzyme
MW 45,000, is inhibited by Trasylol but not by soya bean trypsin
inhibitor (SBTI). It is reactive with and is inhibited by antibodies prepared against pure HUK.

INTRODUCTION

We set out to develop an assay for kallikreins that would com-
bine the sensitivity of the radioassay of Pisano and colleagues
(Beaven et al., 1971) with the high selectivity of the colorimetric
assay of Amundsen et al., (1976). Specifically, we prepared Pro-
Phe-Arg-[^{3}H]anilide (I.) and Pro-Phe-Arg-[^{3}H]benzylamide (II.).
Substrate I. can be used in an assay in which kallikrein activity
is measured by the rate of release of [^{3}H]aniline. Using substrate

115

II., one can measure kallikrein in terms of the rate of release of [^{3}H]benzylamine.

Our substrates, like that of Amundsen et al., were designed to capitalize on the fact that all kallikreins hydrolyze the Arg-Ser bond of kininogen (reaction 3):

- - -Ser-Leu-Met-Lys-Arg-Pro-Pro-Gly-Phe-Ser-Pro-Phe-Arg-Ser- - -
                      ↑   ↑   ↑
                      1   2   3

(cf. Han et al., 1976; Claeson, et al., 1978)

Although the substrate of Amundsen et al., (1976), benzoyl-Pro-Phe-Arg-4-NO$_2$-anilide, works well for measuring plasma kallikrein, it does not appear to be hydrolyzed by human urinary kallikrein. Our substrates I. and II., at low concentrations (below 1 μM) can be used to yield highly sensitive assays for human urinary kallikrein. However, at concentrations >10 μM, substrates I. and II. inhibit urinary kallikrein. Substrate II. can be obtained at high specific radioactivity (∿25 Ci/mmol) and, as a routine, is used at concentrations of 20-40 nM.

MATERIALS AND METHODS

Human urinary kallikrein was prepared as described by Oza and Ryan (1978). Plasmin, trypsin, α-chymotrypsin, urokinase and thrombin were purchased from Sigma Chemical Co. Catalytic tritiations were performed by New England Nuclear Corp. (Pro-Phe-Arg-[^{3}H]anilide) and by Amersham Corp. (Pro-Phe-Arg-[^{3}H]benzylamide). Tritiations were accomplished by dehalogenation in ^{3}H$_2$ using Pro-Phe-Arg-4-iodo-anilide and Pro-Phe-Arg-3-iodo-benzylamide. Iodo-aniline was from Eastman Kodak and iodobenzylamine was obtained from Aldrich Chemical Co. Protected amino acids were obtained from Peninsula Labs, Inc.

The halogenated precursors were prepared by conventional solution phase peptide synthetic methods. In brief, 4-iodo-aniline was coupled to Boc-Arg(NO$_2$)-OH by the mixed anhydride method and then H-Arg(NO$_2$)-4-iodo-anilide was coupled to Boc-Pro-Phe-OH with carbodiimide in the presence of 1-hydroxybenzotriazole. The resulting compound was deprotected with HF. In some syntheses, larger homologs were prepared by selective removal of the N$^\alpha$-Boc group with TFA. Boc-Ser(Bzl)-OH or Boc-Phe-Ser(Bzl)-OH was coupled using carbodiimide. Deprotection was accomplished with HF, The Pro-Phe-Arg-3-iodo-benzylamide was prepared by a similar strategy.

The finished peptides were purified by chromatography on Sephadex G-10 or G-15 developed with 1% acetic acid, by partition chromatography (Sephadex G-25; n-butanol-acetic acid-H_2O, 4:1:5) and by chromatography on Sephadex LH-20 (6% n-butanol in H_2O). The peptides were examined by elemental analysis and amino acid analysis. Each of the peptides behaved as a single substance in four or more thin layer chromatography systems (silica gel) and on paper electrophoresis at pH 1.9 and 5.0. Ninhydrin, o-tolidine/Cl_2 and Sakaguchi reagents were used to visualize compounds separated by tlc and electrophoresis.

Tritium Labelling

For reasons not yet apparent, Pro-Phe-Arg-4-iodo-anilide was not efficiently tritiated (two experiments conducted by New England Nuclear Corp.). In contrast, Pro-Phe-Arg-3-iodo-benzylamide was readily tritiated (Amersham Corp.) using the following protocol: 10 mg of Pro-Phe-Arg-3-iodo-benzylamide was dissolved in 2.0 ml of dimethylformamide and H_2O (1:1). To this solution was added 10% palladium on calcium carbonate and 10 Ci of $^3H_2$ gas. The mixture was stirred at room temperature for 4 h and was filtered. The filtrate was lyophilized repeatedly to remove labile tritium, and the residue (295 mCi) was dissolved in 25 ml of H_2O. The labelled peptide was purified by chromatography on Bio-Rex 70 (gradient elution, 10% to glacial acetic acid). The purified compound could not be separated from authentic Pro-Phe-Arg-benzylamide in four tlc systems nor on electrophoresis at pH 1.9 and 5.0. Specificity of labelling was verified by acid hydrolysis (labelled compound plus added proline, phenylalanine, arginine and benzylamine were reacted with 6N HCl at 115° C for 20 h). The products were separated on silica gel plates developed with $CHCl_3$-methanol-H_2O (12:9:4) and were reacted with ninhydrin. Benzylamine (R_f 0.86) contained 98.5% of the tritium. Phenylalanine (R_f 0.48), proline (R_f 0.20) and arginine (R_f 0.08) each contained less than 0.8% of the total radioactivity.

N^α-acylation of Substrates

N^α-acetyl-, benzoyl- and cyclopentylcarbonyl- derivatives of Pro-Phe-Arg-[^3H]benzylamide were prepared by reacting the respective acid chlorides with the labelled peptide in dioxane and 1 M $NaHCO_3$ (1:1) buffered at pH 8.5 with 1.5 M Na_2CO_3. Succinyl-Pro-Phe-Arg-[^3H]benzylamide was prepared using mono-N-succinimidyl succinate in 1 M $NaHCO_3$ and DMF (1:2). The acylated derivatives were purified by chromatography (1.2 x 95 cm column) on Sephadex G-10 developed with 5% acetic acid.

RESULTS

Tris HCl buffers were used throughout, as we found that, at a given pH and enzyme concentration, the relative rates of formation of [^{3}H]benzylamine were higher using solutions buffered with Tris than with those buffered with Hepes or phosphate. All optimization studies used the human urinary kallikrein preparation of Oza and Ryan (1978).

Unless noted otherwise, each reaction was terminated by adding 0.1 N NaOH, and ^{3}H-labelled product was separated from substrate by extraction with an equal volume (usually 1 ml) of toluene. Ethyl acetate can be used to replace toluene, or substrate and product can be separated by ion exchange.

Effects of pH

The pH optimum was remarkably high (between pH 9.0 and 10.0), and all subsequent studies used 0.05 or 0.1 M Tris·HCl, pH 9.5, as buffer. When 62.5 ng of kallikrein was incubated with Pro-Phe-Arg-[^{3}H]benzylamide ($\sim$20 nM) in a total volume of 100 µl at 37° C for 15 min, the rate of formation of [^{3}H]benzylamine was 2.5-times faster at pH 9.5 than at pH 8.0 or 10.7. Rates at pH 9.0 and 10.0 were approximately 95% of that at pH 9.5. The reaction of kallikrein with Pro-Phe-Arg-[^{3}H]anilide showed the same pH optimum.

At pH 9.5, the reaction of kallikrein with either substrate at 37° C for 15 min is linear when the kallikrein concentration is between 20-700 ng/ml. Much lower amounts of kallikrein can be measured by extending the length of incubation and/or by reducing the volume of the reaction mixture.

Kinetics

V_{max} and K_m values were estimated from Lineweaver-Burk double reciprocal plots. Pro-Phe-Arg-[^{3}H]anilide showed slightly greater affinity having a K_m of 0.8 µM and V_{max} of 0.39 mmol/min/mg of protein versus a K_m of 3.0 µM and V_{max} of 0.88 mmol/min/mg protein for the benzylamide. An important finding arising from these studies is that either substrate inhibits human urinary kallikrein when used at concentrations greater than 10 µM. The result suggests that either substrate or a closely related analog can be used as a reversible inhibitor. Whether these inhibitory effects can be conferred in vivo (e.g., by renal perfusion) remains to be determined.

Structural Requirements

As is well-known, human urinary kallikrein does not appear to be capable of hydrolyzing benzoyl-arginyl-4-NO$_2$-anilide. However, little more is known about its substrate requirements. Therefore, we examined for reactivity of the enzyme with the substrates shown in Table 1.

Within the limits of the study, it appears that the tripeptide anilide is the minimum structure required for hydrolysis by human urinary kallikrein. Detailed kinetic studies have not been performed, and we do not know whether the relatively low rate of reaction obtained with Ser-Pro-Phe-Arg-iodoanilide is owing to increased or decreased affinity of substrate to enzyme.

Specificity

Human urinary kallikrein is only one among many trypsin-like enzymes; enzymes capable of hydrolyzing substrates such as TAME and BAME. Thus, it was important to define the susceptibility of our substrates to hydrolysis by related enzymes. Results are shown in Table 2.

TABLE 1

RELATIVE AFFINITY OF HALOGENATED SUBSTRATES FOR
HUMAN URINARY KALLIKREIN

Substrate	Rate of Hydrolysis
Phe-Arg-4-iodoanilide	Nil
Pro-Phe-Arg-4-iodoanilide	0.73
Ser-Pro-Phe-Arg-4-iodoanilide	0.62
Phe-Ser-Pro-Phe-Arg-4-iodoanilide	1.12

Each substrate, 150 nmol, was incubated with varying amounts of HUK in 0.7 ml of 0.05 M Tris·HCl, pH 8.1, at 37° C. At timed intervals, 100 µl of the reaction mixture was added to 1.0 ml of 0.1 N NaOH. The resulting solution was extracted with CHCl$_3$ and the organic phase was evaporated to dryness. The residue was dissolved in buffer and then examined by UV spectrophotometry (240-300 nm).

As is evident from the results, Pro-Phe-Arg-[^{3}H]benzylamide is hydrolyzed by trypsin and plasmin but only when the latter enzymes are used in several-fold excess. For example, at pH 9.5, a 23-fold excess of trypsin and a 680-fold excess of plasmin are required. Urokinase and thrombin did not hydrolyze the substrate. Reactions of chymotrypsin with substrate were monitored by thin layer chromatography, but formation of the expected reaction product, Arg-[^{3}H]benzylamide, was never observed.

TABLE 2

SPECIFICITY STUDIES: HYDROLYSIS OF PRO-PHE-ARG-[^{3}H]BENZYLAMIDE
BY SERINE PROTEASE ENZYMES

Enzyme	pH	Amount of Enzyme Required for 10% Hydrolysis*
Human Urinary Kallikrein	9.5	45 ng (10 nM)
	7.5	265 ng
Plasmin	9.5	30,600 ng
	7.5	17,200 ng
Trypsin	9.5	1,030 ng
	7.5	400 ng
α-Chymotrypsin	9.5	No hydrolysis**
	7.5	
Urokinase	9.5	No hydrolysis**
	7.5	
Thrombin	9.5	No hydrolysis**
	7.5	

Reactions were conducted in 0.1 M Tris·HCl buffer, at pH 7.5 or 9.5, at 37° C for 15 min.

*Denotes the amount of enzyme required to hydrolyze 10% of the initial substrate over the course of a 15 min reaction.

**No hydrolysis at enzyme concentrations of 0.5 mg/ml.

Effects of N^α-Acylation

Anticipating that Pro-Phe-Arg-[^{3}H]benzylamide or the anilide may be degraded by exopeptidase enzymes of body fluids or tissue homogenates, we examined the effects of adding an N^α-acylating group. In addition, it seemed possible that the apparent inability of urinary kallikrein to hydrolyze benzoyl-Pro-Phe-Arg-4-NO_2-anilide (cf. Amundsen et al., 1976) might be owing to the presence of the benzoyl group. The respective acetyl-, benzoyl-, cyclopentylcarbonyl- and succinyl-derivatives of Pro-Phe-Arg-[^{3}H]benzylamide were prepared as described above and were used at ∿20 nM (without carrier) in reaction with purified urinary kallikrein, 60 ng in 100 μl of 0.1 M Tris·HCl buffer, pH 9.5. Reactions were conducted at 37° C for 15 min. The acetyl- and cyclopentylcarbonyl- groups had no discernable effects. Pro-Phe-Arg-[^{3}H]benzylamide, acetyl-substrate and cyclopentyl-carbonyl-substrate were all hydrolyzed at about the same rate (9-11% of the substrate was hydrolyzed in 15 min). However, the benzoyl-substrate was hydrolyzed at about one-half the rate, and the succinyl-substrate was hydrolyzed at one-tenth of the control rate (cf. Claeson et al., 1978). Our results are consistent with those of Drs. Charles Kettner and Elliott Shaw (personal communication), who have found that Pro-Phe-Arg-CH_2Cl has a lower Ki towards urinary kallikrein than does the N^α-acetyl derivative.

Whether N^α-protection is required is still not clear. Possibly enzymes of plasma or tissue homogenates are capable of attacking Pro-Phe-Arg-[^{3}H]benzylamide, but kallikrein appears to be the only urinary enzyme of concern. Further to clarify the point, we concentrated fresh human and guinea pig urines by ultrafiltration (500 ml to 10 ml) and then applied the washed urinary proteins to a Sephacryl column (2.5 x 110 cm) developed with 0.1 Tris·HCl, pH 8.0, plus 0.5 M NaCl. In terms of hydrolysis of Pro-Phe-Arg-[^{3}H]benzylamide, only one active fraction was found; a fraction corresponding in molecular size (45,000 daltons) to urinary kallikrein (cf. Oza and Ryan, 1978, and Ryan et al., this volume). The active fraction from human urine was inhibited by Trasylol but not by SBTI. Further, it was adsorbed by a Trasylol-sepharose matrix and was inhibited by antibodies to human urinary kallikrein.

Protocol for the Assay of Kallikrein in Human Urine

Pro-Phe-Arg-[^{3}H]benzylamide or Pro-Phe-Arg-[^{3}H]anilide can be used in the following protocol. Each assay is performed in duplicate. Typically, fresh urine samples are dialyzed overnight (vs. 0.9% NaCl), but the urine preparation procedure (separation of protein from small molecular weight substances on Sephadex G-25) of Beaven et al., (1971), can also be used. Reaction mixtures are

prepared using 12 x 75 mm culture tubes. Each mixture contains
50 μl of dialyzed urine and 50 μl (0.1 μCi) of substrate buffered
with 0.1 M Tris·HCl buffer, pH 9.5. The final concentration of
substrate is about 20 nM and is well-below K_m. The latter is important, as the sensitivity of the assay is, in part, a function
of percent substrate utilization (cf. Ryan et al., 1978).

The reaction tubes are incubated at 37° C for 2 h, and the
reactions are stopped by adding 1.0 ml of 0.1 M NaOH. [3H]Benzyl-
amine or [3H]aniline is extracted with 1.0 ml of toluene. Extraction is accomplished by vortex mixing and then centrifugation to
separate phases. A sample, usually 500 μl, of the organic phase
is submitted to liquid scintillation counting. Blanks (reaction
mixtures containing 50 μl of saline instead of dialyzed urine) are
treated identically. Substrate is measured by adding 50 μl of the
stock buffered substrate solution to a scintillation vial. In
general, we use Hydromix or Riafluor, 10 ml/vial. Differential
quenching has not been encountered.

Periodically it is necessary to construct a standard curve,
and this is accomplished by substituting purified kallikrein (2-
70 ng) in saline for dialyzed urine. The activity of a given
urine sample is measured in terms of the rate of release of 3H-
labelled product, and the rate of release is compared with the
standard curve. The results can be expressed in terms of pmoles
of enzyme or as first order units: One unit is that amount of
enzyme required to hydrolyze substrate (at a concentration well-
within the range of first order enzyme kinetics) at an initial rate
of 1%/min at 37° C. In our experience, one first order unit is
equal to 1.17 pmoles of the human urinary kallikrein prepared by
Oza and Ryan (1978).

We use the following equation:

$$\text{units/ml} = \frac{\dfrac{2(\text{Test c.p.m.} - \text{Blank c.p.m.})}{\text{Substrate c.p.m.}} \times 100}{\text{incubation time (min)} \times \text{vol. of enzyme in ml}}$$

(Vol. of enzyme in ml can be substituted by amount of enzyme in mg).

The term 2 is used to correct for the extraction volume (when
500 μl of the toluene phase is used for counting). Using the protocol described above, urine is used at 0.05 ml and incubation is
for 120 min. Hence, the equation can be reduced to:

$$\text{units/ml} = \frac{2(\text{Test c.p.m.} - \text{Blank c.p.m.})}{\text{Substrate c.p.m.}} \times 16.67$$

The technique of the assay is analogous to those described previously for angiotensin converting enzyme (Ryan et al., 1977; 1978).

Comparison with Other Kallikrein Assays

We have just begun to compare the radioassay described above with a radioimmunoassay using antibodies to human urinary kallikrein. While the comparison has just begun, it appears that values obtained by the radioimmunoassay are 1.5 to 2-times higher than those obtained by the radioassay (e.g., 130 ng/ml of human urine vs. 220 ng/ml). Possibly, the difference is owing to inactive or inhibitor-bound kallikrein not measurable by the functional assay.

Our radioassay has been compared to the assay of Beaven et al., (1971) using human urine samples prepared by chromatography on Sephadex G-25. Twelve subjects provided two urine samples, the second collected 24 h after the first. A linear correlation was obtained (r = 0.913; p<0.01). In this limited study, it appeared that 1.0 amidase unit (our assay) was equivalent to 1.24 arginine esterase units. Further correlation tests are required.

In collaborative studies with Drs. John Laragh and Jean Sealey, we have examined eleven urine samples from each of 3 patients treated with SQ 14,225. Each patient was followed for three days and then placed on SQ 14,225. After beginning the drug, eight more 24 h urines were collected. In each case, urinary kallikrein activity fell to less than 25% of control levels within 6 days of beginning SQ 14,225 (from a mean of 67 ng/ml to as low as 8 ng/ml, or from a high of 250 µg/24h to a low of 15 µg/24h).

DISCUSSION

Pro-Phe-Arg-[3H]anilide and Pro-Phe-Arg-[3H]benzylamide appear to be remarkably good substrates for human urinary kallikrein. However, both inhibit the enzyme at concentrations above 10 µM, a point that suggests that either compound, with or without [3H], may be useful as a reversible, competitive inhibitor of kallikrein in pharmacologic or physiologic studies. Because of the low K_m values, it is likely that Pro-Phe-Arg-anilide and the corresponding benzylamide will act as competitive (alternative) substrates for kallikrein when the small molecular compounds are near or above K_m and when kininogen is well-below its K_m.

In view of the usefulness of our compounds for assaying human urinary kallikrein, it is not immediately clear why benzoyl-Pro-Phe-Arg-4-NO_2-anilide is not hydrolyzed by the enzyme. Benzoyl reduces the rate of hydrolysis of our substrates, but the reduction in rate is tolerable and, indeed, could be owing to decreased K_m

and V_{max}. If the latter is correct, the plasma kallikrein substrate of Amundsen et al. (1976) could be an excellent inhibitor
of urinary kallikrein. If it is an inhibitor, then one would not
expect to be able to detect the formation of 4-NO$_2$-aniline when
substrate is used at an initial concentration of 10^{-4} M (Amundsen
et al.).

     A striking finding of our study is that the pH optimum of
human urinary kallikrein is 9.5, a pH level that could not be
tolerated in an arginine esterase assay. Spontaneous hydrolysis
is essentially complete at pH 9.5. pH optimum is, in part, a
function of the substrate as well as the enzyme; thus, the pH optimum for hydrolysis of, e.g., N$^\alpha$-tosyl-L-arginine-methyl ester may
be somewhat lower or higher than that of Pro-Phe-Arg-benzylamide
or -anilide. However, the esterase assays in current use are performed at pH levels that are less than optimal and are therefore
probably subject to large variations in rate as a function of
small changes in pH.

     Once synthesized, there is little to choose between Pro-Phe-
Arg-[^{3}H]benzylamide and Pro-Phe-Arg-[^{3}H]anilide. The latter gives
somewhat lower blank values but has a lower V_{max}. However, we have
found that it is very much easier to prepare the benzylamide than
the anilide. The iodo-precursors are readily prepared, but the
iodo-anilide does not appear to undergo dehalogenation in ^{3}H$_2$ as
well as does the iodo-benzylamide. Thus Pro-Phe-Arg-[^{3}H]anilide
was obtained in a crude yield of ∿2 Ci/mmole, and less than 15% of
the radioactivity was incorporated into the desired compound.
Pure Pro-Phe-Arg-[^{3}H]benzylamide was obtained at approximately
25 Ci/mmole in an overall yield of ∿200 mCi. The pure final
products store well in stock solutions of approximately 1 mCi/ml
of ethanol at -28° C. No radiolysis has been observed over a
period of 12 months.

     As a matter of convenience, we employ a solvent extraction
step to separate product from substrate. As many as 400 assays
can be performed per day by a single technician. With an automatic
pipetter, the procedure can be automated. However, other means can
be employed to separate product from substrate, e.g., ion exchange
or molecular sieve chromatography. Similarly, by selecting a
liquid scintillation mixture having little or no ability to dissolve
aqueous solutions, it should be feasible to conduct an enzyme reaction directly in a scintillation vial and then collect, e.g.,
^{3}H-benzylamide into the scintillation fluid while leaving substrate
at the base of the vial (a method analogous to that of Beaven et
al., 1971). The latter procedure is an important safeguard when
using ^{3}H-TAME, as the radioactive product, methanol, is volatile.
However, neither ^{3}H-aniline nor ^{3}H-benzylamine is particularly
volatile and neither presents the same hazard. Biological hazards
of ^{3}H-aniline and ^{3}H-benzylamine remain to be examined but should

be minimized through the use of substrate at 20-40 nM.   At 10%
hydrolysis of substrate, aniline or benzylamine would occur at no
more than 4 nM.   In a 100 μl reaction mixture, total product
should not exceed 0.4 pmole.

ACKNOWLEDGEMENTS

We thank Dr. Ronald Block of the Papanicolaou Cancer Research
Institute, Miami, Florida, U.S.A., for performing NMR analyses of
peptide intermediates.   This work was supported in part by grants
from the U.S. Public Health Service (HL22087 and HL22896), the John
A. Hartford Foundation, Inc., and the American Heart Association
(Palm Beach County Chapter, Inc.).

REFERENCES

Amundsen, E., L. Svendsen, A.M. Vennerød and K. Laake, Determination
    of plasma kallikrein with a new chromogenic tripeptide derivative,
    1976, in: Chemistry and Biology of the Kallikrein-Kinin System in
    Health and Disease, eds. J.J. Pisano and K.F. Austen (U.S.
    Government Printing Office, Washington, D.C.) p. 215.

Beaven, V.H., J.V. Pierce and J.J. Pisano, 1971, A sensitive iso-
    topic procedure for the assay of esterase activity: Measurement
    of human urinary kallikrein, Clin. Chim. Acta, 32, 67.

Claeson, G., L. Aurell, P. Friberger, S. Gustavsson and G. Karlsson,
    Designing of peptide substrates.   Different approaches exemplified
    by new chromogenic substrates for kallikreins and urokinase,
    Haemostasis, 7, 62.

Han, Y.N., H. Kato and S. Iwanaga, 1976, Identification of Ser-Leu-
    Met-Lys-bradykinin isolated from chemically modified high-
    molecular weight bovine kininogen, FEBS Letters, 71, 45.

Ryan, J.W., A. Chung, L.C. Martin and U.. Ryan, 1978, New substrates
    for the radioassay of angiotensin converting enzyme of endothelial
    cells in culture, Tissue & Cell, 10, 555.

Ryan, J.W., N.B. Oza, L.C. Martin and G.A. Pena (this volume),
    Components of the kallikrein-kinin system in urine.

Oza, N.B. and J.W. Ryan, 1978, A simple high-yield procedure for
    isolation of human urinary kallikreins, Biochem. J., 171, 285.

Ryan, J.W., A. Chung, C. Ammons and M.L. Carlton, 1977, A simple
    radioassay for angiotensin converting enzyme, Biochem. J., 167,
    501.

GLANDULAR KALLIKREIN IN PLASMA AND URINE: EVALUATION OF A

DIRECT RIA FOR ITS DETERMINATION*

S. F. Rabito, V. Amin, A. G. Scicli and O. A. Carretero

Department of Medicine, Henry Ford Hospital

Detroit, Michigan, 48202, U.S.A.

SUMMARY

To determine whether there is glandular kallikrein in plasma, untreated as well as acetone-treated and heated-acidified rat plasmas together with rabbit anti-rat urinary kallikrein were used in counterimmunoelectrophoresis. Precipitation bands were observed with untreated and acetone-treated plasma, suggesting that glandular kallikrein is present in plasma. This enzyme, however, cannot be quantified in the untreated plasma by a new direct RIA since kallikrein inhibitors present in plasma appear to interfere with this assay. Destroying the inhibitors by acetone treatment or by heat and acidification of the plasma partially solves this problem. In the second part of the study, this RIA as well as a kininogenase and an esterase assay were used to measure urinary kallikrein in DOCA-salt treated rats and in control rats. There is a significant correlation between urinary kallikrein measured by the direct RIA and by a kininogenase method ($r = 0.75$, $p < 0.001$) in both DOCA-salt treated and in the control rats. Although the results obtained by the direct RIA and an esterase method significantly correlate in the control rats ($r = 0.67$, $p < 0.001$), they did not in the DOCA-salt rats ($r = -0.048$, $p > 0.1$). This suggests that part of the urinary esterase activity in the DOCA-salt rats is due to urinary enzymes other than kallikrein and that the esterase assay is not reliable for the determination of urinary kallikrein in pathological situations. However, the direct RIA and the kininogenase assay are suitable for this purpose.

* Partially supported by a grant of the National Institutes
  of Health, Grant #HL 15839.

INTRODUCTION

Urinary kallikrein has been implicated in the regulation of local blood flow (13,15), blood pressure and sodium balance (1,18,11), as well as in the pathogenesis of human and experimental hypertension (7,19,20,17,6) and renal diseases (6,12). However, it is not clear whether renal and other glandular kallikreins are excreted only into the exocrine secretion of the gland or whether they are also secreted, or reabsorbed, into the vascular compartment where blood pressure and local blood flow could be more directly affected.

In the first part of this study, the counterimmunoelectrophoresis technique was used with rabbit anti-rat urinary kallikrein and rat plasma to see if there is glandular kallikrein in plasma. In addition, the possibility of measuring glandular kallikrein in rat plasma by using a direct RIA for kallikrein, recently developed in our laboratory (3), was investigated. This assay measures absolute concentration of the enzymic protein (antigen). Since it is well known that plasma has kallikrein inhibitors, the effect of destroying these inhibitors and the effect of the kallikrein inhibitors aprotinin and benzamidine on the direct RIA for kallikrein were also studied.

In the second part of the study, this direct RIA as well as a kininogenase and an esterase assay were used to measure urinary kallikrein in DOCA-salt treated rats and in control rats. The results obtained with these three methods were compared for the purpose of determining whether the conflicting results reported on urinary kallikrein (5) could be explained, in part, by the fact that different methods based on different principles were used to determine urinary kallikrein.

MATERIALS AND METHODS

Glandular kallikrein in plasma. Blood was collected from normal rats in plastic tubes containing disodium ethylenediaminetetraacetate (EDTA). After centrifugation, the plasma was separated and kept frozen until its use. One aliquot was then acidified to pH 2.0 with 5N HCℓ, incubated at room temperature for one hour, brought back to pH 7.4 with 5N NaOH, and then heated at 56°C for one hour (heated-acidified plasma). A second aliquot was treated with acetone (20% v/v) overnight at 4°C, and the solvent was then evaporated under N_2 (acetone-treated plasma). A third aliquot was used without pre-treatment (untreated plasma). An aliquot of each plasma was dialyzed against phosphate-buffered saline pH 7.4. These three plasmas, both dialyzed and non-dialyzed, were used with rabbit anti-rat

urinary kallikrein in counterimmunoelectrophoresis (2,9).
The antiserum was prepared as previously described (28). In
addition, two to twenty microliters of each plasma were also
assayed with a direct RIA for the enzymic protein (3). The
displacement of the labeled kallikrein produced by the plasmas
was compared with the displacement produced by purified urinary
kallikrein (standard curve) by using "logit-log" linearization
of the curves (31).

Effect of inhibitors on the direct RIA. To study the
effect of aprotinin and benzamidine on the direct RIA, different
amounts of aprotinin (Trasylol, Bayer) or 16 mg of benzamidine
hydrochloride hydrate (Aldrich Chemical Company, Inc.) were
added to aliquots of normal rat urine; and the kallikrein activity
was determined by the direct RIA before and after addition of
the inhibitors. Results were expressed as micrograms of enzymic
protein per ml of urine.

Direct RIA for glandular kallikrein. Urinary kallikrein
was measured as previously described (3). In brief, kallikrein
was iodinated by a modification of Hunter and Greenwood's method
(14), and the labeled kallikrein was purified by gel filtration
on Sephadex G-15 and Sephadex G-100. The radioimmunoassay
was done as follows: 1-40 ng of purified urinary kallikrein
(standard curve) or 1-10 µl of rat urine was transferred into
polyethylene tubes. To each tube was also added 100 µl of
^{125}I-kallikrein having approximately 3,000 cpm, 100 µl of a
1:80,000 dilution of kallikrein antiserum and Tris buffer to
keep the final volume in 500 µl. After four hours of incubation at room temperature, 100 µl of a 3:100 dilution of sheep
anti-rabbit gamma globulin was added to each tube to separate
the free from bound ^{125}I-kallikrein. The tubes were incubated
for 18 hours at 4°C and were then centrifuged at 1,700 g for 40
minutes; and the precipitate was counted in a gamma counter. An
internal standard of crude rat urinary kallikrein was run in
every assay. Results were calculated by computer using "logit-
log" linearization of the standard plot (31) and were expressed
as micrograms of enzymic protein per 24-hour urinary volume.

Kininogenase activity. The kininogenase activity of the
urine was determined as we have previously described (4). Results were expressed as micrograms of kinins generated per minute
of incubation per 24-hour urinary volume.

Esterase activity. In this procedure, kallikrein was determined by the capacity of the enzyme to break the ester bond
of p-tosyl-L-arginine methyl ester HCl (TAMe). The unhydrolyzed
ester was measured by a modification of Robert's colorimetric
method (29,24). Results were expressed in micromoles of substrate
consumed per minute per 24-hour urinary volume.

Urinary protein. Urinary protein was determined by the Lowry procedure (16).

Implants of DOCA. Implants were prepared by mixing DOCA with silicone rubber (Dow-Corning) in a ratio of 1:2 (26).

Experimental groups. Six-week-old female Sprague-Dawley rats were unilaterally nephrectomized and were then placed in individual metabolic cages. Ten days later, urine was collected for two 24-hour periods. The rats were then separated into three groups. In the first group, one strip of DOCA-silicone rubber (100 mg of DOCA per kg) was inserted subcutaneously. These rats received 1% sodium chloride as drinking fluid (DOCA-salt rats). In the second and third groups, strips of silicone rubber without DOCA were implanted. The rats of the second group received tap water as drinking fluid (water controls); the rats of the third group, 1% sodium chloride as drinking fluid (saline controls). All rats were fed the same laboratory diet (Rodent Laboratory Chow #5001, Ralston Purina Company). Urine was collected for a 24-hour period once a week for three weeks and was stored at -20°C until assayed for kallikrein. After each collection period, the blood pressure was measured in the unanesthetized animal by the tail-cuff method.

Results are expressed as mean ±SEM and statistical significance was determined by Student's t-test (32).

RESULTS

Figure 1 shows a typical counterimmunoelectrophoresis using antibody anti-rat urinary kallikrein with untreated and acetone-treated plasmas. Precipitation bands were observed with both plasmas. It is important to note, however, that when heated-acidified plasma was used, no precipitation bands were observed. Figure 2 shows a standard curve for the direct RIA, indicating significant displacement of ^{125}I-kallikrein with only 2 ng of purified kallikrein. The slope of the standard curve in the logit-log plot is -2.33.

Table I shows the results obtained when the direct RIA was applied to measure glandular kallikrein in different aliquots of untreated, acetone-treated, and heated-acidified normal rat plasma before and after dialysis. When the results obtained by the different plasma aliquots were plotted and linearized by the logit-log method, the slopes of the curve obtained were -1.40 for the untreated plasma and -2.52 and -2.59 for the acetone-treated and heated-acidified plasmas, respectively.

The effect of aprotinin (Trasylol) and benzamidine on the direct RIA is shown in Figure 3. Whereas aprotinin added to urine produced increases in the values obtained which were three times higher than those of the urine without the inhibitor, benzamidine did not interfere with the RIA.

The values of urinary kallikrein excretion obtained by the three different methods as well as the values of urinary protein excretion of DOCA-salt hypertensive rats and control rats before and during the three weeks of treatment are shown in Table II. Systolic blood pressure increased in the DOCA-salt treated group and differed significantly from both control groups after the second week (Table III).

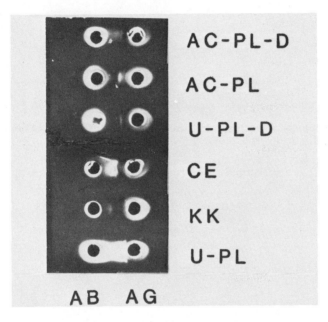

Figure 1: Counterimmunoelectrophoresis using antibodies against rat urinary kallikrein (AB) on the left side and different solutions or plasma containing possible antigen (AG) on the right side. AC-PL indicates acetone-treated plasma; U-PL, untreated plasma; D, dialyzed plasma; CE, crude rat urinary kallikrein; and KK, pure rat urinary kallikrein. The anode was applied to the left side (AB); and the cathode was applied to the right side (AG) of the agar plate.

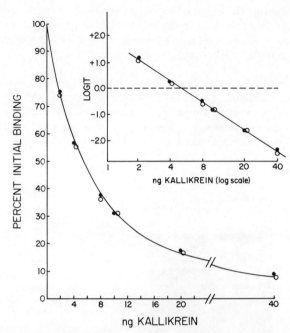

Figure 2:   Standard curve for the direct RIA of kallikrein.
Upper right shows linearization of this plot by using
"logit" scale of B/B_0 in the ordinate and log scale
of standards in the abscissa.

Figures 4 and 5 show the correlation between the results
obtained by the direct RIA and either the kininogenase (Fig. 4)
or esterase (Fig. 5) assay when kallikrein was measured in the
urine of the DOCA-salt treated group and in the water and saline
control groups. No significant correlation was observed between
urinary protein excretion and urinary kallikrein excretion measured by the three methods ($p > 0.05$).

GLANDULAR KALLIKREIN IN RAT PLASMA
(μg/ml of plasma)

Plasma Aliquotes	U-Pl		Ac-Pl		H-A-Pl	
	ND	D	ND	D	ND	D
2 μl	2.35	1.70	0.20	0.75	0.25	0.30
5 μl	1.44	1.02	0.18	0.60	0.24	0.30
10 μl	1.18	0.88	0.20	0.60	0.27	0.29
20 μl	0.91	0.83	0.22	0.60	0.29	0.32

Table I: U-Pl = untreated plasma; Ac-Pl = acetone-treated plasma; H-A-Pl = heated-acidified plasma; ND = non-dialyzed; D = dialyzed. Plasma aliquots indicate amount of plasma used in the RIA. Note that results are expressed in μg of kallikrein/ml of plasma.

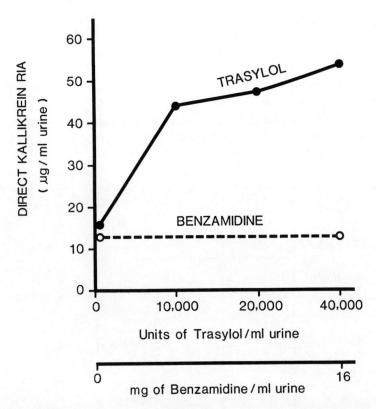

<u>Figure 3</u>: Effect of increasing amount of Trasylol and the effect
            of 16 mg of benzamidine on the direct RIA for the enzymic
            protein. Zero in the abscissa indicates urines to which
            no Trasylol or benzamidine was added.

TABLE II

URINARY KALLIKREIN MEASURED BY THREE DIFFERENT METHODS

AND URINARY PROTEIN EXCRETION IN DOCA-SALT AND WATER AND SALINE CONTROL RATS

	Exp. Groups	Before Treatment*	1 Week of Treatment	2 Weeks of Treatment	3 Weeks of Treatment
Direct RIA (kallikrein µg/24 hs)	DOCA-salt	56.6 ± 2.9	80.3 ± 4.5	85.8 ± 10.2	138.5 ± 15.5
	Water	54.9 ± 5.5	64.4 ± 2.9	82.9 ± 7.3	109.9 ± 5.7
	Saline	38.6 ± 5.8	56.2 ± 5.8	77.9 ± 5.2	90.7 ± 10.8
Kininogenase Method (kinin µg/min/24 hs)	DOCA-salt	35.5 ± 1.6	83.5 ± 6.1	61.5 ± 12.4	86.8 ± 13.4
	Water	43.2 ± 5.1	65.0 ± 7.3	69.1 ± 9.2	99.9 ± 8.5
	Saline	26.6 ± 4.4	66.1 ± 11.5	54.5 ± 5.0	70.7 ± 9.8
Esterase Method (µM/min/24 hs)	DOCA-salt	3.6 ± 0.3	7.1 ± 1.1	8.0 ± 1.0	9.3 ± 1.8
	Water	4.8 ± 0.3	5.7 ± 0.5	9.6 ± 1.9	8.0 ± 0.8
	Saline	2.1 ± 0.3	3.0 ± 0.6	3.7 ± 0.7	7.9 ± 1.2
Urinary Protein (mg/24 hs)	DOCA-salt	49.0 ± 6.4	49.0 ± 4.2	178.1 ± 19.0	120.8 ± 18.7
	Water	48.3 ± 3.9	39.8 ± 1.7	29.9 ± 6.2	37.3 ± 1.6
	Saline	52.8 ± 10.6	48.9 ± 2.2	55.7 ± 15.0	42.1 ± 4.9

* Mean of two 24-hour periods.

TABLE III

Systolic blood pressure (mm Hg) in DOCA-salt and control rats.

	1 Week	2 Weeks	3 Weeks
DOCA (n:14)	130 ± 4.9	148 ± 3.9*	161 ± 6.4*
Water (n:8)	124 ± 4.2	123 ± 2.5	121 ± 2.3
Saline (n:7)	119 ± 5.1	123 ± 2.9	123 ± 2.9

* Differs from both control groups with p < 0.01.

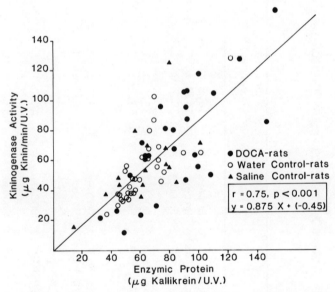

Figure 4: Comparison of 24-hour kallikrein excretion measured by the direct RIA for the enzymic protein and by the kininogenase activity. Closed circles indicate urine from DOCA-treated rats; open circles, urine from water control rats; and triangles, urine from saline control rats.

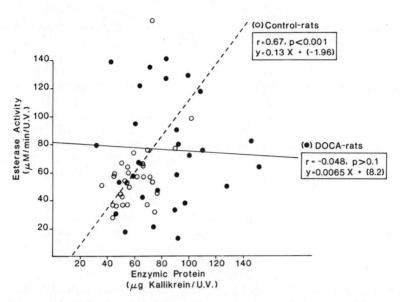

Figure 5:   Comparison of 24-hour kallikrein excretion measured by
the direct RIA for the enzymic protein and by esterase
activity. Closed circles indicate urine from DOCA-treated rats; open circles, urine from control (water and
saline) rats. Solid line is regression line for DOCA
rats; dashed line, regression line for control rats.

DISCUSSION

Since the discovery of kallikrein in 1926 (8), many investigators have suggested that this enzyme, through the release of
kinins, participates in the regulation of local blood flow (13,15).
However, it is not known whether glandular kallikrein reaches the
vascular compartment. The passage of glandular kallikrein into
the systemic circulation has been suggested by Roblero et al (30)
who found that isolated perfused kidneys released kallikrein in
the perfusate, and also by Ørstavik et al (27) who found that
labeled kallikrein, injected into the main duct of the rat submandibular gland appeared in the venous effluent. We investigated the possibility that glandular kallikrein is present in
rat plasma by using antibodies against urinary kallikrein in
counterimmunoelectrophoresis. We found that untreated plasma
and acetone-treated plasma gave a precipitation line, thus
implying that immunoreactive glandular kallikrein is present
in plasma. We also attempted to quantify the amount of glandular

kallikrein found in plasma by using a direct RIA developed in our laboratory (3). When different aliquots of untreated plasma were assayed by this direct RIA and the curve obtained was linearized by the "logit-log" method, the slope obtained (-1.40) was markedly different from that of the standard curve (-2.33). This suggests that plasma contains interfering substances. Since kallikrein inhibitors present in plasma could account for these results, the plasma was either acetone-treated or acidified and heated, two procedures which are known to destroy plasma inhibitors of glandular kallikrein. The slopes of the curves obtained with acetone-treated (-2.52) and heated-acidified plasma (-2.59) were similar to the slope of the standard curve (-2.33). These results suggest that kallikrein inhibitors are partially responsible for the interference observed in untreated plasma. Furthermore, when aprotinin, a polypeptidic inhibitor of kallikrein (MW 6,500), was added to rat urine, the values of kallikrein obtained by the direct RIA were three times higher than those of urine in which the inhibitor had not been added. Benzamidine, a low-molecular weight inhibitor (MW 157), did not modify the results. These findings suggest that plasmatic inhibitors and aprotinin interfere with the binding of the antigen to the antibody and that inhibition of the enzyme per se (benzamidine) does not cause interference in the RIA. It can be deduced from these results that the direct RIA should not be used to measure glandular kallikrein in untreated plasma.

Although treating the plasma with either acetone or heat and acidification seemed to eliminate the inhibitors, it is not clear whether the destruction of the inhibitors is complete and whether or not these treatments also affect glandular kallikrein. Complicating this uncertainty, when the acetone-treated plasma was dialyzed, the values obtained by direct RIA were three times higher than in the non-dialyzed acetone-treated plasma. No differences were observed with dialyzed and non-dialyzed heated-acidified plasma. Using the counter-immunoelectrophoresis technique, we found that untreated plasma as well as dialyzed and non-dialyzed acetone-treated plasma gave a precipitation line. In contrast, heated and acidified plasma did not show any precipitation line, thus suggesting that the treatment altered the antigenic determinants of the kallikrein molecule.

These results imply that until more is known about the influence of plasmatic interference on the direct RIA, results obtained with this technique should be interpreted with caution.

The second part of this study was done to determine if the conflicting results on urinary kallikrein excretion which appear in the literature could be explained, in part, by the different methods used to measure this enzyme. For this purpose, urinary kallikrein was measured using three different methods based on different principles in the urine of DOCA-salt treated rats and control rats receiving either saline or water as a drinking fluid. It was noted that all three groups of rats increased urinary kallikrein excretion and these increases were highly significant three weeks after treatment (p < 0.001). Further-more, the increases were independent of both the treatment that the rats were receiving and the method used for the kallikrein determination (Table II). The lack of a further increase in urinary kallikrein in the DOCA-salt treated rats was unexpected since it has been previously reported that mineralocorticoids produce an increase in urinary kallikrein excretion (11,17,21,23). We do not have an explanation for this. However, a significant increase in urinary kallikrein excretion was observed in both control groups. Since all rats were unilaterally nephrectomized, it is possible that the reduction of the renal mass could stimulate the urinary kallikrein excretion of the remanent kidney. It could be that under this condition, no further increase is possible with the mineralocorticoid treatment. It has been reported that rats with renal damage have a diminished urinary kalli-krein excretion (12). Since the DOCA-salt treated rats showed high proteinuria, some degree of renal damage is possible. This could also explain, in part, the lack of increase in kallikrein excretion in the DOCA-salt rats.

A significant correlation was observed between the results obtained with the direct RIA and those obtained with the kinino-genase method in the three groups of rats (Fig. 4). However, when kallikrein was measured by the esterase method, there was significant correlation with the direct RIA only in the two control groups but not in the DOCA-salt treated rats (Fig. 5). These results suggest that part of the urinary esterase activity in the DOCA-salt rats is due to urinary enzymes other than kalli-krein. We have previously reported a similar lack of correlation between the esterase method and either the direct RIA or the kininogenase assay in the Dahl's salt sensitive rats (3). Furthermore, recent reports also indicate that in rat, dog, and human urine, there are esterases other than kallikrein (24,28,22, 25,10), thus suggesting that esterase methods in these three species are unreliable for the determination of urinary kalli-krein.

In conclusion, it appears that glandular kallikrein is present in plasma. It cannot be quantified in the untreated plasma by a new direct RIA since kallikrein inhibitors normally present in plasma appear to interfere with this assay. Destroying the inhibitors by acetone treatment or heat and acidification of the plasma partially solves this problem. Urinary kallikrein measured by the direct RIA in DOCA-salt treated and in control rats significantly correlates with measurement done by the kininogenase method. However, although the results obtained by this direct RIA and the esterase method significantly correlate in the two control groups, they did not correlate in the DOCA-salt treated rats. Thus the esterase assay appeared to be unreliable for the determination of urinary kallikrein in pathological situations. The direct RIA and the kininogenase assay are suitable for this purpose.

REFERENCES

1. Adetuyibi, A. and I.H. Mills. Relation between urinary kallikrein and renal function, hypertension, and the excretion of sodium and water in man. Lancet. 2:203-207, 1972.
2. Bussard, A. Description d'une technique combinant simultanément l'électrophorèse et la précipitation immunologique dans un gel: L'électrosynerèse. Biochem. Biophys. Acta, 34:358-360, 1959.
3. Carretero, O.A., V.M. Amin, T. Ocholik, A.G. Scicli, J. Koch. Urinary kallikrein in rats bred for their susceptibility and resistance to the hypertensive effect of salt. A new radioimmunoassay for its direct determination. Circ. Res., 42: 727-731, 1978.
4. Carretero, O.A., N.B. Oza, A. Piwonska, T. Ocholik, A.G. Scicli. Measurement of urinary kallikrein activity by kinin radioimmunoassay. Biochem. Pharmacol., 25:2265-2270, 1976.
5. Carretero, O.A. and A.G. Scicli. The renal kallikrein-kinin system in human and in experimental hypertension. Klin. Wochenschr., 56 (Suppl. I): 113-125, 1978.
6. Croxatto, H.R. and M. San Martin. Kallikrein-like activity in the urine of renal hypertensive rats. Experientia, 26: 1216-1217, 1970.
7. Elliot, A.H. and F.R. Nuz-m. Urinary excretion of a depressor substance (kallikrein of Frey and Kraut) in arterial hypertension. Endocrinology, 18: 462-474, 1934.
8. Frey, E.K. Zusammenhänge zwischen Herzarbeit und Nierentatigkeit. Langenbecks Arch. klin. Chir., 142: 66, 1926.
9. Gajos, E. Electroimmunoprécipitation des proteines anodiques et cathodiques à pH 8.2. Experientia, 26: 1007-1008, 1970.

10. Geiger, R., K. Mann, T. Bettels. Isolation of human urinary
    kallikrein by affinity chromatography. Determination of
    urinary kallikrein. J. Clin. Chem. Clin. Biochem., 15: 479–
    483, 1977.
11. Geller, R.G., H.S. Margolius, J.J. Pisano, H.R. Keiser.
    Effects of mineralocorticoids, altered sodium intake and
    adrenalectomy on urinary kallikrein in rats. Circ. Res.,
    31: 857–861, 1972.
12. Glasser, R.J. and A.F. Michael. Urinary kallikrein in ex-
    perimental renal disease. Lab. Invest., 34: 616–622, 1976.
13. Hilton, S.M. The physiological role of glandular kallikreins.
    In: Handbook of Experimental Pharmacology, ed. E. Erdos,
    Vol. 25 (Bradykinin, Kallidin, and Kallikrein), Springer-
    Verlag, New York, pp. 389–399, 1970.
14. Hunter, W.M. and F.C. Greenwood. Preparation of iodine-131
    labeled human growth hormone of high specific activity.
    Nature, 194: 495–496, 1962.
15. Levy, S.B., J.J. Lilley, R.P. Frigon, R.A. Stone. Urinary
    kallikrein and plasma renin activity as determinants of
    renal blood flow. J. Clin. Invest., 60: 129–138, 1977.
16. Lowry, O.H., N.J. Ro-ebrough, A.L. Farr, R.J. Randall.
    Protein measurement with the folin phenol reagent. J. Biol.
    Chem., 193: 265–275, 1951.
17. Margolius, H.S., R.G. Geller, W. deJong, J.J. Pisano, A.
    Sjoerdsma. Altered urinary kallikrein excretion in rats with
    hypertension. Circ. Res., 30: 358–362, 1972.
18. Margolius, H.S., R.G. Geller, W. deJong, J.J. Pisano, A.
    Sjoerdsma. Urianry kallikrein excretion in hypertension.
    Circ. Res., 31 (Suppl. II): 125–131, 1972.
19. Margolius, H.S., R.G. Geller, J.J. Pisano, A. Sjoerdsma.
    Altered urinary kallikrein excretion in human hypertension.
    Lancet, II: 1063–1065, 1971.
20. Margolius, H.S., D. Horwitz, J.J. Pisano, H.R. Keiser.
    Urinary kallikrein excretion in hypertensive man. Relation-
    ships to sodium intake and sodium retaining steroids. Circ.
    Res. 35: 820–825, 1974.
21. Marin-Grez, M., N.B. Oza, O.A. Carretero. The involvement of
    urinary kallikrein in the renal escape from the sodium re-
    taining effect of mineralocorticoids. Henry Ford Hosp. Med.
    J. 21: 85–90, 1973.
22. Moriya, H., Y. Matsuda, K. Miyasaki, C. Moriwaki, Y. Hojima.
    Some aspects of urinary and renal kallikreins. In:
    Kininogenases, Kallikrein. ed. G.L. Haberland, et al. Vol. 4,
    Schattauer Verlag, Stuttgart-New York, pp. 29–34.
23. Nasjletti, A., J.C. McGiff, J. Colina-Chourio. Interrelations
    of the renal kallikrein-kinin system and renal prostaglandins
    in the conscious rat. Influence of mineralocorticoids.
    Circ. Res., 43: 799–807, 1978.

24. Nustad, K. and J.V. Pierce. Purification of rat urinary
     kallikreins and their specific antibody. Biochemistry,
     13: 2312-2319, 1974.
25. Ole-MoiYoi, O., K.F. Austen, J. Spragg. Kinin-generating
     and esterolytic activity of purified human urinary kalli-
     krein (urokallikrein). Biochem. Pharmacol., 26: 1893-1900,
     1977.
26. Ormsbee, H.S. and C.F. Ryan. Production of hypertension
     with desoxycorticosterone acetate-impregnated silicone
     rubber implants. J. Pharmaceut. Sci., 62: 255, 1973.
27. Ørstavik, T.B., K.M. Gautvik, K. Nustad, J. Hedemark-Poulsen.
     Diffusion of ^{125}I-glandular kallikrein after local admini-
     stration in the rat submandibular gland. Microvasc. Res.,
     15: 115, 1978.
28. Oza, N.B., V.M. Amin, R.K. McGregor, A.G. Scicli, O.A. Carre-
     tero. Isolation of rat urinary kallikrein and properties
     of its antibodies. Biochem. Pharmacol., 25: 1607-1612, 1976.
29. Roberts, P.S. Measurement of the rate of plasmin action on
     synthetic substrates. J. Biol. Chem., 232: 285-291, 1958.
30. Roblero, J., H.R. Croxatto, R. Garcia, J. Corthorn, E. DeVito.
     Kallikrein-like activity in perfusates and urine of isolated
     rat kidneys. Am. J. Physiol., 231: 1383-1389, 1976.
31. Rodbard, D., P.L. Rayford, J.A. Cooper, G.T. Ross. Statis-
     tical quality control of radioimmunoassays. J. Clin. Endo-
     crinol. Metab., 28: 1412-1418, 1968.
32. Steel, R.G.D. and J.H. Torrie. Principles and Procedures of
     Statistics. New York: McGraw-Hill, 1960.

METHOD FOR MEASUREMENT OF HUMAN URINARY KININASE ACTIVITY

Porcelli G., Di Jorio M., Ranieri M., Ranalli L.,
D'Acquarica L.

Istituto di Chimica, Facoltà di Medicina, Università
Cattolica S. Cuore, Roma-Centro Chimica Recettori del
C.N.R., Roma, Italy

ABSTRACT

A method was developed to measure kininase activity in human
urine. The method consists of dialysis of human centrifuged urine
sample against phosphate buffer and partial fractionation of A-50
Sephadex column. The enzymatic property of urinary kininase, which
destroys bradykinin when incubated, is estimated from its effect on
a definite amount of bradykinin, using rat uterus.

INTRODUCTION

Kininases are the enzymes which inactivate kinins (Erdös and
Yang, 1970). Bradykinin and kallidin are very rapidly inactivated
by circulating and lung peptidases which are the major factors in the
duration of kinin actions. The importance of the kinin-destroying
mechanism in man is not really clear at the present time nor is the
effect on this mechanism of various hypertensive or hypotensive diseases states known (Levine et al., 1973). From human urine a 160.000
molecular weight kininase has been separated and partially characterized (Porcelli et al.). To clarify the role of urinary kininase it
is necessary to develop a reliable, sensitive method to measure it.
In the present study, a method was developed, which permits the measurement of kininase activity in 5 ml of urine. The method described
here is based of the enzymatic properties of the urinary kininase
which, when incubated with bradykinin destroys it. The amount of
destroyed bradykinin/min. is estimated on isolated rat uterus.

METHODS

Human urine was collected over a 24h period, covered by toluene
and stored in cold room at 4°C until sample preparation. Buffered
1 M NaCl was prepared by dissolving 58.6 g of NaCl in 1 lt of 0.005 M
disodium/monosodium phosphate solution (pH 7.3). This buffer was
used, diluted to 12%, to wash the column A-50 Sephadex and, concentrated, to separate human urinary kininase from the same column.
0.1 M disodium/monosodium phosphate buffer (pH 7.5) was used to
dilute bradykinin vials and 0.01 M to dialyze the human urinary samples. The standard of bradykinin was prepared dissolving 0.08 mg of
synthetic bradykinin in vials (Sandoz BRS 640) in 100ml of 0.1 M sodium phosphate buffer (pH 7.5) and stored at -20°C in 3 ml siliconized vials. The following procedure was adopted to prepare urinary
samples: 5 ml of a 24 h urine sample, after centrifugation at 5,000
rpm for 20 min., was dialyzed overnight against 200 ml of 0.01 M
sodium phosphate (10 samples in 2 lt of buffer), with magnetic stirring. The urinary sample was then introduced into a A-50 Sephadex
column (0.6 x 6 cm) equilibrated in H_2O. When the urinary sample was
adsorbed, 100 ml of 12% of buffered 1 M NaCl were used to wash the
column. The remaining material on the column containing all kininase activity was then eluted by 1.5 ml of concentrated buffered 1 M
NaCl. The sample was added of 0.5 ml of 0.1 M sodium phosphate pH
7.5 containing 400 ng of bradykinin, and incubated for 15 min. at
37°C. The reaction was stopped at -3°C in ice-NaCl bath and the destroyed kinin was calculated by comparing the activity of a same
sample of bradykinin diluted with 1.5 ml of buffered 1 M NaCl instead of the urinary enzyme solution. Biological activity of bradykinin was determined on the isolated rat uterus, suspended in an
oxygenated tyrod solution at 34°C. The isotonic contractions were
registered with the help of an instrument which is basically formed
by a transductor (Basile, Italy), a signal conditioner (Mod. 5100,
BLH, England) and by an automatic recorder (Mod. CR 555, JJ, Instruments, England). The incubation mixture of substrate (bradykinin)
and enzyme (urinary chromatographic fraction) was diluted to the
point at which 4 ng of bradykinin remained active on the rat uterus.
Samples of the incubated mixture containing respectively 4 ng, 12
ng, 20 ng, 60 ng and 100 ng of bradykinin were progressively injected into the muscle bath. From the enzymatic hydrolyzed bradykinin corresponding to 5 ml of urine sample in 15 min., the amount
of destroyed peptide in ng/min. and then for 24 h urine sample was
calculated.

RESULTS

Five samples of 5 ml were prepared using the same urine from
healthy subjects and 400 ng of bradykinin. The samples were incubated as previously described. A destruction of 4 ng of bradykinin
for each sample was observed after 15 min. of incubation, corres-

ponding to 80 ng of destroyed bradykinin/min. for 1150 ml of 24 h
urine. Dialysis procedure of urinary sample with different ratio
than 5 ml urine against 200 ml of 0.01 M sodium phosphate buffer altered the urinary kininase activity. Co^{++} and Zn^{++} potentiate kininase activity, Cd^{++}, phenantroline, EDTA and TRIS inhibit the urinary enzyme. The method is capable of detecting different amounts
of enzyme obtained from different amounts of the same urine: 5 ml,
3.75 ml, 2.5 ml and 1.25 ml, respectively, by incubation for 15
min. of the same amount of bradykinin (400 ng). The influence of
time was studied by incubating a mixture containing kininase corresponding to 5 ml of urine and 400 ng of bradykinin. Kininase reaction was stopped after 5, 10 and 15 min., as mentioned earlier. The
kinin destruction was proportional to the time incubation.

DISCUSSION

A method was developed for the measurement of kininase activity in human urine which allows urinary kininase to act on bradykinin
"in vitro". The undestroyed residues of bradykinin are subsequently
bioassayed. The method is based on a partial purification of urinary kininase by dialysis and chromatographic procedure, to separate
some inhibitor or activator components, as well as to remove endogenous kinins contained in human urine. Some questions might be
raised about the specificity of this method. However, it was evident that bradykinin was destroyed only when the kinin and urinary
sample obtained after chromatographic fractionation were incubated
together. Other methods for measuring kininase activity in human
urine have not been developed at the present time. The incubation
period demonstrated a significant increase of urinary kininase in
hypertensive subjects (Greco et al.) and a net reduction of the
same enzyme in urine of infarctuated patients (Greco et al.) in comparison to normals.

REFERENCES

Erdös, E.G. and Yang, H.Y.T. (1970) Kininases - in: Hdb of Exp.
Pharmacol., Vol. XXV, Ed. by Erdös, E.G., Springer Verlag, N.Y.,
p. 289.
Greco, A., Porcelli G., Di Jorio, M., Ranieri M., D'Acquarica, L.
    and Ranalli L., Altered urinary Excretion of human kininase ac-
    tivity in hypertension; same issue
Greco, A., Porcelli, G., Rebuzzi, A.G., Di Jorio, M., Ranieri, M.
    and Ranalli L., Altered urinary excretion of human kininase ac-
    tivity in acute myocardial infarction; same issue
Levine, B.W., Talamo, R.C. and Kazemi, H. (1973), Action and metabo-
    lism of bradykinin in the dog lung, J.Appl.Physiol., 34, 821
Porcelli, G., Marini-Bettòlo, G.B., Di Jorio, M., Ranieri, M.,
    Ranalli, L., D'Acquarica, L., Preliminary purification and bio-
    chemical characterization of human urinary kininase; same issue.

FLUOROGENIC PEPTIDE SUBSTRATES FOR PROTEASES IN BLOOD COAGULATION, KALLIKREIN-KININ AND FIBRINOLYSIS SYSTEMS

S. Iwanaga*, T. Morita, H. Kato, T. Harada, N. Adachi,
T. Sugo, I. Maruyama, K. Takada**, T. Kimura**, and
S. Sakakibara**
*Department of Biology, Faculty of Science, Kyushu
University, Fukuoka 812, Japan
Institute for Protein Research, Osaka University, Suita
Osaka 565 and ** Peptide Institute, Protein Research
Foundation, Minoh, Osaka 565, Japan

INTRODUCTION

Mammalian plasmas contain a number of "serine-active site" trypsin-like proteinases, which participate in blood coagulation, kallikrein-kinin, fibrinolysis and complement systems. The proteinases have an ability to cleave selectively proteins, that is, limited proteolysis, and catalyze the cascade reactions, which involve several sequential transformations of proenzymes to enzymes (Davie et al. 1969). Table 1 shows the amino acid sequences around the scissile bonds of natural substrates attacked by these proteinases. It has been well known that the amino acid residues preceding the scissile bond, P2 and P3 sites, in the substrates, are of importance for the enzyme-substrate interaction (Blomback, 1970). For instance, a part of the sequence, Asp-Asp-Asp-Lys, which is located in the NH_2-terminal portion of trypsinogen, has been known to comprise the substrate recognition sites and specificity sequence for enterokinase (Ottesen, 1967). Similarly, Factor Xa is presumed to recognize the tetrapeptide sequence Ile-Glu-Gly-Arg located close to the cleavage site required for the activation of bovine prothrombin (Magnusson et al. 1975). Based on this idea, several peptidyl-p-nitroanilides, so called "chromogenic substrate", which suit a specificity requirement of proteinases, have recently been introduced and proved to be useful for specific assay of blood coagulation factors, kallikreins, plasmin and urokinase (Claeson et al. 1977). Peptide amides of 7-amino-4-methylcoumarin (MCA), originally developed for the sensitive assay for α-chymotrypsin (Zimmerman et al. 1976) and an

147

TABLE 1. APPARENT PRIMARY AND SECONDARY SPECIFICITES OF TRYPSIN-LIKE PROTEINASES

Enzymes	Natural substrates	Sequences required for cleavage
		P4 P3 P2 P1 ▏P1' P2' P3'
Enterokinase (Hog)	Trypsinogen (Bovine)	-Asp-Asp-Asp-Lys-Ile-Val-Gly-
α-Thrombin (Human)	Fibrinogen (Human)	-Phe-(X)₇-Val-Arg-Gly-Pro-Arg-
	Factor XIII (Bovine)	-Leu-Val-Pro-Arg-Gly-Phe-Asx-
	Prothrombin (Bovine)	-Val-Ile-Pro-Arg-Ser-Gly-Gly
Factor Xa (Bovine)	Prothrombin (Bovine)	-Ile-Glu-Gly-Arg-Thr-Ser-Glu-
Factor IXa (Bovine)	Factor X (Bovine)	-Gln-Val-Val-Arg-Ile-Val-Gly-
Factor XIa (Bovine)	Factor IX (Bovine)	-Lys-Leu-Thr-Arg-Ala-Glu-Thr-
	Factor IX (Bovine)	-Glu-Phe-Ser-Arg-Val-Val-Gly-
Factor XIIa (Bovine)	Factor XI (Bovine)	X-Ile-Val-Gly-
	Prekallikrein (Bovine)	-Arg-
Plasma Kallikrein (Bovine)	HMW Kininogen (Bovine)	-Ser-Leu-Met-Lys-Arg-Pro-Pro-
		-Ser-Pro-Phe-Arg-Ser-Val-Gln-
		-Tyr-Asp-Trp-Arg-Thr-Pro-Tyr-
Tissue Kallikreins (Hog)	LMW Kininogen (Bovine)	-Ser-Leu-Met-Lys-Arg-Pro-
Urokinase (Human)	Plasminogen (Human)	-Cys-Pro-Gly-Arg-Val-Val-Gly-
Plasmin (Bovine)	Plasminogen (Human)	-Phe-Glu-Lys-Lys-Val-Tyr-Leu-
	Fibrinogen (Human)	-Ser-Tyr-Lys-Met-Ala-Asp-
		-Gly-Tyr-Lys-Ala-Arg-Pro-
Limulus Clotting Enzyme	Coagulogen (Tachypleus)	-Val-Leu-Gly-Arg-Thr-Gln-Ile-
		-Val-Ser-Gly-Arg-Gly-Phe-Ser-

aminopeptidase (Kanaoka et al. 1977), have also proven useful for
the assay of proteases including elastase (Zimmerman et al. 1977),
X-prolyl dipeptidase (Kato et al. 1977) and pyroglutamyl peptidase
(Fujiwara and Tsuru 1978). This assay method is more sensitive
than the chromogenic assay, becuase the reaction product, 7-amino-
4-methylcoumarin is highly fluorescent (Zimmerman et al. 1976).

To extend further the availability of fluorogenic substrates,
we have newly synthesized 36 peptidyl-MCA's and tested for their
possible use as specific substrates for assay of proteolytic enzymes
with limited specificity (Morita et al. 1977). The results indicate
that the peptidyl-MCA substrate, which fits preferentially the
specificity requirements of α-thrombin, Factor Xa, kallikreins,
horshoe crab clotting enzyme (Harada et al. 1978), and urokinase,
is valuable for specific enzyme assay. The new substrates for
plasmin and Factor XIa will also be reported.

MATERIALS AND METHODS

Peptidyl-MCA substrates were synthesized by standard chemical
procedures, using L-amino acids. Purity of all intermediates and
products was confirmed by thin layer chromatography, elemental
analysis and amino acid analysis. The experimental details of the
peptide synthesis will be reported elsewhere. Highly purified
α-thrombin (2,000-2,500 NIH units per mg)(Morita et al. 1974),
Factor Xa (Morita and Iwanaga, 1978), plasma kallikrein (Takahashi
et al. 1972) from bovine source and horseshoe crab clotting enzyme
(Nakamura et al. 1978) were prepared according to the previous
methods. Bovine Factor IX was kindly supplied by Dr. K. Fujikawa,
Dept. of Biochemistry, University of Washington, Seattle, and was
activated by Russell's viper venom activator (Fujikawa et al. 1972).
Factor XIIa and Factor XI were prepared from bovine plasma by the
previous methods (Kato et al. 1978), and the latter was activated
by trypsin or Factor XIIa. Bovine plasminogen, which was purified
by the lysine-Sepharose method (Deutsch and Mertz, 1970), was
activated by human urokinase (a product of Mochida Pharmaceutical
Co., Ltd., Tokyo). Hog urinary kallikrein was a generous gift
from Prof. H. Tschesche, Lehrstuhl fur Org. Chemie und Biochemie
der Technischen Universitat Munchen. Hog pancreatic kallikrein
was purified according to the previous method (Han et al. 1978).
Highly purified human urokinase, which has a molecular weight of
34,000 (Ogawa et al. 1975), was a kind gift from Dr. N. Ogawa,
Mochida Pharmaceutical Co.

As shown in Fig. 1, a proteinase with limited specificity
hydrolyzes a peptidyl-MCA substrate, releasing 7-amino-4-methyl-
coumarin (AMC). Because the reaction product, AMC, is highly
fluorescent, the rate at which AMC is released can be measured
fluorometrically with excitation at 380 nm and emmision at 460 nm

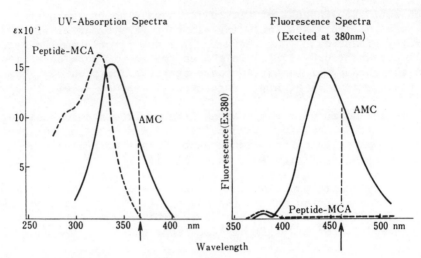

Fig. 1. Ultraviolet and fluorescence spectra of peptide MCA and AMC.

(Fig. 2). Moreover, UV absorption difference between peptidyl–MCA
and free AMC at 370 nm (ε=6,200) was applicable for estimation of
enzyme activity.

Preparation of Substrate Solution: A water–insoluble peptidyl–MCA
was first dissolved in dimethylsulfoxide (DMSO, analytical grade)
and the solution diluted to give a final concentration of 0.1 mM,
using 50 mM Tris–HCl buffer, pH 8.0, containing 100 mM NaCl and 10
mM $CaCl_2$. The substrate solution (0.1 mM) thus prepared gave an
absorbance of 1.60 at 325 nm.

Procedures for Enzyme Assay: Two methods were used to determine
enzyme activity. Initial rate method; A fluorescence spectrophotometer, Hitachi Model MPF 2A, was set up with excitation at
380 nm and emission at 460 nm. A recorder was connected to the
spectrophotometer and 2.5 ml of 0.1 mM substrate solution was added
to a cuvette. After preincubation at 37°C for 3 min, 5 to 10 µl
of enzyme was added and mixed immediately. The increase of the
relative fluorescence (%) was read at regular time intervals. The
instrument was standarized so that a 10 µM solution of AMC in 0.1%
DMSO gave 1.0 relative fluorescence unit. The absolute amount
(nmole) of AMC released per min was calculated as follows:

$$\text{AMC (nmole)} = \frac{10 \text{ nmole}}{\text{ml}} \times \frac{\%}{100\%} \times 2.5 \text{ (ml)} \times \frac{60 \text{ sec}}{100 \text{ sec}}$$

$$= \Delta \times 0.15 \text{ nmole}$$

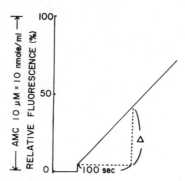

Fig. 2.   Initial-rate measurement from the increase of relative
          fluorescence.

Fig. 2 shows an example for the initial-rate measurement from the
increase of relative fluorescence.

   For end-point method; 1.0 ml of 0.1 mM substrate-buffer solution used in the initial-rate method is added to a test tube (1.0
x 10 cm) and preincubated at 37°C for 2.5 min. Ten to 50 µl of
enzyme is added and mixed immediately. The reaction is carried
out at 37°C for appropriate times (1 to 10 min) and terminated by
adding 1.5 ml of 17% acetic acid to give a final concentration of
10%. The estimation of the relative fluorescence on test samples
was made as that used in the initial-rate method. Under the conditions described above, the linearities of the rate of AMC
released versus incubation time (within 10 min) and various enzyme
concentrations (at least 10-fold range) were satisfactory.
Enzyme activity was expressed as the amount of AMC (µmole) liberated
per min per mg protein or absorbance unit = 1.0 at 280 nm.

                         RESULTS

Specific Substrates for α-Thrombin, Factor Xa, Various Kallikreins
and Urokinase

   Table II shows a comparison of the rates of hydrolysis of
different peptidyl-MCA substrates by various serine-proteinases
with limited specificity. For α-thrombin, Boc-Val-Pro-Arg-MCA
(A-1 in Table II) was specific and no detectable hydrolysis was
observed with plasma and tissue kallikreins, and urokinase.
Factor Xa showed activity of less than 1% of that of α-thrombin.
This tripeptide sequence was based on the information from the
COOH-terminal part of the "activation peptide", which is released

TABLE II.
HYDROLYSIS[a] OF PEPTIDE-MCA's BY PROTEINASES WITH LIMITED SPECIFICITY.

Group	Substrates	α-Thrombin	Factor Xa	Kallikreins			Urokinase	Plasmin
				Plasma	Pancreatic	Urinary		
A-1	Boc-Val-Pro-Arg-MCA	60.0	0.4	ND[b]	ND	ND	ND	0.3
A-2	Z-Pro-Arg-MCA	6.8	ND	ND	ND	ND	ND	ND
B-1	Boc-Ile-Glu-Gly-Arg-MCA	0.2	2.4	ND	ND	ND	0.6	ND
B-2	Acetyl-Glu-Gly-Arg-MCA	0.1	0.7	ND	ND	ND	1.5	ND
B-3	Boc-Val-Leu-Gly-Arg-MCA	0.3	1.7	0.3	ND	ND	0.4	ND
B-4	Boc-Leu-Gly-Arg-MCA	0.8	1.7	0.1	ND	ND	0.9	ND
B-5	Z-Leu-Gly-Arg-MCA	1.1	2.2	0.5	ND	—[c]	0.8	ND
B-6	Boc-Val-Ser-Gly-Arg-MCA	0.2	0.4	0.1	ND	ND	2.5	ND
B-7	Boc-Ser-Gly-Arg-MCA	0.8	2.8	0.3	ND	ND	0.8	ND
B-8	Boc-Ser(0-Bzl)-Gly-Arg-MCA	1.3	3.0	0.3	ND	ND	0.5	ND
C-1	Pro-Gly-Arg-MCA	0.1	0.1	0.1	ND	ND	0.4	ND
C-2	Z-Pro-Gly-Arg-MCA	0.8	0.2	0.1	ND	ND	ND	ND
C-3	Glutaryl-Gly-Arg-MCA	ND	0.1	ND	ND	ND	6.2	ND
C 4	Glu-Gly-Arg-MCA	0.1	0.2	ND	ND	ND	5.5	ND
C-5	Z-Gly-Arg-MCA	0.2	0.1	ND	ND	ND	0.6	ND
C-6	Gly-Arg-MCA	ND	ND	ND	ND	ND	0.5	ND
D 1	Z-Pro-Phe-Arg-MCA	0.1	0.1	2.9	2.9	4.3	ND	0.2
D-2	Pro-Phe-Arg-MCA	0.1	0.2	3.3	6.3	9.7	ND	0.4
D-3	Z-Phe-Arg-MCA	ND	0.2	4.6	0.8	0.5	ND	0.3
D-4	Phe-Arg-MCA	ND	—[c]	0.2	0.2	0.2	ND	ND

[a] Values are expressed as μmoles hydrolyzed per min per mg protein (α-thrombin, factor Xa, urinary kallikrein and urokinase) or absorbance unit=1.0 at 280 nm (plasma kallikrein, pancreatic kallikrein, and plasmin). [b] ND not detectable; Boc, *tert*-butoxycarbonyl; Z, carbobenzoxy; Bzl, benzyl. [c] —, not determined.

during the conversion of plasma Factor XIII into its active transglutaminase in the presence of α-thrombin (Mikuni et al. 1973; Nakamura et al. 1974). The importance of the Pro-Arg sequence as P1 and P2 binding sites for α-thrombin has been suggested (Graf et al. 1976).

Factor Xa hydrolyzed all the peptidyl-MCA's having the COOH-terminal Gly-Arg sequence, although these substrates were essentially resistant to plasmin and various kallikreins, and also to Factor IXa and XIIa, as described later. Of the substrates, Boc-Ile-Glu-Gly-Arg-MCA (B-1), Boc-Ser-Gly-Arg-MCA (B-7) and Boc-Ser (0-Bzl)-Gly-Arg-MCA (B-8) seemed to be the most specific for Factor Xa. The tetrapeptide sequence of B-1 originates

from the sequence located close to the cleavage site required for
the activation of bovine prothrombin by Factor Xa (Magnusson et al.
1975). It should be noted that Glu (P3 site) and Ile (P4 site) in
B-1 are not essential requirements for Factor Xa, because B-7 and
B-8, which are substituted with Ser residue at P3 site and did not
contain Ile residue at P4 site, respectively, are easily hydrolyzed
by Factor Xa.

Substrates containing the COOH-terminal Pro-Phe-Arg sequence
of bradykinin were all susceptible to hydrolysis by plasma and
tissue kallikreins, although there is a significant difference in
the rates of hydrolysis by the different kallikreins. These peptidyl-MCA's were slightly hydrolyzed by α-thrombin, Factor Xa and
plasmin but not urokinase. Plasma kallikrein hydrolyzed Z-Phe-
Arg-MCA (D-3) more readily than Z-Pro-Phe-Arg-MCA (D-1), while
the inverse was observed with tissue kallikreins. Thus, best
substrate for plasma kallikrein seemed to be D-3 and the Km value
estimated by the Lineweber-Burk plots for this substrate was lowest
(2.4×10^{-4} M) among these peptidyl-MCA's (Table III). On the
other hand, Pro-Phe-Arg-MCA (D-2) was good substrate for pancreatic
and urinary kallikreins, and there was no specificity difference
between them towards these peptide substrates (Table II and III).

TABLE III.

THE K_m AND Vmax VALUES OF PLASMA AND TISSUE KALLIKREINS
TOWARDS PEPTIDE-MCA's

Substrate	Kallikrein	Km(M)	Vmax (μmoles·min^{-1}·mg^{-1})	Vmax / Km
Z-Pro-Phe-Arg	Bovine Plasma	4.7×10^{-4}	7.2[*]	15.3
Pro-Phe-Arg	Bovine Plasma	6.1×10^{-4}	12.5[*]	18.4
Z-Phe-Arg	Bovine Plasma	2.4×10^{-4}	8.0[*]	33.5
Z-Pro-Phe-Arg	Hog Pancreatic	1.8×10^{-4}	4.6[*]	25.6
Pro-Phe-Arg	Hog Pancreatic	1.6×10^{-4}	11.9[*]	74.4
Z-Phe-Arg	Hog Pancreatic	5.3×10^{-4}	0.3[*]	0.5
Z-Pro-Phe-Arg	Human Urinary	1.7×10^{-4}	7.5	44.1
Pro-Phe-Arg	Human Urinary	2.2×10^{-4}	30.0	136.4
Z-Phe-Arg	Human Urinary	2.8×10^{-4}	1.1	3.96

[*] μmoles per min per A_{280} = 1.0

The substrates from C-1 to C-6 shown in Table II were synthesized for urokinase. To develop a best substrate for urokinase, we first synthesized Z-Pro-Gly-Arg-MCA and Pro-Gly-Arg-MCA, referring to the information of COOH-terminal sequence located at the cleavage site for both activation of human plasminogen by urokinase. However, both substrates were almost unsusceptible to human urokinase. As shown in Table II, urokinase similar to Factor Xa showed a broad specificity towards all the peptidyl-MCA substrates having the COOH-terminal Gly-Arg sequence. The Km and Vmax values of human urokinase towards a few of peptidyl-MCA's are shown in Table IV. Among them, glutaryl-Gly-Arg-MCA (C-3) was found to be the best substrate for urokinase. This substrate was very useful for uro-kinase assay and the analytical use in clinical field is now being developed (Nakabayashi et al. 1978).

Peptidyl-MCA Substrates for Plasmin

Bovine plasmin hydrolyzed some of the substrates shown in Table II. However, all the substrates containing COOH-terminal arginine were essentially resistant to plasmin except the sub-strates (D-1, D-3 and D-3) for kallikreins. To find out a good fluorogenic substrate for plasmin, we have synthesized peptidyl-MCA's containing COOH-terminal lysine residue and tested for their susceptibilities to bovine plasmin. The results are shown in Table V. Among six peptidyl-MCA's, Boc-Val-Leu-Lys-MCA and Boc-Glu-Lys-Lys-MCA were found to be good substrates for the assay of plasmin. The tripeptide sequence of the former was based on the data, which is generously found in the COOH-terminal sequence of early plasmic fragments (fibrinogen degradation product, FDP) de-rived from human fibrinogen, and that of the latter originated from the COOH-terminal sequence of the NH_2-terminal fragment re-leased in the plasmin-mediated transformation of Glu-plasminogen to Lys-plasminogen (Wiman, 1973). The Km and Vmax values estimated by the Lineweber-Burk plots for these substrates are also shown in Table V.

The plasmin substrate, Boc-Glu-Lys-Lys-MCA, contains two lysine residues. Thus, there is a possibility that plasmin hydro-lyses not only the lysyl-MCA linkage but also the lysyl-lysyl linkage during prolonged incubation. Using thin-layer chromato-graphy, we identified the hydrolytic products derived from the peptidyl-MCA after digestion with bovine plasmin. As shown in Fig. 3, a ninhydrinpositive spot of the substrate decreased rapidly with increase in a fluorescence spot with AMC, and in parallel of formation of AMC, another ninhydrin-positive spot was newly detected on the thin-layer plate. This material consisted of Glu and Lys residues in a mole ratio of 1 to 2, as revealed with its amino acid composition. Moreover, free lysine was unde-tectable (Fig. 3). These results indicate that plasmin hydrolyzes only the COOH-terminal lysyl-MCA linkage of Boc-Glu-Lys-Lys-MCA

TABLE IV.

THE Km and Vmax VALUES OF HUMAN UROKINASE TOWARDS PEPTIDE—MCA's

SUBSTRATE	KM(M)	VMAX (μMOLES$\cdot$MIN$^{-1}\cdot$MG^{-1})	VMAX / KM
BOC-VAL-SER-GLY-ARG	3.3×10^{-4}	9.6	19
GLU-GLY-ARG	3.2×10^{-4}	18.1	55
GLUTARYL-GLY-ARG	4.2×10^{-4}	18.4	42

TABLE V.

AMIDASE ACTIVITY OF BOVINE PLASMIN TOWARDS PEPTIDE MVA's

SUBSTRATE	SPECIFIC ACTIVITY (μMOLES/MIN/MG PROTEIN)	KM (M)	VMAX (μMOLES/MIN/CU)	VMAX / KM
BOC-VAL-LEU-LYS	1.25	2.5×10^{-4}	0.62	0.24×10^4
BOC-GLU-LYS-LYS	0.75	6.7×10^{-4}	0.62	0.09×10^4
BOC-PHE-GLU-LYS-LYS	0.23	4.0×10^{-4}	0.28	0.07×10^4
BOC-PHE-GLU-LYS	0.12			
BOC-ILE-GLU-LYS	0.11			
BOC-GLU-LYS	ND			
Z-PHE-ARG	0.44			
BOC-VAL-SER-GLY-ARG	0.01			
Z-GLY-GLY-ARG	0.003			
Z-PRO-GLY-ARG	ND			
PRO-GLY-ARG	ND			
GLUTARYL-GLY-ARG	0.005			
BOC-PHE-SER-ARG	0.04			
BOC-GLY-SER-ARG	0.02			

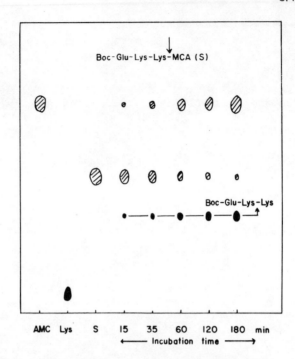

Fig. 3.   Identification of hydrolytic products derived from
           Boc-Glu-Lys-Lys-MCA(s) by bovine plasmin, using thin-
           layer (cellulose plate, Merck) chromatography.

substrate. The fact that Boc-Glu-Lys-MCA shown in Table V was
unsusceptible to plasmin, seems to also support the above result.
The optimum pH of bovine plasmin was compared using various buffers
with Boc-Glu-Lys-Lys-MCA and a chromogenic peptide, H·D-Val-Leu-
Lys-p-nitroanilide, as the substrates. As shown in Fig. 4, maximum
activity was observed at neutral pH either with the former or the
latter.

Table VI shows the results for Boc-Glu-Lys-Lys-MCA and Boc-
Val-Leu-Lys-MCA, in comparison with the hydrolytic rates of various
serine-proteinases. Plasma kallikrein hydrolyzed the former with
a rate less than one-tenth to that of bovine plasmin, and also the
latter was susceptible to tissue kallikreins. However, both
peptidyl-MCA's were essentially resistant to urokinase, α-thrombin,
Factors Xa, IXa and XIIa. These results suggest that a specific
assay for plasmin is possible even in the presence of urokinase
and several coagulation factors. As shown in this paper, urokinase-

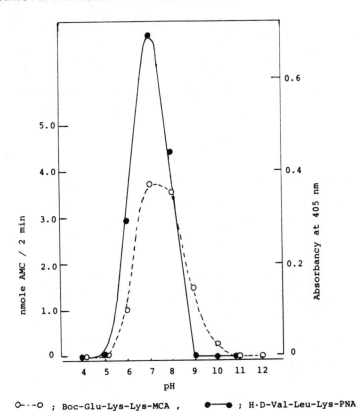

O---O ; Boc-Glu-Lys-Lys-MCA ,   ●—● ; H·D-Val-Leu-Lys-PNA

Fig. 4.   Effect of pH on amidase activity of bovine plasmin.
Buffers used were 0.1 M sodium acetate, pH 4.0 to 6.0;
0.1 M potassium phosphate, pH 6.5; 0.1 M Tris-HCl,
pH 7.0 to 9.0; and sodium borate, pH 10 to 12.

activated plasmin from human plasminogen showed almost the same
activity toward both Boc-Val-Leu-Lys-MCA and Boc-Glu-Lys-Lys-MCA.
However, a streptokinase-activated human plasmin did not hydrolyze
Boc-Glu-Lys-Lys-MCA, indicating that streptokinase-plasmin complex
has the activity to hydrolyze Boc-Val-Leu-Lys-MCA, but no activity
toward Boc-Glu-Lys-Lys-MCA (Kato et al. unpublished results). The
following table summarizes a best substrate selected for α-thrombin,
Factor Xa, plasma kallikrein, tissue kallikreins, urokinase, Limulus
clotting enzyme (Harada et al. 1978), and plasmin, and their K_m
and Vmax values toward these peptidyl-MCA. The apparent Michaelis
constants for each substrate appeared to be good, since their Km
values fall in the millimolar range. Especially, Boc-Val-Pro-Arg-
MCA and Boc-Leu-Gly-Arg-MCA were found to have the greatest affinity to α-thrombin and Limulus clotting enzyme (Table VII).

TABLE VI.

AMIDASE ACTIVITY OF PLASMIN AND OTHER SERINE PROTEINASES
TOWARD Boc-Glu-Lys-Lys-MCA AND Boc-Val-Leu-Lys-MCA

	Boc-Glu-Lys-Lys-MCA	Boc-Val-Leu-Lys-MCA
	μmole AMC/min/mg enzyme	
Bovine plasmin	0.75	1.25
Human plasmin	0.4	0.37
Hog urinary kallikrein	0.0001	0.046
Human urinary kallikrein	0	0.022
Bovine plasma kallikrein	0.05	0.002
Hog pancreatic kallikrein	0	0.03
Urokinase	0.008	0.008
Thrombin	0	0.0045
Factor Xa	0	0
Factor IXa	0	0
Factor XIIa	0	0

TABLE VII.

THE Km AND Vmax VALUES OF PROTEINASES TOWARDS
PEPTIDE-MCA's

Substrate	Enzyme	$K_M(M)$	V_{MAX} ($\mu moles \cdot min^{-1} \cdot mg^{-1}$)
Boc-Val-Pro-Arg-MCA	α-Thrombin	2.1×10^{-5}	78.1
Boc-Ile-Glu-Gly-Arg-MCA	Factor Xa	1.6×10^{-4}	6.1
Z-Phe-Arg-MCA	Plasma Kallikrein	2.4×10^{-4}	8.0[*]
Pro-Phe-Arg-MCA	Pancreatic Kallikrein	1.6×10^{-4}	11.9[*]
Pro-Phe-Arg-MCA	Urinary Kallikrein	2.2×10^{-4}	30.0
Glutaryl-Gly-Arg-MCA	Urokinase	4.4×10^{-4}	18.4
Boc-Val-Leu-Gly-Arg-MCA	Limulus Clotting Enzyme	6.0×10^{-5}	4.3[*]
Boc-Leu-Gly-Arg-MCA	Limulus Clotting Enzyme	2.7×10^{-5}	4.8[*]
Boc-Val-Ser-Gly-Arg-MCA	Limulus Clotting Enzyme	1.1×10^{-4}	3.1[*]
Boc-Ser-Gly-Arg-MCA	Limulus Clotting Enzyme	2.4×10^{-5}	4.3[*]
Boc-Glu-Lys-Lys-MCA	Plasmin	5.0×10^{-4}	25.0
Boc-Val-Leu-Lys-MCA	Plasmin	1.3×10^{-4}	20.0

[*] μmoles per min per A_{280} = 1.0

Peptidyl-MCA Substrates for Factor XIa

A need for a specific assay of Factors XII and XI, which contribute in the contact phase of intrinsic blood coagulation, is
quite apparent, since present methods based on clotting test using
a deficient plasma are difficult to standarize and quantitate these
proteinase activities. For assay of Factor XII, we have recently
established a new method, which estimates the kallikrein activity
induced by the kaolin-mediated activation of Factor XII in the
presence of HMW kininogen and prekallikrein (Kato et al. in this
proceedings). The kallikrein activity can be measured quantitatively, using Z-Phe-Arg-MCA. The subsequent approach was to
develop a specific substrate for Factor XIa, and we have newly
synthesized four peptidyl-MCA's, Boc-Phe-Ser-Arg, Boc-Leu-Thr-Arg,
Boc-Leu-Ser-Thr-Arg- and Boc-Gly-Ser-Arg. These peptide sequences
mainly originate from the sequence located close to the split
sites required for the activation of Factor IX by activated Factor
XI (Titani et al. 1978). Table VIII shows a comparison of the
rates of hydrolysis of these substrates, in addition to others, by
Factor IXa, XIa and XIIa. Factor XIa hydrolyzed preferentially
the peptide-MCA's having the COOH-terminal Thr(Ser)-Arg sequence,
although these substrates were relatively resistant to Factor IXa
and XIIa. Of the substrates, Boc-Leu-Thr-Arg-MCA and Boc-Phe-Ser-
Arg-MCA, seemed to be the best for Factor XIa. Factor XIa similar
to Factor Xa (Table II) showed a broad specificity towards peptidyl-
MCA's. On the other hand, for Factor IXa and XIIa, Boc-Glu(OBz)-
Gly-Arg-MCA was found to be one of the good substrates. However,
the hydrolytic rates of this substrate by these proteinases were
relatively slow, comparing with that of the specific substrate
(Boc-Val-Pro-Arg-MCA) for α-thrombin. Thus, further studies to
find a best substrate for Factor IXa and Factor XIIa will be required.

DISCUSSION

During the past few years, many kinds of peptide substrates
including peptidyl(X)-p-nitroanilide (Svendsen et al. 1972), X-7-
methylcoumarin amide (Morita et al. 1977), X-β-naphthylamide
(Nieuwenhuizen et al. 1977) and X-4-methoxy-β-naphthylamide (Huseby
et al. 1977; Clavin et al. 1977) have been developed for a specific
assay of various proteinases. Some of them are now commercially
available and proved to be very useful for the assay of plasma and
urine proteinases.

Our synthetic substrates described here are also valuable and
the assay utilizing the fluorogenic peptide has several advantages
over other commonly used methods. It is a one step reaction releasing the fluorogenic product, AMC, at high rate and with high
sensitivity. The substrate seems to show a specificity towards

TABLE VIII.
RELATIVE REACTION RATES OF FACTORS IXa, XIa and XIIa TOWARDS PEPTIDE MCA's

Substrates	IXa	XIa	XIIa
Boc-Val-Pro-Arg	<u>100</u>	86	16
Boc-Phe-Ser-Arg	29	<u>100</u>	14
Boc-Leu-Thr-Arg	ND	<u>182</u>	10
Boc-Gly-Ser-Arg	14	62	11
Boc-Leu-Ser-Thr-Arg	–	56	ND
Boc-Glu(OBz)-Gly-Arg	<u>178</u>	52	<u>100</u>
Boc-Glu-Gly-Arg	ND	48	70
Glu-Gly-Arg	ND	56	ND
Z-Gly-Gly-Arg	–	56	11
Boc-Val-Leu-Gly-Arg	ND	52	ND
Boc-Leu-Gly-Arg	ND	51	16
Boc-Ile-Glu-Gly-Arg	ND	32	33
Boc-Val-Ser-Gly-Arg	ND	25	24
Glutaryl-Gly-Arg	ND	28	ND
Pro-Phe-Arg	ND	ND	33

The following substrates were essentially resistant to these proteinases:
Z-Pro-Arg, Acetyl-Glu-Gly-Arg, Z-Leu-Gly-Arg, Boc-Ser-Gly-Arg, Z-Gly-Arg,
Gly-Arg, Pro-Gly-Arg, Z-Phe-Arg, and Phe-Arg. ND: not detectable

individual enzyme. Furthermore, the method is rapid, accurate and simple to perform. Therefore, these new substrates may be a useful tool to measure the enzyme activity in biological fluid as well as the proteinase inhibitors by a direct measurement of its proteolytic activity. In fact, a specific assay method for urokinase (Naka-bayashi et al. 1978), plasma kallikrein (Sugo et al. 1978), urinary kallikrein (Kato et al. 1978) and Factor XIIa (Kato et al. 1978, in this proceeding), using the corresponding fluorogenic substrates (Table VII) has recently been established. Moreover, the sub-strate, Boc-Leu-Gly-Arg-MCA, for Limulus clotting enzyme is applic-able for the detection and quantitation of bacterial endotoxins, because the latent proclotting enzyme contained in Limulus hemocyte lysate is activated depending on the concentration of the endotoxins added to the lysate (Iwanaga et al. 1978, Nakamura et al. 1977). This new method for the endotoxin assay is a fifty times more sensitive than that of so called "Limulus gelation test" and is very reproducible.

The peptidyl-MCA may be also useful in localization of enzyme activity on electropherograms, fluorometrically.

ACKNOWLEDGEMENTS

We express our thanks to Dr. K. Titani, Dept. of Biochemistry, University of Washington, Seattle, for his kind information about the specificity site of Factor XIa towards Factor IX. This work was supported in part by grants from The Scientific Research Fund of the Ministry of Education, Science and Culture, of Japan.

REFERENCES

Blombäck, B. (1970) In: The Hemostatic Mechanism in Man and Other Animals (ed. by R. G. Macfarlane), pp. 169-182, Academic Press, New York.

Claeson, G., Aurell, L., Karlsson, G., and Fiberger, P. (1977) In: New Methods for the Analysis of Coagulation Using Chromogenic Substrates (ed. by Witt, I.), pp. 251-259, Walter de Gruyter, Berlin, New York.

Clavin, S. A., Bobbitt, J. L., Shuman, R. T. and Smithwich, E. L. Jr. (1977). Use of peptidyl-4-methoxy-2-naphthylamides to assay plasmin. Anal. Biochem. 80, 355-365.

Davie, E. W., Hougie, C. and Lundblad, R. L. (1969) In: Recent Advances in Blood Coagulation (ed. by L. Poller), pp. 13-27, J. & A. Churchill Hill Ltd., London.

Deutsch, D. G. and Mertz, E. T. (1970). Plasminogen: Purification from human plasma by affinity chromatography. Science, 170, 1095-1096.

Fujikawa, K., Legaz, M. E. and Davie, E. W. (1972). Bovine Factor X_1 (Stuart factor). Mechanism of activation by a protein from Russell's viper venom. Biochemistry, 11, 4892-4899.

Fujiwara, K. and Tsuru, D. (1978). New chromogenic and fluorogenic substrates for pyrorridonyl peptidase. J. Biochem. 83, 1145-1149.

Graf, L., Barat, E., Borvendeg, J., Hermann, J. and Patthy, A. (1976). Action of thrombin on ovine, bovine and human pituitary growth hormones. Eur. J. Biochem. 64, 333-340.

Han, Y. N., Kato, H., Iwanaga, S. and Komiya, M. (1978). Primary structure of bovine plasma high-molecular-weight kininogen, characterization of carbohydrate-free fragment 1·2 (fragment X) and its biological activity. J. Biochem. 83, 223-235.

Harada, T., Morita, T. and Iwanaga, S. (1978). A new assay method for bacterial endotoxins using horseshoe crab clotting enzyme. J. Med. Enz. (in Japanese), 3, 43-60.

Huseby, R. M., Clavin, S. A., Smith, R. E., Hull, R. N. and Smitheick, E. L. Jr. (1977). Studies on tissue culture plasminogen activator II. The detection and assay of urokinase and plasminogen activator from LLC-PK1 cultures (porcine) by the synthetic substrate Nα -benzyloxycarbonyl-glycyl-glycyl-arginyl-4-methoxy-2-naphthylamide. Thrombosis Research, 10, 679-687.

Iwanaga, S., Morita, T., Harada, T., Nakamura, S., Niwa, M., Takada, K., Kimura, T., and Sakakibara, S. (1978). Chromogenic substrates for horseshoe crab clotting enzyme. Its application for the assay of bacterial endotoxins. Haemostasis, 7, 183-188.

Kanaoka, Y., Takahashi, T. and Nakayama, H. (1977). A new fluorogenic substrate for aminopeptidase. Chem. Pharm. Bull. 25, 362-363.

Katayama, K., Ericsson, L. H., Wade, R. D., Fujikawa, K., Walsh, K. A., Neurath, H. and Titani, K. (1978). Structural studies of bovine Factor IX. Fe. Proc. 37, 1617.

Kato, T., Nagatsu, T., Kimura, T. and Sakakibara, S. (1977). Seikagaku (in Japanese), 49, 990.

Kato, H., Adachi, N., Iwanaga, S., Abe, K., Takada, K., Kimura, T. and Sakakibara, S. (1978) In: Abstract, New assay method for kallikrein in urine, using fluorogenic peptide substrate. The 98th Congress on Pharmaceutical Society of Japan held in Okayama on April 5 to 9, p. 485.

Magnusson, S., Sottrup-Jensen, L. and Petersen, T. E. (1975) In: Prothrombin and Related Coagulation Factors (ed. by Hemker, H. C. & Veltkamp, J. J.) pp. 25-46, Leiden University Press, Leiden.

Mikuni, Y., Iwanaga, S. and Konishi, K. (1973). A peptide released from plasma fibrin stabilizing factor in the conversion to the active enzyme by thrombin. Biochem. Biophys. Res. Communs. 54, 1393-1402.

Morita, T., Iwanaga, S. and Suzuki, T. (1974). Studies on the activation of bovine prothrombin. Isolation and characterization of the fragments released from the prothrombin by activated factor Xa. J. Biochem. 76, 1031-1048.

Morita, T. and Iwanaga, S. (1978). Purification and properties of prothrombin activator from the venom of Echis carinatus. J. Biochem. 83, 559-570.

Nakabayashi, M., Chin, N., Ogino, M., Kaneko, Y., Sato, K. and Sakamoto, M. (1978) In: Abstract (in Japanese), The 1st Congress of Japanese Society on Thrombosis and Hemostasis. p. 60.

Nakamura, S., Iwanaga, S., Suzuki, T., Mikuni, Y. and Konishi, K. (1974). Amino acid sequence of the peptide released from bovine factor XIII following activation by thrombin. Biochem. Biophys. Res. Communs. 58, 250-256.

Nakamura, S., Morita, T., Iwanaga, S., Niwa, M. and Takahashi, K. (1977) Seikagaku (in Japanese) 49, 759.

Nakamura, S., Morita, T., Iwanaga, S., Niwa, M. and Takahashi, K. (1977). A sensitive substrate for the clotting enzyme in horseshoe crab hemocytes. J. Biochem. 81, 1567-1569.

Nieuwenhuizen, W., Wijngaads, G. and Groeneveld, E. (1977). Fluorogenic peptide amide substrates for the estimation of plasminogen activators and plasmin. Anal. Biochem. 83, 143-148.

Ogawa, N., Yamamoto, H., Katamine, T. and Tajima, H. (1975). Purification and some properties of urokinase. Thrombosis Diathes. Haemorrh. (Stuttg.), 34, 194-209.

Ottesen, M. (1967).   Induction of biological activity by limited
proteolysis.   Ann. Rev. Biochem. 36, 55-76.
Sugo, T., Kato, H., Iwanaga, S., and Fujii, S. (1978).   Seikagaku
(in Japanese) 50, 763.
Svendsen, L., Blombäck, B., Blombäck, M. and Olsson, P. (1972).
Synthetic chromogenic substrates for determination of trypsin,
thrombin, and thrombin-like enzymes.   Thrombosis Research, 1, 267-
278.
Takahashi, H., Nagasawa, S. and Suzuki, T. (1972).   Studies on prekallikrein of bovine plasma. I. Purification and properties.   J.
Biochem. 71, 471-483.
Wiman, B. (1973).   Primary structure of peptides released during
activation of human plasminogen by urokinase.   Eur. J. Biochem.
39, 1-9.
Zimmerman, M., Yurewicz, E. C. and Patel, G. (1976).   A new fluorogenic substrate for chymotrypsin.   Anal. Biochem. 70, 258-262.

Zimmerman, M., Ashe, B., Yurewicz, E. C. and Patel, G. (1977).
Sensitive assays for trypsin, elastase, and chymotrypsin using
new fluorogenic substrates.   Anal. Biochem. 78, 47-51.

DETERMINATION OF HAGEMAN FACTOR (HG, FACTOR XII) AND PLASMA

PREKALLIKREIN (FLETCHER FACTOR) BY RADIOIMMUNOASSAYS

Hidehiko Saito

Department of Medicine, Case Western Reserve University
School of Medicine and University Hospitals of Cleveland
Cleveland, Ohio 44106

ABSTRACT

The titers of components of the plasma kallikrein-kinin
system have been measured conventionally by their biological
functions. The functional assays are, however, antagonized by
the presence of inhibitors and/or the absence of potentiators in
test samples. Immunologic assays obviate these difficulties. We
have developed specific, sensitive and reproducible radioimmunoassays (RIA) for HF and prekallikrein, and have applied these
assays to some clinical conditions. Normal pooled human plasma
contained approximately 40 µg of HF and 50 µg of prekallikrein per
ml. RIA were able to measure concentrations of HF and prekallikrein
as low as 0.1% and 0.3% that of normal pooled plasma respectively.
A good correlation existed between titers measured by clotting and
radioimmunoassays among 40 normal subjects (correlation co-efficient
= 0.82 for HF and 0.71 for prekallikrein). There was no significant
difference between the levels of HF and prekallikrein in plasma
and those in serum. Both HF and prekallikrein were significantly
reduced in plasmas of patients with advanced liver cirrhosis or
disseminated intravascular coagulation (DIC) and in cord serums,
but they were normal in plasmas obtained after strenuous physical
exercise and in plasmas of patients under treatment with warfarin.

INTRODUCTION

Both Hageman factor (HF, factor XII) and plasma prekallikrein
(Fletcher factor) are plasma proteins that participate both in
plasma kinin-generating and blood clotting systems (Ratnoff and

Colopy, 1955; Margolis, 1958; Hathaway et al., 1965; Wuepper, 1973).
The titers of these proteins have been measured conventionally by
their biological functions. The titer of HF is usually assayed by
measuring the effect of a test sample on the prolonged partial
thromboplastin time (PTT) of Hageman trait (factor XII deficiency)
plasma. The titer of prekallikrein is measured by the esterolytic
or amidolytic activity of contact-activated plasma (Colman, et al.,
1969; Amundsen, et al., 1977; Kluft, 1977) or by procoagulant
activity for Fletcher trait (prekallikrein-deficient) plasma
(Hathaway et al., 1965).

These functional assays are however, interfered with by the
presence of inhibitors and/or the absence of potentiators in test
samples. The clotting assay may give an erroneous titer if the
sample contains an anticoagulant such as heparin that interferes
with coagulant assays. The esterolytic or amidolytic assay requires
the presence of other proteins (HF and high molecular weight-kini-
nogen) for optimal activation of prekallikrein in the test sample.
Immunologic assays obviate these difficulties. We have developed
specific, sensitive and reproducible radioimmunoassays for HF and
prekallikrein and have applied these assays to some clinical
conditions.

MATERIALS AND METHODS

Citrated plasmas from normal individuals and patients were
prepared as described earlier (Saito et al., 1978a). High molecular weight kininogen-deficient (Fitzgerald trait) plasma was
obtained through the courtesy of Dr. R. Waldmann, Henry Ford
Hospital, Detroit, Michigan.

Radioimmunoassays of HF and prekallikrein were performed by a
double-antibody technique (Fig. 1 and 2) (Saito et al., 1976a;
Saito et al., 1978a). A standard curve was prepared by plotting
the percentage of bound (precipitated) radioactivity against the
logarithm of the concentration of purified proteins or normal
pooled plasma. Titers were expressed as units per ml plasma,
one unit of HF or prekallikrein being arbitrarily defined as that
amount present in one ml of a standard pool of 24 normal plasmas
of male adults.

The amounts of HF and prekallikrein in normal pooled plasma
were estimated to be approximately 40µg and 50 µg protein per ml,
respectively as judged by comparison to a standard curve using
purified HF and kallikrein. The minimum concentration of HF and
prekallikrein detectable by RIA were approximately 0.1% and 0.3%
that of normal pooled plasma (Saito et al., 1976a; Saito et al.,
1978a).

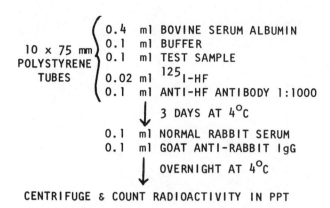

Figure 1.   Procedures for HF radioimmunoassay. From Saito et al.,
            1976 a. Reproduced with permission.

          ┌ 0.5 ml Bovine Serum Albumin
10 x 75   │ 0.02ml ^{125}I-Kallikrein
POLY-   ┤ 0.1 ml Test Sample
STYRENE   │ 0.1 ml Anti-Kallikrein
TUBES   └   serum 1:200
            ↓ 3 DAYS AT 4° C
        0.1 ml NORMAL RABBIT SERUM
        0.1 ml Goat Anti-Rabbit IgG
            ↓ OVERNIGHT AT 4° C
    CENTRIFUGE AND COUNT RADIOACTIVITY
              IN PPT

Figure 2.   Procedures for prekallikrein radioimmunoassay. From
            Saito, et al., 1978a. Reproduced with permission.

        Simultaneous clotting and radioimmune assays for HF were per-
formed on 40 normal plasmas. There was good correlation between
both assays (correlation co-efficient 0.82). Similarly, a good
correlation existed between titers of prekallikrein measured by
Fletcher factor clotting assays and RIA (correlation co-efficient
0.71, Fig. 3) (Saito et al., 1978a).

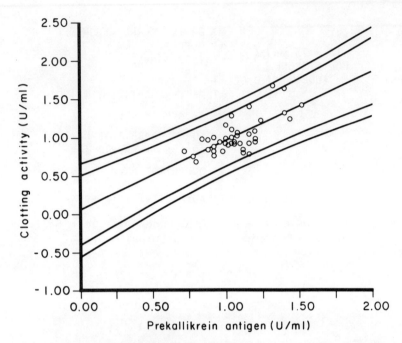

Figure 3. Correlation between prekallikrein clotting assays and
           radioimmunoassays. From Saito et al., 1978b. Re-
           produced with permission.

The concentrations of HF and prekallikrein in citrated plasma
were essentially the same as these in serum, suggesting that in
vitro clotting does not significantly alter the level of HF and
prekallikrein (Saito et al., 1976a; Saito et al., 1978a). Thus,
serum samples can be used for assay.

RESULTS AND DISCUSSION

Plasma HF and prekallikrein levels in some physiological
conditions.

HF antigen was determined by radioimmunoassay in plasmas of
43 normal adults (22 males and 21 females). The mean ± S.D. in
males were 1.02 ± 0.24 U/ml and that in females, 1.09 ± 0.26 U/ml,
indicating that there is no sex difference. No change in HF antigen was found after strenuous physical exercise. HF antigen was
significantly lower in 36 cord serums than in normal adults (0.61
± 0.24 U/ml, P < 0.001) (Saito et al., 1976a). This is consistent

with the report that HF activity is reduced in the neonatal period
(Kurkcuoglu and McElfresh, 1960).

Prekallikrein antigen was slightly higher in female subjects
than in male subjects. There was no difference between the concentration of prekallikrein antigen of normal non-pregnant females and
that during pregnancy (Saito et al., 1978a). No change in prekallikrein antigen was detected after strenuous physical exercise,
although the titer of antihemophilic factor (AHF, factor VIII)
activity rose significantly. Prekallikrein antigen was strikingly
reduced in 12 cord serums as compared to serums of normal adults
(0.33 ± 0.12 U/ml P < 0.001).

Plasma HF and prekallikrein levels in some pathological
conditions.

HF antigen was greatly diminished in plasmas of 10 patients
with advanced liver cirrhosis (P < 0.001) and six patients with
disseminated intravascular coagulation (P < 0.001), but was normal
in plasmas of patients treated with warfarin (Fig. 4). The low HF
levels in liver cirrhosis suggests that HF may be produced in the
liver. Direct evidence, however, remains to be obtained.

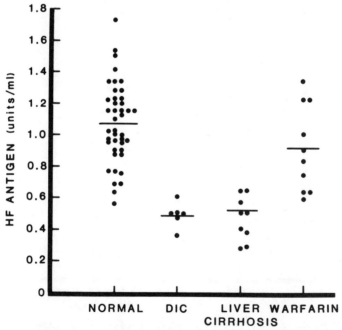

Figure 4. Plasma HF antigen titers in some pathological
          conditions. The transverse lines indicate mean
          values for each group.

Prekallikrein antigen was markedly decreased in plasmas of seven patients with severe hepatic cirrhosis (P < 0.001) and six patients with DIC (P < 0.001) (Fig. 5). In contrast, it was normal in plasmas of 12 patients treated with warfarin, 12 patients with systemic lupus erythematosus (SLE), 12 patients with rheumatoid arthritis, and four patients with sarcoidosis (Saito, et al., 1978a). These data are in good agreement with previous reports supporting the hypothesis that the liver may be the site of the production of plasma prekallikrein (Hathaway, et al., 1965; Colman et al., 1969; Bagdassarian et al., 1974).

The reduced plasma HF and prekallikrein titers in the patients with DIC suggest that the decreased prekallikrein concentration was mediated through activation of HF in these patients. It is interesting to point out that high molecular weight kininogen (Fitzgerald factor) titers were also low in these patients (Saito et al., 1976b). Low HF activity and prekallikrein activity as measured by the esterolytic activity of contact-activated plasma, was previously reported in gram-negative bacteremia (Mason et al., 1970).

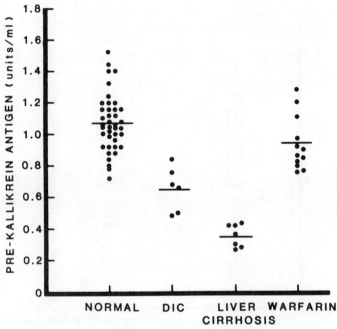

Figure 5.   Plasma prekallikrein antigen titers in some pathological conditions. The transverse lines indicate mean values for each group.

Plasma HF and prekallikrein levels in some congenitally deficient plasmas.

HF antigen was undetectable in most individuals with homozy-
gous Hageman trait (factor XII deficiency) (less than 0.001 U/ml).
But in two unrelated individuals with Hageman trait, non-functional
material immunologically indistinguishable from normal HF was
detected in plasma by radioimmunoassay (Saito et al., 1978b).
This suggests the molecular heterogeneity of Hageman trait.

Normal amount of HF antigen was present in all other congenitally deficient plasmas tested including plasma thromboplastin
antecedent (PTA, factor XI) deficiency, Christmas factor (factor
IX) deficiency, classic hemophilia, von Willebrand's disease,
Fletcher trait and Fitzgerald trait (Saito et al., 1976a).

Prekallikrein antigen was measured in plasmas of seven individuals with Fletcher trait (plasma prekallikrein deficiency), all of
which contained less than 1% of prekallikrein clotting activity.
In two cases, material immunologically indistinguishable from
normal prekallikrein was detected in plasmas by radioimmunoassay,
suggesting the molecular heterogeneity of human prekallikrein
deficiency (Saito and Ratnoff, 1977).

High molecular weight kininogen-deficient plasma contained
reduced level of prekallikrein antigen (Donaldson, et al., 1977),
but all other clotting factor-deficient plasmas had normal amounts
of prekallikrein in plasmas.

ACKNOWLEDGEMENTS

I thank Dr. Oscar D. Ratnoff for his support and encouragement,
and Ms. Janet Shlaes and Ms. Ellen Strecker for their invaluable
technical help.

This work was supported in part by research grant HL 01661, The
National Heart, Lung and Blood Institute of the National Institutes
of Health, U.S. Public Health Service and in part by grants from
the American Heart Association and its Northeast Ohio Affiliate.

REFERENCES

Amundsen, E., L. Svendsen, A.M. Vennerd, and K. Laake. 1977.
    Determination of plasma kallikrein with a new chromogenic
    tripeptide derivative. In: Chemistry and Biology of Kallikrein-
    Kinin System in Health and Disease. Pisano, J.J. and Austen,
    K.F. (eds.) (DHEW Pub. No. 76-791, Washington, D.C. p. 215).

Bagdassarian, A., B. Lahiri, R.C. Talamo, P. Wong and R.W. Colman.
    1974. Immunochemical Studies of Plasma Kallikren. J. Clin.
    Invest. 54: 1444.
Colman, R.W., J.W. Mason and S. Sherry. 1969. The kallikreinogen-
    kallikrein enzyme system of human plasma. Assay of components
    and observations in disease states. Ann. Intern. Med. 71: 763.
Donaldson, V.H., J. Kleniewski, H. Saito and J.K. Sayed. 1977.
    Prekallikrein deficiency in a kindred with kininogen deficiency
    and Fitzgerald trait clotting defect. Evidence that high
    molecular weight kininogen and prekallikrein exist as a complex
    in normal human plasma. J. Clin. Invest. 60: 571.
Hathaway, W.E., L.P. Belhasen and H.S. Hathaway. 1965. Evidence for
    a new plasma thromboplastin factor I. Case report, coagula-
    tion studies and physico-chemical properties. Blood. 26: 521.
Kluft, C. 1978. Determination of prekallikrein in human plasma:
    Optimal conditions for activating prekallikrein. J. Lab. Clin.
    Med. 91: 83.
Kurkcuoglu, N. and A.E. Mc Elfresh. 1960. The Hageman factor:
    Determination of its concentration during the neonatal period
    and presentation of a case of Hageman factor deficiency. J.
    Pediatr. 57: 61.
Margolis, J. 1958. Activation of plasma by contact with glass:
    Evidence for a common reaction which releases plasma kinin
    and initiates coagulation. J. Physiol. (Lond.) 144: 1.
Mason, J.W., U.R. Kleeberg, P. Dolan and R.W. Colman, 1970.
    Plasma kallikrein and Hageman factor in gram-negative bacte-
    remia. Ann. Intern. Med. 73: 545.
Ratnoff, O.D. and J.E. Colopy. 1955. A familial hemorrhagic trait
    associated with a deficiency of a clot-promoting fraction of
    plasma. J. Clin. Invest. 34: 602.
Saito, H., O.D. Ratnoff and J. Pensky. 1976a. Radioimmunoassay
    of human Hageman factor (factor XII). J. Lab. Clin. Med.
    88: 506.
Saito, H., G.H. Goldsmith and R. Waldmann. 1976b. Fitzgerald factor
    (high molecular weight kininogen) clotting activity in human
    plasma in health and disease, and in various animal plasmas.
    Blood. 48: 941.
Saito, H. and O.D. Ratnoff. 1977. Molecular heterogeneity of human
    plasma prekallikrein deficiency (Fletcher trait). Clin. Res.
    25: 347A.
Saito, H., M.C. Poon, W. Vicic, G.H. Goldsmith and J.E. Menitove.
    1978a. Human plasma prekallikrein (Fletcher factor) clotting
    activity and antigen in health and disease. J. Lab. Clin. Med.
    92: 84.
Saito, H., J.G. Scott, H.Z. Movat and S.J. Scialla. 1978b. CRM+
    Hageman trait. Blood. 52: (supplement 1): 194.
Wuepper, K.D. 1973. Prekallikrein deficiency in man. J. Exp. Med.
    138: 1345.

ASSAY METHODS FOR PREKALLIKREIN AND KININOGENS AND THEIR

APPLICATIONS

Yasuhiro Uchida, Sachiko Oh-Ishi, Kunio Tanaka,
Yoshiteru Harada, Akinori Ueno, Makoto Katori and
Shuji Funahashi*, Takenori Hashimoto*, Takami Ueno*,
Junzo Kodama*

Department of Pharmacology, Kitasato University School
of Medicine, Sagamihara 228, Japan and *Osaka National
Hospital, Osaka 540, Japan

ABSTRACT

Prekallikrein activity in plasma was assayed using a synthetic peptidyl fluorogenic substrate (carbobenzoxy-L-phenylalanyl-
L-arginine 4-methylcoumarinyl-7-amide), after activation of prekallikrein by acetone and kaolin. For total kininogen assay, the
pretreatment of plasma at pH 2.0 was the best to eliminate bradykinin potentiators and kininase activity, before addition of trypsin
to convert kininogen to bradykinin. Assay method of high molecular
weight (HMW) kininogen was established by conversion of HMW-kininogen to bradykinin through activation of Hageman factor by glass
powder and that of low molecular weight (LMW) kininogen was also
by treatment of HMW-kininogen-depleted plasma in the same way as
that for total kininogen.
The marked reduction of prekallikrein and HMW-kininogen, not
of LMW-kininogen, was found in pleural fluid of rat carrageenin
pleurisy, and in plasma after i.v. injection of bromelain in rats.
Members of the pedigree of hereditary angioneurotic edema patients
also show low levels of prekallikrein and kininogens in plasma.

INTRODUCTION

The detection of the increased levels of free kinin and plasma kallikrein activity in plasma or body fluid in pathological states may be one of the way to prove the involvement of the plasma kallikrein-kinin system. It may, however, be difficult, since inactivation of kallikrein by plasma inhibitors and destruction of kinin by kininases occurred rapidly in the tissues. The reduced levels of prekallikrein and high molecular weight (HMW)-kininogen may provide the evidence for the involvement of plasma kallikrein-kinin system, since plasma kallikrein-kinin system is once activated, prekallikrein and HMW-kininogen are consumed and do not recover before 72 hrs in rats (Oh-ishi et al., in press).

The present paper describes the assay methods of prekallikrein and HMW- and low molecular weight (LMW)-kininogens, and their applications to certain inflammatory models and hereditary angioneurotic edema.

MATERIALS AND METHODS

Blood collection. For the development of prekallikrein assay method, normal human plasma was collected from antecubital vein of healthy subjects with a plastic syringe and needle into plastic tubes containing 1/10 volume of 3.8% sodium citrate and immediately centrifuged at 1,000 g at 25°C for 15 min. Plasma was distributed into small plastic tubes and was kept at -70°C until use.

For the development of kininogen assay method, male albino rabbits (2.5 – 3.5 kg of body weight) were slightly anesthetized with ether. Blood was collected from carotid artery through a polyethylene cannula to plastic tubes containing 2 units of heparin (Sigma Co., St. Louis, Mo.)/ml of blood. Human blood was collected from antecubital vein of healthy subjects with a plastic syringe and needle into plastic tubes containing heparin (2 units/ml blood). Blood was immediately centrifuged at 1,000 g at 25°C for 15 min. Plasma was distributed into plastic tubes and was kept at -20°C until use. All contact with glass or negative charge surfaces was carefully avoided during the whole procedure.

Bioassay of bradykinin. Kininogens were converted to bradykinin, which was bioassayed on esterus rat uterus. Virgin rats weighing 150-250 g were injected i.p. and s.c. with 5 mg of hexestrol (Hexron, Teikoku Zoki, Tokyo). Contractions of the isolated rat uterus were recorded using an isotonic transducer (ME Commercials Ltd., Tokyo), connected to a pen recorder (Rikadenki Kogyo Ltd., Tokyo). Synthetic bradykinin (Peptide Institute Inc., Osaka) was used as a standard.

Rat pleurisy. Male rats (8-10 weeks old) of Sprague Dowley (specific pathogen free) were slightly anesthetized with ether and 0.1 ml of 2% λ-carrageenin (Pasco International Corp., Tokyo) in sterile physiological saline was injected into the right pleural cavity through the chest skin sterilized by 70% ethanol. After three hr, the rats were sacrificed by exasanguination under ether anesthesia and the levels of prekallikrein and kininogens in pleural fluid and plasma were determined (Katori et al., in press).

Experiment with stem bromelain. Stem bromelain (Jintan Dolf, Tokyo), a SH protease from stem of pineapples, was injected into rats (10 mg/kg, i.v.). Blood was collected through the carotid artery under ether anesthesia 15 min after bromelain injection and the levels of prekallikrein and kininogens in plasma were determined.

Agents. Carbobenzoxy-L-phenylalanyl-L-arginine 4-methyl-coumarinyl-7-amide (Z-Phe-Arg-MCA) and 7-amino 4-methylcoumarin (AMC) (Peptide Institute Inc., Osaka), soybean trypsin inhibitor (SBTI) and limabean trypsin inhibitor (LBTI) (Worthington Biochem. Co., New Jersey) and kaolin (K-5, Fisher Sci. Co., New Jersey) were purchased. Trypsin was a product of National Biochemical Corp. (twice crystalized, salt free, bovine pancreas). Highly purified hog pancreas kallikrein was a gift of Dr. C. Kuzback (Bayer AG., Germany) (1290 kallikrein units/mg) and highly purified snake venom kininogenase (Agkistrodon halys blomhoffii) was a gift of Drs. H. Kato and S. Iwanaga (Protein Research Institute, Osaka University, Osaka) (10 TAME units/mg protein).

RESULTS

Fig. 1 shows the assay method of plasma prekallikrein (Oh-ishi and Katori, in press). The assay of plasma prekallikrein consists of both activation process and amidolysis of the substrate. Plasma was activated with acetone and kaolin. The activity of plasma kallikrein generated was assayed using Z-Phe-Arg-MCA, a peptidyl fluorogenic substrate. Tube A contained 40 µg of LBTI and tube B contained 40 µg of SBTI. The fluorescence of AMC released was measured by fluorometer (Hitachi, MPF-3) in such a way that excitation was at 380 nm and emission at 460 nm. The difference between the values from tube A and tube B was considered as prekallikrein activity. Fig. 2 shows the comparison of the activities of plasma kallikrein, glandular kallikrein (KZC) and plasmin using Z-Phe-Arg-MCA with the esterase activity which were determined by ^{3}H-TAME. Z-Phe-Arg-MCA was specific for plasma kallikrein, compared with the activities of glandular kallikrein and plasmin.

When Fletcher trait plasma, a plasma deficient in prekallikrein, was substituted with normal plasma in various ratios, the

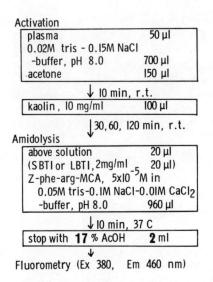

Fig. 1. A schematic diagram showing assay method for prekallikrein.

This assay method is composed of the activation of prekallikrein by acetone and kaolin and the amidolysis of Z-Phe-Arg-MCA by plasma kallikrein.   r.t.: room temperature.

activity, expressed as an arbitrary unit (1 unit = 10^{-7} M AMC for 10 min), showed a linear relationship to prekallikrein contents.

Kininogen levels in plasma were widely determined by Diniz's method (Diniz and Carvalho, 1963), but this method is known to produce bradykinin potentiators with bradykinin (Aarsen, 1968, Hamberg et al., 1969). Thus, this method was improved by comparing the different ways of pretreatment of plasma (Uchida and Katori, 1978).

Table 1 shows the pretreatment of rabbit or human plasma. In Diniz's method, 0.2 ml of plasma was added to 1.8 ml of 0.2% acetic acid (pH 3.5) and boiled (98°C) for 30 min. The pretreated plasma was then neutralized with 0.05 ml of 1 N NaOH (monitored with universal pH paper) and incubated with 200 μg trypsin in 0.04 M tris buffer pH 7.8 for 30 min. The incubation was terminated using

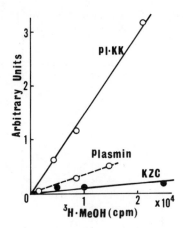

Fig. 2. Specificity of the substrate compared with TAME activity.

Ordinate shows the amounts of AMC released (one arbitrary unit = 10^{-7} M). Abscissa indicates the counts (cpm) of ^{3}H–MeOH released from ^{3}H–TAME (N^α–tosyl–L–arginine ^{3}H–methyl ester hydrochloride). Pl·KK: partially purified human plasma kallikrein. KZC: highly purified hog pancreas kallikrein.

warm ethanol and heating for 10 min at 70°C. After evaporation of the supernatant fluid, the dried residue was dissolved in 2 ml of physiological saline and then bradykinin in the saline was assayed on rat uterus. This pretreated plasma was compared with five other pretreatments shown in Table 1; nontreated, boiled (at 98°C) or heated (at 60°C) in distilled water and acidified by 0.2% acetic acid (at pH 3.5) or by 0.03 N HCl (at pH 2.0) at 37°C for 15 min. The acidified plasmas were neutralized with 1 N NaOH. These plasmas, pretreated in different ways, were incubated with 200 µg of trypsin and the released bradykinin was assayed in the same manner as that in Diniz's method.

Fig. 3 indicates the amounts of bradykinin released from kininogen in plasma pretreated differently. When the amounts of bradykinin released by hog pancreas kallikrein or snake venom kininogenase were calculated as the amount/ml of the original plasma, the calculated amounts were 2.9 ± 0.1 or 3.0 ± 0.1 µg bradykinin eq/ml of plasma, respectively (mean ± S.E.), and was constant even if the volume of the sample solutions added to the organ bath was increased

Table 1. Different ways of pretreatment of plasma.

Diniz	Non-treated	Heated		Acidified	
		98°C	60°C	pH 3.5	pH 2.0
0.2 ml Plasma					
1.8 ml acet. acid pH 3.5	1.8 ml H2O	1.8 ml H2O	1.8 ml H2O	1.8 ml acet. acid pH 3.5	1.8 ml 0.03 N HCl pH 2.0
98°C, 30' neutral-ized		98°C, 30'	60°C, 30'	37°C, 15' neutral-ized	37°C, 15' neutral-ized

Incubation → 0.2 M Tris buffer (0.5 ml)
Trypsin (200 μg)

←5 ml of absolute alcohol

Extraction

Bioassay

(from Biochem. Pharmacol. 27, 1463, 1978 with permission)

from 0.05 to 0.2 ml. On the other hand, the amounts of BK eq/ml
plasma in the sample solution from Diniz and 98°C-treated plasma
were increased with the increased volumes of the sample solution
added to the organ bath. The bradykinin levels after addition of
0.2 ml of the sample solution was significantly higher than that of
0.05 ml ($P < 0.05$). This result indicates clearly that bradykinin
potentiators exist in the sample solution with bradykinin. The nontreated, and the pH 3.5 and pH 2.0 treated plasmas did not contain
bradykinin potentiators. The amounts of bradykinin released from
the pH 2.0 and 60°C treated plasmas were not different from those
released by hog pancreas kallikrein and by the snake venom kininogenase, whereas the amounts of bradykinin from the nontreated and the
pH 3.5 treated plasmas were lower even in the presence of a sufficient amount of o-phenanthroline, a kininase inhibitor.

The pretreatment of Diniz, pH 2.0 and 98°C destroyed the kininase activity in plasma, whereas the kininase activity still remained
after the pretreatment at pH 3.5 and 60°C. Therefore, it could be
concluded that the pretreatment of pH 2.0 was the best in rabbit and
human plasmas. For human plasma, the pretreatment of 60°C was also
suitable, since kininase was inactivated by the pretreatment of 60°C.

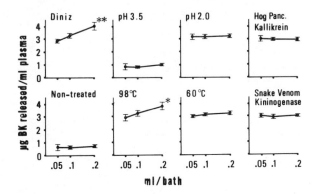

Fig. 3.   Presence of bradykinin potentiators and the amounts of bradykinin released from differently pretreated rabbit plasma.

Ordinate shows the amounts (μg) of bradykinin (BK) expressed as the amounts in terms of ml of the original plasma.   Abscissa indicates the volumes of sample solutions added to the organ bath.   The values are mean of nine plasmas from three rabbits with S.E.   The presence of bradykinin potentiators was indicated, when the apparent amounts of bradykinin eq/ml of the original plasma were increasing amounts of the sample solution added to the organ bath from 0.05 to 0.2 ml, as shown in Diniz and 98°C-treated plasmas.

(from Biochem. Pharmacol. <u>27</u>, 1463, 1978 with permission)

Fig. 4 shows the differential assay method of HMW- and LMW-kininogens (Uchida and Katori, in press).   For assay of HMW-kininogen, glass powder was added to plasma (0.5 g/0.2 ml plasma) in 1.8 ml of 0.06 M tris buffer in siliconized tube in the presence of o-phenanthroline at the final concentration of 2 mg/ml plasma.   The mixture was incubated for 30 min at 37°C.   The incubation was stopped by addition of warm ethanol (5 ml).   The released bradykinin was separated and assayed.

For assay of LMW-kininogen, plasma was incubated with glass powder in the absence of o-phenanthroline and this HMW-kininogen-depleted plasma was treated in the same manner to that for the total kininogen.   The amounts of bradykinin released by trypsin was considered as the level of LMW-kininogen.   The normal plasma levels of HMW-, LMW- and total kininogens were 0.98, 3.08 and 4.11 μg BK eq/ml of plasma for human (n=10) and 0.96, 0.94 and 1.93 μg

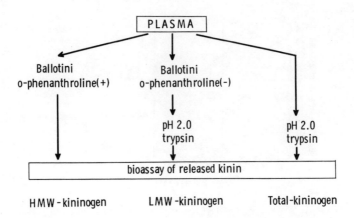

Fig. 4. A schematic diagram showing differential assay method of high molecular weight (HMW) and low molecular weight (LMW) and total kininogens.

BK eq/ml of plasma for rats (n=10). Thus, human LMW-kininogen level was three times as high as that of HMW-kininogen, but HMW-kininogen level in rats was the same as that of LMW-kininogen.

These assay methods were applied to an inflammatory model of rat carrageenin-induced pleurisy, the activation of plasma kallikrein-kinin system by bromelain and plasma kallikrein-kinin system in hereditary angioneurotic edema (HANE).

Carrageenin-pleurisy was induced in rats by intrapleural injection of 0.1 ml of 2% λ-carrageenin (Katori et al., 1978). The volume of the pleural exudate increased rapidly 1-3 hr after the injection and reached the maximum at 19 hr. As shown in Table 2, prekallikrein and kininogen levels in plasma at 3 hr were not different from those in plasma of control rats. On the contrary, the level of prekallikrein in pleural fluid of 3 hr was markedly reduced and that of HMW-kininogen was almost depleted, whereas LMW-kininogen level was not different from that in plasma (Table 2). These results strongly indicate that 1) plasma kallikrein-kinin system was activated and 2) this activation occurred only in the pleural cavity, but not in plasma (Katori et al., in press).

When bromelain, a SH protease from pineapples, was injected intravenously into rats, prekallikrein and HMW-kininogen were almost

Table 2. Levels of kininogens and prekallikrein in plasma and pleural fluid of rats affected by carrageenin-induced pleurisy. The each value shows means of 5-14 animals with S.E.

		Kininogen (ng BK eq/mg protein)			Prekallikrein
		HMW	LMW	TOTAL	$(cpm \times 10^{-3})$
Normal plasma		13.8 ± 0.8	11.1 ± 1.5	25.2 ± 2.2	4768.2 ± 267.9
Pleurisy	plasma	12.9 ± 0.4	11.2 ± 1.0	24.3 ± 1.5	3839.2 ± 614.5
	pleural fluid	< 1.1	11.4 ± 0.8	12.4 ± 1.0	762.0 ± 109.3

depleted 15 min after the injection. This depletion was found to be due to the activation of plasma kallikrein-kinin system through activation of Hageman factor (Oh-ishi et al., in press). When rats, in which prekallikrein and HMW-kininogen were depleted previously by intravenous injection of bromelain, were exposed to carrageenin pleurisy, dye exudation into the pleural cavity in 1-3 hr was significantly reduced and the accumulation of the pleural fluid was markedly suppressed at the first 3 hrs (Katori et al., 1978).

In HANE, the levels of prekallikrein and kininogens in plasma were found to be low in the most members of the pedigree.

DISCUSSION

Prekallikrein activity in plasma was assayed using carbobenzoxy-L-phenylalanyl-L-arginine 4-methylcoumarinyl-7-amide (Z-Phe-Arg-MCA), a synthetic peptidyl fluorogenic substrate, after activation of plasma prekallikrein by acetone and kaolin (Oh-ishi and Katori, in press). The specificity of this substrate showed very specific to plasma kallikrein, compared with glandular kallikrein (KZC) and plasmin (Fig. 2). The sensitivity was also very high so that 1 µl of plasma was sufficient to assay the activity of prekallikrein. When Fletcher trait plasma or heated human plasma (60°C, 1 hr) was substituted with normal plasma at different ratios, a linear relationship was obtained between prekallikrein contents and kallikrein activity after kaolin activation. Thus, prekallikrein levels could be assayed quantitatively by this method. Hageman factor and HMW-kininogen were required for the activation

of prekallikrein and the complete deficiency of each factor produced no prekallikrein activity, even if a sufficient amount of
prekallikrein was contained in plasma. When Fujiwara trait plasma,
a plasma deficient in HMW- and LMW-kininogen (Oh-ishi et al., this
proceeding), was substituted with normal plasma, it was known that
10% of Hageman factor or HMW-kininogen was required to get the full
activation of prekallikrein (Oh-ishi and Katori, in press).

For assay of kininogens, it is necessary to convert kininogens
to bradykinin and thus to eliminate bradykinin potentiators and
kininase activity when bradykinin was assayed by bioassay. As
trypsin does not induce the full release of bradykinin from unde-
natured plasma, plasma must be denatured before addition of trypsin.
As shown in Fig. 3, treatment of plasma at pH 2.0 is most suitable
for this purpose, since two factors, bradykinin potentiators and
kininase activity, were eliminated and the full conversion of kininogen to bradykinin was obtained as shown in comparison with the
amounts of bradykinin released by two standard kininogenases, purified hog pancreas kallikrein and purified snake venom kininogenase (Fig. 3).

The differential assay method of HMW- and LMW-kininogens is
also necessary to prove the involvement of plasma kallikrein-kinin
system. As the assay of HMW-kininogen was initiated by the activation of Hageman factor in plasma by addition of glass powder,
deficiency in Hageman factor and prekallikrein in plasma does not
allow to release bradykinin from HMW-kininogen. When heated plasma
(60°C, 1 hr) was substituted with 10% of normal plasma, the full
convertion of HMW-kininogen to bradykinin was obtained for 30 min
incubation (Uchida and Katori, in press).

In vivo experiments, detection of free bradykinin in plasma
or body fluid is good evidence to show the involvement of plasma
kallikrein-kinin system, but bradykinin is destroyed very rapidly
and is difficult to detect. On the other hand, the reduced levels
of prekallikrein and HMW-kininogen, but not LMW-kininogen, are very
convincing evidence to indicate the activation of plasma kallikrein-kinin system. This was proved in an inflammatory model, rat
carrageenin-induced pleurisy, in which the prekallikrein activity
was markedly reduced and HMW-kininogen was depleted in pleural
fluid 3 hr after carrageenin injection. No reduction of prekallikrein and HMW-kininogen levels in plasma indicates that the activation of the system is localized only in the pleural cavity (Katori
et al., in press).

The markedly reduced levels of prekallikrein and HMW-kininogen
were also found after intravenous injection of bromelain, showing
that plasma kallikrein-kinin system was activated.

Plasma of HANE patients contained the reduced levels of pre-kallikrein and HMW-kininogen. The significance of the facts is under investigation in relation to clinical symptoms.

In any case, the assays of prekallikrein and HMW-kininogen, with that of LMW-kininogen, are recommended as one of the best ways to prove the involvement of plasma kallikrein-kinin system in certain pathological states.

ACKNOWLEDGEMENT

This work was supported partly by Naito Research Grant for 1976 (76-108) and by Scientific Research Grants from the Ministry of Education, Sciences and Cultures for 1975 (067158), and for 1978 (310507).

REFERENCES

Aarsen, P.N., 1968. Sensitization of guinea-pig ileum to the action of bradykinin by trypsin hydrolysate of ox and rabbit plasma. Br. J. Pharmacol. Chemother. 32: 453.

Diniz, C.R. and I.F. Carvalho, 1963. A micromethod for determination of bradykininogen under several conditions. Ann. N.Y. Acad. Sci. 104: 79.

Hamberg, V., P. Elg and P. Stelwagen, 1969. Tryptic and plasmic peptide fragments increasing the effect of bradykinin on isolated smooth muscle. Scand. J. Clin. Lab. Invest. 24: Suppl. 107, 21.

Katori, M., K. Ikeda, Y. Harada, Y. Uchida, K. Tanaka and S. Oh-ishi, 1978. A possible role of prostaglandins and bradykinin as a trigger of exudation in carrageenin-induced rat pleurisy. Agents & Actions. 8: 108.

Katori, M., Y. Uchida, S. Oh-ishi, Y. Harada, A. Ueno and K. Tanaka, Involvement of plasma kallikrein-kinin system in rat carrageenin-induced pleurisy. Europ. J. Reumatol. (in press).

Oh-ishi, S. and M. Katori, Fluorogenic assay for plasma kallikrein using peptidylmethyl-coumarinyl-amide as a substrate. Thromb. Res. (in press).

Oh-ishi, S., A. Ueno, Y. Uchida, M. Katori, H. Hayashi, H. Koya, K. Kitajima and I. Kimura. Fujiwara trait: The first case of kininogen deficiency in Japan. (this volume).

Oh-ishi, S., Y. Uchida, A. Ueno and M. Katori. Bromelain, a thiol-protease from pineapple stem, depletes high molecular weight kininogen through the activation of Hageman factor. Thromb. Res. (in press).

Uchida, Y. and M. Katori, 1978. An improved method for determination of the total kininogen in rabbit and human plasma. Biochem. Pharmacol. 37: 1463.

Uchida, Y. and M. Katori. Differential assay method for high mole-
    cular weight and low molecular weight kininogens. Thromb.
    Res. (in press).

SYNTHETIC BRADYKININ-LIKE PEPTIDES

C. Yanaihara, M. Sakagami, M. Kubota, H. Sato,
T. Mochizuki, A. Inoue, N. Yanaihara, T. Yasuhara,*
T. Kanajima,* and T. Hashimoto**

Laboratory of Bioorganic Chemistry, Shizuoka College
of Pharmacy, Shizuoka 422, Institute of Pharmaceutical
Sciences, Hiroshima University, Hiroshima 734*, and
Faculty of Pharmaceutical Sciences, Hokuriku University
Kanazawa 920-11**, Japan

Several bradykinin-like peptides have recently been isolated
from frog skin or wasp venom extracts. These include bradykinyl-
Val-Ala-Pro-Ala-Ser-OH (I)(Nakajima, 1968), bradykinyl-Gly-Lys-
Phe-His-OH (II)(Yasuhara et al., 1973), [Thr^6]-bradykinyl-Ile-Ala-
Pro-Glu-Ile-Val-OH (III)(Yasuhara et al., 1975), vespakinin-X (IV)
(Yasuhara et al., 1977) and vespakinin-M (V)(Kishimura et al.,
1976). Table 1 shows the amino acid sequences of these bradykinin-
like peptides.

In the present investigation, we have carried out the syntheses of III, IV and V in order to confirm their primary structures.
In addition, some biological and immunological properties of these
peptides and the related fragments are described. The syntheses
of I (Yanaihara et al., 1973) and II (Yasuhara et al., 1973) were
reported previously.

Synthesis

The syntheses of the kinin analogues were carried out by the
conventional method for peptide synthesis.

Synthesis of III: Scheme 1 shows the synthetic route employed for
preparation of III. The C-terminal undecapeptide was prepared by
using protected dipeptide azides such as the azides of Z-Ile-Ala,
Z-Pro-Phe, and Z-Phe-Thr. Introduction of the Glu, Pro and Arg

185

TABLE 1.

AMINO ACID SEQUENCES OF VARIOUS BRADYKININ-LIKE PEPTIDES.

H-Arg-Pro-Pro-Gly-Phe-Ser-Pro-Phe-Arg-OH

H-Arg-Pro-Pro-Gly-Phe-Ser-Pro-Phe-Arg-<u>Val-Ala-Pro-Ala-Ser</u>-OH   (Rana nigromaculata)

H-Arg-Pro-Pro-Gly-Phe-Ser-Pro-Phe-Arg-<u>Gly-Lys-Phe-His</u>-OH   (Bombina orientalis)

H-Arg-Pro-Pro-Gly-Phe-<u>Thr</u>-Pro-Phe-Arg-<u>Ile-Ala-Pro-Glu-Ile-Val</u>-OH   (Rana rugosa)

Vespakinin X   H-<u>Ala</u>-Arg-Pro-Pro-Gly-Phe-Ser-Pro-Phe-Arg-<u>Ile-Val</u>-OH   (Vespa xanthoptera)

Vespakinin M   H-<u>Gly</u>-Arg-Pro-<u>Hyp</u>-Gly-Phe-Ser-Pro-Phe-Arg-<u>Ile-Asp</u>-OH   (Vespa manderenea)

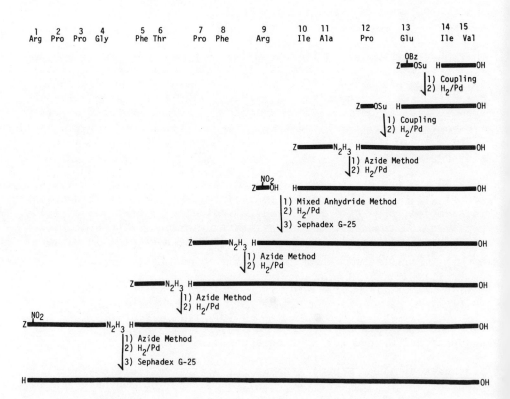

Scheme 1.   Synthesis of [Thr[6]]-Bradykinyl-Ile-Ala-Pro-Glu-Ile-Val-OH

moieties was carried out by the mixed anhydride (Anderson et al.,
1966) or the active ester method (Anderson et al., 1964).
Benzyloxycarbonyl (Z) group used for α-amino protection was removed
by hydrogenolysis over Pd. After removal of the Z group from the
undecapeptide, the ensuing peptide was acylated with Z–Arg(NO_2)–
Pro-Pro-Gly-azide derived from the corresponding hydrazide (Yānai-
hara et al., 1973) to give the protected pentadecapeptide, which
was hydrogenated in diluted acetic acid for removal of the Z and
NO_2 protections. The resulting pentadecapeptide acetate was
purified by gelfiltration on Sephadex G-25.

Synthesis of IV: The synthetic route employed for preparation of
IV is shown in Scheme 2. The C-terminal protected heptapeptide was
prepared by successive chain elongation of H–Arg(H^+)–Ile–Val–OH
using the azides derived from Z–Pro–Phe–$NHNH_2$ and Z–Phe–Ser–$NHNH_2$,
respectively. Hydrogenolysis of the ensuing protected heptapeptide,
followed by acylation with Z–Ala–Arg(H^+)–Pro–Pro–Gly–azide gave
the protected dodecapeptide, which was deprotected by hydrogenolysis.
The ensuing crude IV was purified by gelfiltration on Sephadex G–25,
followed by droplet counter current distribution using solvent
system 1–BuOH:AcOH:H_2O = 4:1:5.

Synthesis of V: The synthesis of V was carried out in a manner
similar to that used for the synthesis of IV as shown in Scheme 3.
The C-terminal heptapeptide which was prepared by successive chain
elongation was coupled with Z–Gly–Arg(H^+)–Pro–Hyp–Gly–azide to
give the protected dodecapeptide, which was deprotected by hydrogenolysis. The resulting crude V was purified in the manner
described in the preparation of IV.

     The products prepared in the present study were proved to be
homogeneous by tlc with different solvent system and acid hydrolysates of the peptides contained the constituent amino acid in
the ratios predicted by theory. The chromatographic patterns of
dansylated products of synthetic III, IV and V were identical
with those of the dansylated derivatives of the natural materials,
respectively. In addition, contracting activity of the synthetic
peptides III, IV and V on isolated rat uterus was found to be
identical with that of the corresponding natural products. Fig.
1 shows the dose-response curves of III of natural origin, synthetic
III and synthetic bradykinin with respect to contracting activity
on rat uterus.

     N^{α}-Tyrosyl-bradykinin and kallidin were also synthesized in
this study which were used for development of bradykinin radioimmunoassay. The tyrosylated bradykinin was used as substrate of
radioiodination and the synthetic kallidin as heptenic immunogen
for preparation of antisera to bradykinin.

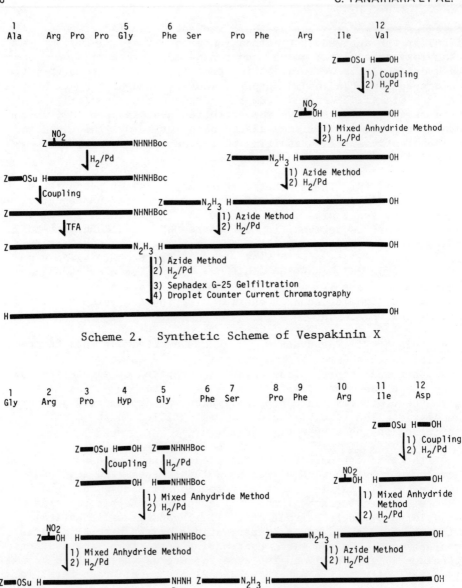

Scheme 2.   Synthetic Scheme of Vespakinin X

Scheme 3.   Synthesis of Vespakinin M

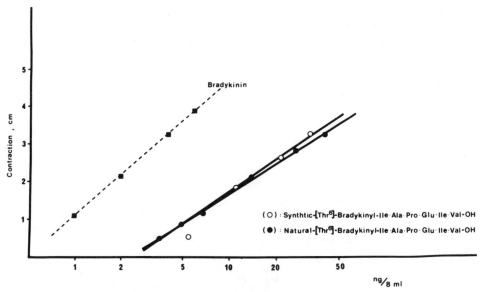

Fig. 1. Contracting effect of synthetic and natural preparations
of [Thr[6]]-bradykinyl-Ile-Ala-Pro-Glu-Ile-Val-OH (III)
on rat uterus.

Biological property

Biological properties of the synthetic bradykinin–like peptides
and their fragments were examined in terms of contracting effect on
the isolated guinea pig ileum and colon, and the activities were
compared with that of synthetic bradykinin. Compound I and the
fragments of compound II, which had been prepared previously, were
also examined in this respect. The results are summarized in
Table 2. Both N^α-tyrosyl-bradykinin and vespakinin (IV) were
found to possess significant contracting activities in guinea pig
iluem as well as in the colon. The activity of N^α-tyrosyl-bradykinin
was slightly higher than that of kallidin in either preparation.
The relative potency of IV on the guinea pig colon preparation
was nearly identical with that of N^α-tyrosyl-bradykinin. In
contrast, vespakinin M (V) having the amino acid sequence similar
to that of IV showed a considerably weak activity on the guinea
pig colon preparation as compared with IV. Bradykinin analogues
I and III in which penta- or hexa-peptide connects to the C-
terminus of the bradykinin molecule also showed lower activities
on both preparations than those of N^α-tyrosyl-bradykinin and
kallidin having an additional amino acid residue at the N-terminus
of the bradykinin molecule. All synthetic fragments of bradykinin-
like peptides exhibited significantly reduced activities.

TABLE 2.

RELATIVE CONTRACTING ACTIVITIES OF BRADYKININ-RELATED
PEPTIDES ON GUINEA PIG INTESTINE

Compound	Ileum	Colon
Bradykinin	Accepted as 100	Accepted as 100
N^{α}-Tyrosyl-bradykinin	106.0	96.9
Kallidin	78.8	83.1
Bradykinyl-Val-Ala-Pro-Ala-Ser-OH (I)	6.3	28.6
Bradykinyl-Val-Ala-Pro-Ala-Ser-OH (5-14)	1.8	4.5
Bradykinyl-Val-Ala-Pro-Ala-Ser-OH (7-14)	4.2	4.8
[Thr^6]-Bradykinyl-Ile-Ala-Pro-Glu-Ile-Val-OH (III)	9.8	21.9
Bradykinyl-Gly-Lys-Phe-His-OH (5-13)	-	33.4
Bradykinyl-Gly-Lys-Phe-His-OH (5-13) (ε-Boc)	4.0	tonus reduction
Bradykinyl-Gly-Lys-Phe-His-OH (11-13) (ε-Boc)	-	7.5
Vespakinin X (IV)	72.0	95.6
Vespakinin X (6-12)	-	12.1
Vespakinin M (V)	-	28.8
Vespakinin M (6-12)	-	13.8
Bradykinin (5-9)	-	3.4

Magnus's Method (Tyrode sol.   36.5°C)

TABLE 3.

RELATIVE CROSSREACTIVITIES OF BRADYKININ-RELATED PEPTIDES
IN BRADYKININ RIA

Bradykinin	Accepted as 100
N^{α}-Tyrosyl-bradykinin	100
Kallidin	100
Bradykinyl-Val-Ala-Pro-Ala-Ser-OH (I)	0.1
Bradykinyl-Val-Ala-Pro-Ala-Ser-OH (7-14)	0.1
[Thr^6]-Bradykinyl-Ile-Ala-Pro-Glu-Ile-Val-OH (III)	0.1
Vespakinin X (IV)	0.1
Vespakinin M (V)	0.1

Immunological property

The radioimmunoassay was performed by the dextran-coated charcoal method using synthetic bradykinin as standard and ^{125}I-N^{α}-tyrosyl-bradykinin as tracer. The labelled compound was prepared by radioiodinated of N^{α}-tyrosyl-bradykinin according to the method of Hunter and Greenwood (1962). Anti-bradykinin serum R-3601 conjugate was used in the assay. Bradykinin radioimmunoassay using ^{125}I-N^{α}-tyrosyl-bradykinin as tracer has been described by Odya et al. (1978). The dose-response curve of N^{α}-tyrosyl-bradykinin and kallidin were superimposable on that of standard bradykinin. On the other hand, none of the bradykinin-like peptides such as I, III, IV and V competed with the tracer at the concentrations employed, although the nonapeptide sequence of bradykinin is embodied in their molecules. The results are summarized in Table 3.

DISCUSSION

In the present investigation, [Thr^6]-bradykinyl-Ile-Ala-Pro-Glu-Ile-Val-OH (III) which had been isolated from frog (Rana rugosa) shin extract was synthesized by the conventional method for peptide synthesis. The resulting pentadecapeptide with a high degree of purity was found to be identical with that of the natural origin with respect to chemical and biological properties. Vespakinin-X and vespakinin-M were also synthesized according to manners similar to that employed for preparation of III. Both synthetic dodeca-peptides were proved to possess chemical and biological properties identical to those of naturally occurring vespakinin-X and M, respectively. In addition, N^{α}-tyrosyl-bradykinin and kallidin were synthesized to use for development of bradykinin radioimmunoassay system.

The bradykinin-like peptides prepared in the present study were assayed in vitro on isolated guinea pig ileum and colon. The activites of bradykinyl-Val-Ala-Pro-Ala-Ser-OH (I) and the fragments of bradykinyl-Gly-Lys-Phe-His-OH (II) were also compared. N^{α}-Tyrosyl-bradykinin and vespakinin-X were found to be very active in both assay systems, while I, III and V and the fragments of these peptides possessed considerably weak activites. Bradykinyl-Ile-Tyr-OH, desulfated phyllokinin, was also reported to be less active than bradykinin on all preparations tested (Anastasi et al., 1966). It is of interest that vespakinin-X possesses higher activity on guinea pig colon than vespakinin-M containing hydroxyproline (Hyp) residue in position 4. [Hyp^3]-Bradykinin was described to possess rather high potency on guinea pig ileum (Stewart et al., 1974). Although the bradykinin-like peptides with amino acid residues attached at the C-terminus of the bradykinin molecule were less

active than bradykinin, these peptides exhibited significant stimu-
lant action on guinea pig colon rather than on the ileum.

Striking observations are that any of the synthetic peptides
of the present study having lengthened peptide chains with exception
of kallidin and N$^\alpha$-tyrosyl-bradykinin did not displace the tracer
in the radioimmunoassay system developed. The result suggests
that the antigenic determinants of bradykinin may be masked by the
extension of the peptide chains.

The synthetic bradykinin-related peptides and their fragments
prepared in the present investigation may be useful substrates for
study of kinin-kininogen system.

REFERENCES

Anastasi, A., G. Bertaccini and V. Erspamer, 1966, Pharmacological
    data on phyllokinin (bradykinylisoleucyltyrosine O-sulfate) and
    bradykinylisoleucyltyrosine, Brit.J.Pharmacol., 27,479.
Anderson, G.W., J.E. Zimmerman and F.M. Callahan, 1964, The use of
    esters of N-hydroxysuccinimide in peptide synthesis, J.Amer.Chem.
    Soc., 86,1839.
Anderson, G.M., J.E. Zimmerman and F.M. Callahan, 1966, Racemiza-
    tion control in the synthesis of peptides by the mixed carbonic-
    carboxylic anhydride method, J.Amer.Chem.Soc., 88,1338.
Hunter, W.M., and F.C. Greenwood, 1962, Preparation of iodine-131
    labelled human growth hormone of high specific activity, Nature
    (London), 194,495.
Kitamura, H., T. Yasuhara, H. Yoshida and T. Nakajima, 1976,
    Vespakinin-M, a novel bradykinin analogue containing hydroxy-
    proline, in the venom of Vespa mandarinia Smith, Chem.Pharm.Bull.,
    24,2896.
Nakajima, T., 1968, On the third active peptide on smooth muscle in
    the skin of Rana nigromaculata, Chem.Pharm.Bull., 16,2088.
Odya, C.E., T.L. Goodfriend, J.M. Stewart and C. Pena, 1978, Aspects
    of bradykinin radioimmunoassay, J.Immunological Methods, 19,243.
Stewart, J.M., J.W.Ryan and A.H. Brady, 1974, Hydroxyproline analogs
    of bradykinin, J.Med.Chem., 17,537.
Yanaihara, N., C. Yanaihara, M. Sakagami, T. Nakajima, T. Nakayama
    and K. Matsumoto, 1973, Synthesis of bradykinyl-Val-Ala-Pro-Ala-
    Ser-OH and its biological properties, Chem.Pharm.Bull., 21,616.
Yasuhara, T., M. Hira, T. Nakajima, N. Yanaihara, C. Yanaihara,
    T. Hashimoto, N. Sakura, S. Tachibana, K. Araki, M. Bessho and
    T. Yamanaka, 1973, Active peptides on smooth muscle in the
    skin of Bombina orientalis Boulenger and characterization of a
    new bradykinin analogue, Chem.Pharm.Bull., 21,1388.

Yasuhara, T., O. Ishikawa, T. Nakajima and S. Tachibana, 1975.
    The active substances on smooth muscle in the skin of Rana
    rugosa, Proceedings of the 12th Symposium on Peptide Chemistry,
    ed. H. Yajima, Protein Research Foundation, Osaka, pp 168 (in
    Japanese).
Yasuhara, T., H. Yoshida and T. Nakajima, 1977. Chemical investi-
    gation of the hornet (Vespa xanthoptera Cameron) venom. The
    structure of a new bradykinin analogue "vespakinin-X",
    Chem. Pharm. Bull, 25: 936.

ENZYME IMMUNOASSAY OF BRADYKININ

Akinori Ueno, Sachiko Oh-Ishi, Tsunehiro Kitagawa* and
Makoto Katori
Department of Pharmacology, Kitasato University, School
Of Medicine, Sagamihara, Kanagawa 228 and *Faculty of
Pharmaceutical Sciences, Nagasaki University, Nagasaki
852, Japan

ABSTRACT

An enzyme immunoassay of bradykinin was developed by using β-
D-galactosidase as a labeling enzyme. Bradykinin was conjugated
to β-D-galactosidase with a new coupling agent of a hetero bis-
functional type, N-(m-maleimidobenzoyloxy)-succinimide (MBS).
Antisera were obtained from rabbits immunized with bradykinin linked to albumins (ovalbumin or bovine serum albumin) with toluene-
2,4-diisocyanate. Double antibody method was employed to separate
the antibody-bound antigen from free. The enzyme activity in the
precipitate was measured with a fluorogenic substrate, 4-methyl-
umbelliferyl-β-D-galactoside. This assay is based on heterogeneous
competitive binding between unlabeled and labeled antigens, so that
unlabeled bradykinin reduces binding of bradykinin-enzyme conjugates to the antibody. A standard inhibition curve was linear between 3 and 300 ng bradykinin/assay tube.

Bradykinin, Kininogen, Enzyme immunoassay, β-D-galactosidase,
N-(m-maleimidobenzoyloxy)-succinimide, Fluorometry.

INTRODUCTION

For the determination of bradykinin (BK), bioassay is widely
used, but radioimmunoassay (RIA) has lately taken a place of bioassay, since the sensitivity and specificity of RIA have been improved to be comparable to bioassay (Spragg et al., 1966; Rinderknecht
et al., 1967; Talamo et al., 1968; Goodfriend and Ball, 1969,
Webster et al., 1970; Odya et al., 1978). More recently, an enzyme

195

immunoassay (EIA), in which enzymes are used as labeling antigens, has been developed for the measurement of the concentration of hormones and drugs in biological fluids (Schuurs and Van Weeman, 1977). EIA, using β-D-galactosidase from E. coli (EC 3.2.1.23), has been developed for insulin (Kitagawa and Aikawa, 1976), viomycin (Kitagawa et al., 1978) and angiotensin I (Suzuki et al., 1978) and is used for clinical applications. The working ranges of these assays were reported as 20 - 200, 1.5 - 200 and 100 - 4,000 pg, respectively. In this report, the authors describe the development of EIA of bradykinin, using the same enzyme (β-D-galactosidase) as a labeling enzyme.

MATERIALS AND METHODS

Preparation of the BK-β-D-galactosidase conjugate. Preparation of the BK-β-D-galactosidase conjugate was carried in the way similar to that reported previously (Kitagawa and Aikawa, 1976; Kitagawa et al., 1978; Suzuki et al., 1978) (Fig. 1). Briefly, a solution of bradykinin triacetate (1.5 μmole) (Peptide Institute Inc., Minoh, Osaka, Japan) in 75 mM phosphate buffer (pH 7.0, 1 ml) was mixed with 0.375 ml of a solution of N-(m-maleimidobenzoyloxy)-succinimide (MBS) in the presence of tetrahydrofuran. The MBS-acylated bradykinin (3.6 nmole of maleimide) was conjugated to β-D-galactosidase (Boehringer Mannheim, W. Germany) (0.93 nmole) in 1/15 M phosphate buffer (pH 7.0). The solution of β-D-galactosidase-BK conjugate was stable over a year at 4°C. The enzyme activity of β-D-galactosidase was not interfered by the conjugation with bradykinin.

Preparation of antisera to bradykinin. a) Immunogens. Bradykinin triacetate (32.7 mg) reacted with toluene-2,4-diisocyanate (75 μl) (Nakarai Chemicals Ltd., Nagoya, Japan) and then bovine serum albumin (Fraction V, Sigma, St. Louis, Mo.) (20 mg) or ovalbumin (Grade VI, Sigma) (20 mg) was added to the mixture as described by other reports (Talamo et al., 1968; Spragg et al., 1966). Amino acid analysis of the immunogens and albumins or all amino acids except cystein was performed. b) Immunization of animals. Two mg of the BK-albumin conjugates per animal was injected into foot pads of four male rabbits. Two of them were immunized with BK-ovalbumin (OA) conjugate and others were with BK-bovine serum albumin (BSA) conjugate. After 5 months, the emulsion of incomplete Freund's adjuvant (Difco Labs., Detroit, Mich.) containing 1 mg of the conjugates was injected into multiple subcutaneous sites on the backs of the rabbits. The second and the third booster injections (100 μg/animal) were performed at 2-4 weeks intervals. Rabbit blood was collected for testing titer from the ear artery into a plastic tube (#2006, Falcon, Oxnard, Calif.). Serum was centrifuged at 2,000 g for 20 min at 4°C and stored at -70°C until used.

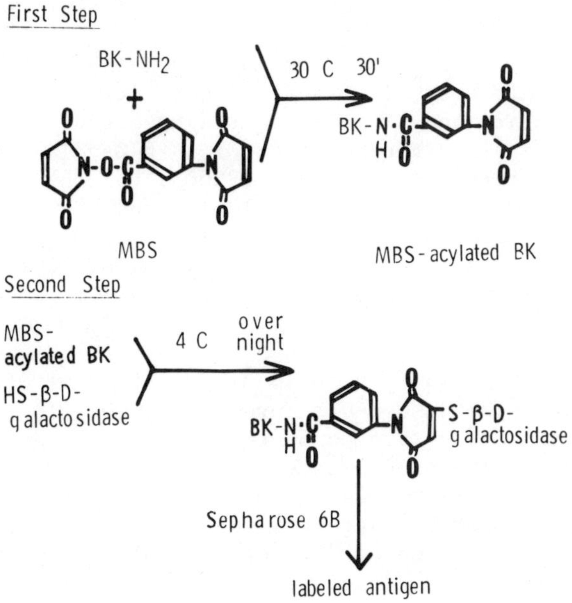

Fig. 1. The preparation of the BK-β-D-galactosidase conjugate with N-(m-maleimidobenzoyloxy)-succinimide (MBS). BK: bradykinin.

Assay of the activity of β-D-galactosidase. The activity of β-D-galactosidase was measured using 4-methylumbelliferyl-β-D-galactoside (Nakarai Chemicals Ltd., Nagoya, Japan) as a substrate. The amount of the released fluorescence was measured by fluorescence spectrophotometer (MPF-3, Hitachi Ltd., Tokyo).

Preparation of ^{125}I-Tyr[1]-kallidin. Tyr[1]-kallidin (Peptide Institute Inc., Minoh, Osaka) was iodinate with Na[125]I (The Radiochemical Centre, Amersham, England) by using chloramin-T method (Odya et al., 1978). ^{125}I-Tyr[1]-kallidin (10,000 cpm/tube) in Buffer B, was used for radioimmunoassay and other conditions were the same as that reported by Odya et al. (1978).

Determination of total kininogen in normal human plasma. Citrated normal human plasma was heated at 60°C for 30 min and then incubated with trypsin as reported (Uchida and Katori, 1978). In this method, as total kininogen is known to be converted to bradykinin, the released bradykinin was assayed by this EIA.

Buffers. Buffer A. 0.02 M sodium phosphate buffer, pH 7.0, containing 0.1 M NaCl, 0.1% NaN$_3$, 0.1% bovine serum albumin and 2 mM MgCl$_2$. Buffer B. 0.02 M sodium phosphate buffer, pH 7.0, containing 0.1 M NaCl, 0.1% NaN$_3$, 0.1% bovine serum albumin, 2.7 mM EDTA-2Na and 0.003 M 1,10-phenanthroline.

RESULTS

Assay procedure of enzyme immunoassay (EIA) of bradykinin (BK).
A principle of this assay is based on competitive binding between
unlabeled bradykinin and BK-β-D-galactosidase conjugate to anti-BK
antiserum. Fifty μl of the solution of BK-β-D-galactosidase (4
μunit) was mixed in a plastic tubes (#2005, Falcon) with 50 μl of
sample or unlabeled BK (3-300 ng) solution and 50 μl of the anti-
BK antiserum in Buffer B. The total volume was 0.25 ml. After the
mixture was incubated for 18 hr at 4°C, 10 μl of 10-fold diluted
solution of non-immunized rabbit IgG antiserum from goat were added
to each tube.

After further incubation for 6 hr at 4°C, 2 ml of Buffer A was
added, throughly mixed and centrifuged at 2,000 g for 30 min at
4°C. The supernate was removed by decanting. The activity of β-
D-galactosidase in the precipitate was assayed by adding 300 μl of
0.2 mM 4-methylumbelliferyl-β-D-galactoside in Buffer A. The mixture was incubated for 2 hr at 37°C with shaking. The reaction
was terminated by addition of 3 ml of cold 0.2 M sodium phosphate
buffer (pH 10.3). Fluorescence was read at 365 nm (excitation) and
448 nm (emission).

Amino acid analysis of BK-albumin conjugates in comparison
with albumin. For production of anti-BK antibody, BK-bovine serum
albumin or BK-ovalbumin conjugates were injected into rabbit foot
pads as immunogens. Preliminary result on amino acid analysis of
these BK-albumin conjugates is shown in comparison with that of
albumins in Table 1. The differences of number of amino acids between bovine serum albumin (BSA) and BK-BSA indicates that 3 to 11
moles of BK was conjugated to BSA. If one would consider that the
coupling agent, toluene-2,4-diisocyanate, reacts with arginine of
N-terminal of BK and lysine of BSA, the reduced number of arginine
of BK (3.7 mole) and lysine of BSA (10.9 mole) could be explained.
Thus, the number of BK conjugated to BSA might be at least 7 to 8
moles per mole of BSA. In the same way, that of bradykinin conjugated to ovalbumin (OA) might be 4 to 5 moles per mole of OA.

Characteristics of antisera to bradykinin. Antisera to BK
were obtained from rabbits immunized with BK-bovine serum albumin
or BK-ovalbumin. Antibody was slowly developed in all rabbits and
reached to the peak levels 2 months after the initial injection.
An antiserum which was obtained from a rabbit (AS-4) 9 months after
the initial immunization of BK-bovine serum albumin and the subsequent booster injections, showed 20-40% binding of the labeled
antigen in dilution of 1 : 200,000.

Binding of the labeled antigen in various dilution rates was
tested using AS-4. Four μunits of BK-β-D-galactosidase was incubated with 50 μl of the antiserum diluted at various rates (Fig. 2).

Table 1. Amino acid analysis of bradykinin-albumin conjugates in comparison with albumin.
Bovine serum albumin (BSA) contains 17 His and 54 Asp residues and ovalbumin (OA) contains 8 His and 32 Asp residues, in one molecule of each albumin. Parenthesis indicates moles of amino acid content of bradykinin (BK).

	BSA	BSA-BK	molar excess	BK calculated	OA	OA-BK	molar excess	BK calculated
Lys	55.8	44.9	-10.9		23.8	19.2	-4.6	
His	17	17			8	8		
Arg(2)	20.6	27.9	7.3	3.7	17.0	19.8	2.8	1.4
Asp	54	54			32	32		
Ser(1)	21.4	32.2	7.8	7.8	33.6	37.1	3.5	3.5
Pro(3)	24.7	48.0	23.3	7.8	14.4	27.5	13.1	4.4
Gly(1)	12.9	24.5	11.6	11.6	17.9	22.4	4.5	4.5
Phe(2)	22.3	38.9	16.6	8.3	17.0	27.1	10.1	5.1

The enzyme activity in the bound complex was well related to the dilution rates of the antiserum. This indicates specific binding of the antiserum to BK-β-D-galactosidase.

Standard curve of bradykinin. Competitive binding between un-labeled bradykinin and BK-β-D-galactosidase occurred in proportion to the amount of bradykinin added. A linear relationship was obtained when plotted on logit scale in ordinate (Fig. 3). In the case of rabbit No. AS-4, at least 3 ng/tube of bradykinin could be detected and 50% inhibition of binding was achieved at 30 ng/tube of unlabeled bradykinin.

The application to the measurement of total kininogen. Human kininogen level was measured by conversion of kininogens to BK. The value estimated by this EIA was 3.7 µg BK eq/ml plasma and that by RIA was 4.4 µg. Usually normal human plasma contains 4.1 µg BK eq/ml plasma by Uchida's method using bioassay (Uchida and Katori, 1978).

A standard curve was made on logit scale in ordinate. B_o = the enzyme activity in the absence of unlabeled BK, B = the enzyme activity in the sample or in the presence of the known amount of bradykinin as a standard. Abscissa: ng of unlabeled bradykinin/tube on logarithmic scale.

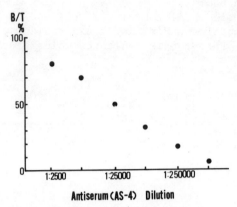

Fig. 2. Binding of enzyme-labeled bradykinin to progressive dilution of the antiserum of rabbit No. AS-4.
Abscissa: Final dilution of the serum. Ordinate: Percentage of the
antibody-bound antigens (B) in the total antigens added (T) (20
μunits of β-D-galactosidase). For the routine assay, the serum
dilution which bound about 30% of B/T was used.

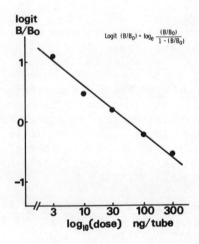

Fig. 3. Standard curve of bradykinin.

DISCUSSION

An enzyme immunoassay (EIA), using an enzyme for labeling of the compounds instead of isotope, would be harmless from the ecological point of view. Other merit of the EIA is that the method could measure bradykinin (BK) itself. A bi-unifunctional type of coupling agents is generally used for the EIA. It reacts with amino groups, thus making it difficult to avoid polymerization. On the contrary, N-(m-maleimidobenzoyloxy)-succinimide (MBS) was used as a hetero bis-functional type of coupling agents which has an active ester group on the one side and maleimide residues on the other side. Thus, using MBS method, no polymerization could occur if a hapten reacts at the first step contains no SH group. In the case of viomycin (Kitagawa et al., 1978) and antiotensin I (Suzuki et al., 1978), one mole of ligand was shown to be conjugated to one mole of β-D-galactosidase. Further, the labeled compound, BK-β-D-galactosidase, is stable over a year at 4° C. Whereas in RIA, ^{125}I-labeled antigen decays rapidly so that the assay may be expensive and troublesome.

The number of bradykinin conjugated to bovine serum albumin of ovalbumin were important as an immunogen for production of high quality of the anti-BK antibody. The numbers of bradykinin were estimated by amino acid analysis. Seven to eleven moles of bradykinin was found to be conjugated to bovine serum albumin and three to four moles to ovalbumin. These numbers were different from those reported in other papers, in which one mole of bradykinin is coupled to ovalbumin (Talamo et al., 1968) or two moles of bradykinin to ovalbumin (Webster et al., 1970), although the preparation method of the conjugates in the present paper was the same as that in the report (Talamo et al., 1968; Spragg et al., 1966). This effective BK immunogen may have produced the high quality of the antibody in rabbit No. AS-4 in this study, so that 20-40% of binding percentages was obtained by the diluted serum of 1 : 200,000.

The sensitivity of the method to detect 3 ng of bradykinin was not sufficient enough to detect free bradykinin in plasma or body fluid in pathological states. The improvement of this method is certainly required.

ACKNOWLEDGEMENT

Authors are indebted to Ms. Etsuko Nagata, Kitasato University School of Medicine, for amino acid analysis.

This work was supported partly by Scientific Research Grants from the Ministry of Education, Sciences and Culture (310507 and 387061).

REFERENCES

Goodfriend, T.L. and D.L. Ball, 1969, Radioimmunoassay of bradykinin: chemical modification to enable use of radioactive iodine,
J. Lab. Clin. Med. 73, 501.

Kitagawa, T. and T. Aikawa, 1976, Enzyme coupled immunoassay of
insulin using a novel coupling reagent, J. Biochem. 79, 233.

Kitagawa, T., T. Fujitake, H. Taniyama and T. Aikawa, 1978, Enzyme
immunoassay of viomycin; new cross-linking reagent for the enzyme
labeling and a preparation method for antiserum to viomycin, J.
Biochem. 83, 1493.

Odya, C.E., T.L. Goodfriend, J.M. Stewart and C. Pena, 1978, Aspects of bradykinin radioimmunoassay, J. Immunol. Method 19, 243.

Rinderknecht, H., B.J. Haverback and F. Aladjem, 1967, Radioimmunoassay of bradykinin, Nature 213, 1130.

Sohuurs, A.H.W.M. and B.K. Van Weeman, 1977, Enzyme immunoassay,
Clin. Chim. Acta 81, 1.

Spragg, J., K.F. Austen and E. Haber, 1966, Production of antibody
against bradykinin: Demonstration of specificity by complement
fixation and radioimmunoassay, J. Immunol. 96, 865.

Suzuki, S., M. Murayama, K. Hashiba, T. Aikawa and T. Kitagawa,
1978, Measurement of plasma renin activity by enzyme immunoassay
of angiotensin I, Igaku no Ayumi 101, 723 (in Japanese).

Talamo, R.C., E. Haber and K.F. Austen, 1968, Antibody to bradykinin: effect of carrier and method of coupling on specificity
and affinity, J. Immunol. 101, 333.

Uchida, Y. and M. Katori, 1978, An improved method for determination of the total kininogen in rabbit and human plasma, Biochem.
Pharmacol. 27, 1463.

Webster, M.E., J.V. Pierce and M.U. Sampaio, Studies on antibody
to bradykinin, 1970, in: Advances in Experimental Medicine and
Biology, Vol. 8, eds. F. Sicuteri, M. Rocha e Silva and N. Back
(Plenum Press, New York - London) p. 57.

ASSAY OF ANGIOTENSIN I BY FLUORESCENCE POLARIZATION METHOD

Hiroshi Maeda*, Mahito Nakayama, Daisuke Iwaoka and
Tatsuo Sato

Departments of Microbiology* and Internal Medicine
Kumamoto University Medical School, Kumamoto, Japan 860

ABSTRACT

Fluorescence polarization technique was applied for the assay
of angiotensin I (Al) in human plasma. In this assay system, fluorescein labeled Al (F-Al), which retained the original antigenicity,
and antibody to Al was allowed to interact in a cuvette in the
instruments yielding an increase in the fluorescence polarization
(P) value. Non-labeled Al in the sample blocked the binding of
F-Al to the antibody resulting lower P value. Log of antigen
concentration and P value was found to exhibit reverse linear
proportionality between 0.05 ng to 2 ng/ml of antigen (Al) concentration. The present method was compared with standard radioimmunoassay method and the result showed that data were compatible
with each other. The calculation of P value is automated and three
cavity filter and optics of the instrument gave reliable results.
The method is fast (<2 min), sensitive (<10 picomole/ml) and simple
(no separation step before readout of the results).

INTRODUCTION

Fluorescence polarization (FP) pioneered by Perrin (1926),
was extended by Weber (1953) and others and applied to the study
of the physicochemical behavior of proteins. Later, Dandliker
et al.(1961), Kierszenbaum et al. (1969), Watson et al. (1976),
McGregor et al. (1978) and Maeda (1978) have applied FP method
for the determination of albumin, insulin, ovalbumin, phenytoin,
gentamycin and neocarzinostatin based on the antigen-antibody
reaction. In this system increased molecular weight of the labeled
molecules is reflected as a higher P value of the complex thus

203

formed, which is determined by the fluorescence polarization spectrophotometer. We have shown that such P values are indeed reflecting
respective molecular weight (Maeda, 1979). Using automated FP
instrument, the measurement of a P value is carried out very easily
within 82 seconds without separation process. The value is an
average of an integrated reading of one hundred times for a period
of 50 seconds, thus the improved instrument exhibited very high
accuracy and reproducibility (Maeda, 1978). Despite of this
progress, general application of the FP method is, however, limited
until now. The purpose of the present report is to extend an
application of FP method further for the determination of Al.

MATERIALS AND METHODS

Chemicals

Angiotensin I (Al) is a synthetic product (cat. No. 4007-V)
obtained from Protein Research Foundation, Osaka, Japan. FITC
(fluorescein isothiocyanate) was obtained from Sigma Chemical Co.,
St. Louis, Mo. 63178, or Dojindo Chemical Co., Ltd., Kumamoto 860
Japan. Anti-angiotensin I antibody (anti-Al) was obtained from
Calbiochem. San Diego, Calif. 92037; (rabbit serum, cat. No. 869093,
Lot. 420037). All other chemicals were obtained from commercial
sources.

Instrumental Information

JIMCO (Japan Immunoresearch Co. Ltd., Takasaki, 370 Japan)
fluorescence polarization spectrophotometer, Model MAC-2, type HR-
1, was employed for the measurement of P value. The instrument is
equipped with a primary polarizer, an excitation filter for about
490 nm, a cell housing, an analyser-polarizer that is driven by a
synchronous motor at 1,800 rpm, an emission filter for 520 nm and
a photomultiplier (Hamamatsu Televi Co., Ltd., R105 UH) which
responds as low as 30 µA/Lm on cathode with standing time of 2.6 n
sec. Both filters were a product of Ditric Optics Inc. (Marborough,
Mass. 02176) and they yield almost monochromatic spectra band with
small loss in transmission. A diagram is shown to represent the
instruments in Fig. 1. A built-in microcomputer is also furnished
in the instrument which will calculate the P value as defined in
the next equation.

$$P = \frac{IA - IB}{IA + IB} \quad ------ \quad (1)$$

Where IA is the fluorescence polarization intensity measured with
the secondary polarizer at parallel position (to the primary polarizer), while IB is that at perpendicular position.

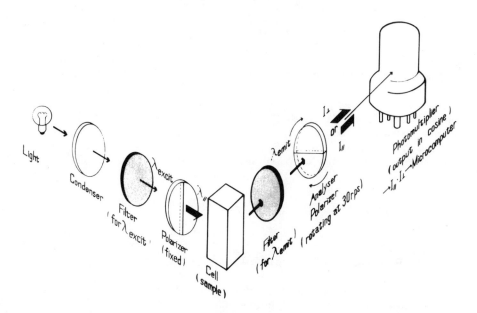

Figure 1.   Diagram of polarization fluorophotometer JIMCO Model
            MAC-2, type HR-1. The light source is a 30W/110V
            tungsten bulb. The second polarizer (analyser)
            rotates at 1,800 rpm and thus the output of the
            photomultiplier is a cosine function of the angle of
            rotation. From this DC-output, P value in eq. (1)
            is calculated with a built-in microcomputer. Three
            cavity filters used in the instrument for both
            excitation and emission spectra yield near mono-
            chromatic wavelength and free from depolarization
            as is a case of grating-type monochrometer and they
            eliminate effectively back-ground noise.

Temperature Control

     The main cause of the error of FP method resides on this
point. Thus the temperature of the instrument must be kept
constant during measurement. "U-cool" constant temperature cir-
culator (± 0.02°C) (Neslab Ist. Inc., Portsmouth, N.H.) was used
for this purpose. Operating room is air-conditioned.

FITC-labeling and Stability of the Labeled Al

The antigen was labeled with FITC as described (Maeda et al., 1969) in 0.5 M carbonate buffer at pH 9.0 and room temperature for about four hours. Primary amino group of the N-terminal Asp residue is the target of the reaction and the fluorescein thiocarbamyl Al (F-Al) was separated by Sephadex G-25 or G-50 and lyophilized. Prolonged standing and excessive exposure to light resulted in a gradual release of free chromophore, perhaps spontaneous hydantoin formation and cleavage of aspartyl residue (Maeda and Kawauchi, 1968). Therefore, unnecessary acidic pH and exposure to light were avoided and F-Al was stored at -20°C (frozen) until use. F-Al retained original antigenicity.

Preparation of Assay Samples (Angiotensin I: antigen)

The method was adapted from the method of Oparil (1976) with some modifications as shown in Fig. 2. Isolation of renin-generated Al is as follows: Sample plasma (1 ml) was adjusted to have pH 6.0 with 1 M acetic acid and the volume was made up to 2 ml with 0.1 M Na acetate buffer, pH 6.0. The two fold diluted plasma was incubated at 37°C for 2 hours at first in order to generate Al by renin in the plasma, in which Al destroying enzymes were inhibited by excess EDTA (0.03 M) and 15 mM phenyl methyl sulfonyl fluoride (PMSF). Then, renin activity was stopped by boiling at

EDTA-Plasma (1 ml)

   Add EDTA and PMSF* to give
   final conc. of 30 mM and
   15 mM respectively

Boil, 100°C, 10 min.

Centrifuge, 2,500 rpm, 20 min.

Remove supernatant for assay

Figure 2.   Preparation of a sample of angiotensin I:
Renin activity in plasma.
*PMSF: phenyl methyl sulfonyl fluoride.

about 100°C for 10 min, followed by centrifugation. The supernatant thus obtained was used as the assay sample. Standard curve of AI was obtained similarly using synthetic AI and diluted with normal serum in the presence of the inhibitors followed by boiling and centrifugation. The serum concentration of AI is negligibly small (<5 pg/ml).

Assay of Antibody to Angiotensin I

An aliquot of F-AI (about 0.13 ng/ml) was placed in a cuvette containing 2 ml of 0.05 M tris-HCl buffer (pH 7.4) at 20.0°C. With such amount of fluorochrome, the anode voltage of the photomultiplier indicated about 680. Then the antibody, dissolved in 0.01 M phosphate buffered saline (pH 7.4) to give a 100 fold dilution of the antiserum (Calbiochem), was added in 40 μl aliquot. P value was obtained for each addition of antibody in 82 sec. directly.

Assay of Antigen (Angiotensin I: AI)

Three components were employed in the experiment: a sample or antigen preparation, F-AI and anti-AI antibody. To a cuvette containing 1 ml of 0.3 M tris-HCl buffer (pH 7.4), 1 ml of AI containing sample (supernatant) followed by the diluted antibody (40 μl) were added and they were allowed to react for 5 min at 20°C. Then F-AI (0.5 ng) was added to the cuvette similarly. The amount of fluorochrome added yielded the anode voltage no more than 730 (maximum operational capacity; 1,000 V). A standard curve was obtained for the supernatant of the boiled serum with appropriate amount of added AI in the presence of inhibitors and a linear increment of P value was observed in accordance with the amount of synthetic material added.

RESULTS

Assay of Antibody to Angiotensin I

In Figure 3, the result of stepwise addition of the anti-AI antibody is shown. The increase of P value paralleled with each addition of the antibody until all F-AI was consumed by the antibody, where further addition of antibody resulted in little increase in P value (plateau).

Assay of Angiotensin I in Plasma: Renin Activity

Standard cruve of synthetic AI which was diluted with normal serum is shown in Figure 4. This data was compared with that of radioimmunoassay and appears compatible with each other. The amount of AI determined by FP method is between 0.1 to 10 ng in

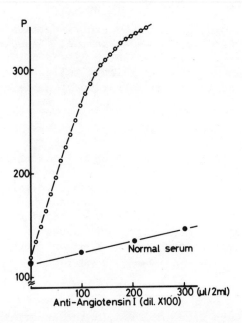

Figure 3.   Titration of fluorescein-labeled antigen (angiotensin I)
             with its antibody. P value increases when more antigen-
             antibody complex is formed with increasing amount of
             antibody (abscissa). A lower (closed circles) indicates
             normal serum (no antibody). P value : arbitrary unit.

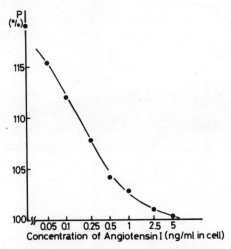

Figure 4.   Determination of angiotensin I in plasma. Dose response
             between P value (% of change) and the concentration of
             the antigen (Al). About 40 µl of 100x-diluted antisera
             (rabbit) is used.

the cuvette. One ml plasma was found to be adequate in amount and
it appears to be a practical method. Twenty samples from healthy
and hypertensive persons were chosen at random and subjected for
both FP and radioimmunoassay and the result indicated reliable
(P<0.05) if A1 concentration is below 1 ng/ml in plasma.

DISCUSSION

Assay of renin activity, based on the antigenicity of A1, in
human plasma was determined by FP method. The data corresponded
well with that obtained by radioimmunoassay below 1 ng/ml. Furthermore, assay of antibody is very simple if a labeled antigen is
available. These results can be obtained almost immediately.
Thus, FP method is advantageous over other methods which require
usually an incubation period of overnight. The labeling procedure
in FP method is much easier than radio isotope labeling and a
shelf-life of the derivative is longer than, for example, that of
^{125}I when stored properly. The assay of either antigen or antibody is rapid because P value is printed out in 82 sec, and simple
because no separation step of the bound or unbound is necessary.
The operation of the instrument is very simple due to automation;
no calculation of the equation (1) is required. The accuracy and
reproducibility is high owing to the integration of one hundred
readings before printout of a P value (Maeda, 1968). The interference of serum protein to the P value due to its variable
viscosity of plasma was eliminated by deproteination (heat denaturation and centrifugation) in case of A1.

The three cavity filters, which are free from depolarization,
used in the instrument, appear very effective to eliminate scat-
tered light or Raman effect (peak at 581 nm) (Jameson and Weber,
1978) becuase of the near monochromatic performance of the filters.
The emission spectrum (520 nm) of FITC is far from excitation wavelength (490 nm), and they are remote from autofluorescence of
proteins.

All the above data appears very promising, although we have
not pursued all possible deviations in the practical plasma samples
such as that from cancer patients, or patients with complications
from different plasma preparations - old heparinized or two days
old EDTA plasma etc. We have obtained so far reliable results
when A1 concentration is less than 1 ng/ml but more than 0.05 ng/ml
in plasma. FP method appears more convenient and sensitive than
radioisotope derivatization assay (Gregerman and Kowatch, 1972).
Dilution of high A1 concentration in the supernatant should be
carried out with supernatant of heat denatured serum as a diluent.
If a buffer solution is used, variations of the viscosity may
affect P value. More extensive studies will warrant general
practice.

Present results will encourage further application of this
method to other peptide hormones in general.

REFERENCES

Dandliker, W.B. and G.A. Feigen, 1961. Quantification of the anti-
    gen-antibody reaction by the polarization of fluorescence.
    Biochem. Biophys. Res. Comm. 5: 299.
Gregerman, R.I. and M. A. Kowatch, 1972. Isotope derivative assay
    of nanogram quantities of angiotensin I: Use for renin measu-
    rement in plasma. Chemistry and Biology of Peptide, ed. J.
    Meienhofer, (Ann Arbor Science Pub. Inc., Ann Arbor, Mich).
    p. 533.
Haber, E. and J.C. Bennett, 1962. Polarization of fluorescence as
    a measurement of antigen-antibody interaction. Proc. Nat.
    Acad. Sci. USA. 48: 1935.
Jameson, R.D. and G. Weber, 1978. Fluorescence polarization: Measu-
    rements with a photon counting photometer. Rev. Sci. Instrum.
    49: 510.
Kierszenbaum, F., J. Dandliker and W.B. Dandliker, 1969. Investi-
    gation of the antigen antibody reaction by fluorescence
    polarization: Measurement of the effect of the fluorescent
    label upon the bovine serum albumin (BSA) and anti-BSA equili-
    brium. Immunochem. 6: 125.
Maeda, H. and H. Kawauchi, 1968. A new mehtod for the determination
    of N-terminus of peptide chain with fluorescein isothio-
    cyanate. Biochem. Biophys. Res. Comm. 31: 188.
Maeda, H., H. Kawauchi, N. Ishida and K. Tsuzimura, 1969. Reaction
    of fluorescein isothiocyanate with proteins and amino acids.
    I. Covalent and non-covalent binding of fluorescein isothio-
    cyanate and fluorescein to proteins. J. Biochemistry (Tokyo)
    65: 777.
Maeda, H., 1978. Assay of an antitumor protein, neocarzinostatin,
    and its antibody by fluorescence polarization. Clin. Chem.
    24: December issue.
Maeda, H., 1979. Assay of proteolytic enzymes by fluorescence
    polarization. Anal. Biochem. (January issue, in press).
McGregor, A.R., J.O. Crokall-Greening, J. Landon and D.S. Smith,
    1978. Polarization fluoroimmunoassay of phenytoin. Clin.
    Chim. Acta 83: 161.
Oparil, S., 1976. Theoretical approaches to estimation of renin
    activity: A review and some original observations. Clin. Chem.
    22: 583.
Perrin, M.F., 1926. Polarization de la lumiere de fluorescence.
    Vie myenne des molecules dans l'etat excité. J. Phys. Radium.
    7: 390.
Spencer, R.D., F.B. Toledo, T.B. Williams and N.L. Yoss, 1973.
    Design, construction and two applications for an automated
    flow-cell polarization fluorometer with digital read out:

Enzyme-inhibitor (antitrypsin) assay and antigen-antibody (insulin-anti-insulin) assay. Clin. Chem. 19: 838.

Watson, R.A.A., J. Landon, E.J. Shaw and D.S. Smith, 1976. Polarization of fluoroimmunoassay of gentamycin. Clin. Chim. Acta 72: 51.

Weber, G., 1953. Rotational Brownian motion and polarization of the solution. Adv. Protein Chem. 8: 415.

A SYSTEM FOR THE STUDY OF KALLIKREINS

John M. Stewart and Dan H. Morris

University of Colorado School of Medicine

Denver, Colorado 80262

The formation of kallidin (lysyl-bradykinin) by the action of glandular kallikreins upon plasma kininogen shows that the substrate specificity of these enzymes is very different from that of trypsin and plasma kallikrein, which yield bradykinin from the same substrate. Although one of the bonds cleaved by glandular kallikrein (Arg-Ser, at the carboxyl end of bradykinin and kallidin) is a typical trypsin substrate cleavage site, and is also cleaved by plasma kallikrein, the other site (Met-Lys, at the amino end of kallidin) is not cleaved by trypsin and plasma kallikrein. This unique second cleavage site has led to considerable work and discussion as to whether the enzyme has one or two active sites (see Fiedler and Leysath, and Prado and Araujo-Viel, this volume). In order to study glandular kallikreins more exactly and as an aid to development of specific inhibitors for glandular kallikreins, a new set of substrates has been synthesized and used for initial studies with rat urinary kallikrein (RUK).

MATERIALS AND METHODS

Three substrates for kallikrein were synthesized by the solid phase method as previously described (Morris and Stewart, 1979). The structures of the substrates are:

KS-1: Acetyl-Ser-Leu-Met-Lys-Arg-Pro-Pro-Gly-
-Phe-Ser-Pro-Phe-Arg-Ser-Val-Gln-Val-Ser-NH$_2$

KS-2: Acetyl-Ser-Leu-Met-Lys-Arg-Pro-Pro-Gly-NH$_2$

KS-3: Acetyl-Phe-Ser-Pro-Phe-Arg-Ser-Val-Gln-Val-Ser-NH$_2$

KS-1 contains the entire sequence of bradykinin extended at each end with the four amino acids known to occur in the bovine kininogen

213

(Kato, et al., 1977) and further modified by acetylation and amida-
tion so as to resemble more closely the natural protein substrate
and to be resistant to the action of exopeptidases. KS-1 was designated to yield biologically active kinin upon treatment with kinin
liberating enzymes; in this process it must be cleaved at two sites.
KS-2 and KS-3 each contain only one of the kallikrein substrate
sites, and should be particularly useful for design of inhibitors
specific for one or the other of these two cleavage sites. Inhibitors of the Met-Lys cleavage site, if found, would be expected to
have a high degree of specificity for glandular kallikrein and
would probably not be inhibitors of trypsin and other enzymes with
trypsin-like substrate specificity. When KS-2 is used as a substrate
for trypsin- or glandular kallikrein-like enzymes, the point of
cleavage of the substrate is easily determined by analysis of the
new amino-group-bearing products formed. An additional substrate,
benzoyl-Pro-Phe-Arg-p-nitroanilide (BPNA) was used as a convenient
aid to purification of RUK.

Rat urinary kallikrein was purified by a modification of the
methods of Nustad and Pierce (1974) and Silva et al. (1974). Rat
urine, 300 ml, collected under toluene, was filtered, centrifuged,
dialyzed exhaustively against distilled water at 5°, diluted with
an equal volume of 0.05 $\underline{M}$ phosphate buffer, pH 7.0, and applied to
a 3.6 x 4 cm column of DEAE-Sephadex A-50 which had been equilibrated
in the same buffer. The column was eluted at 5° successively with
200 ml of the starting buffer, 250 ml of the same buffer containing
0.2 $\underline{M}$ KCl, and 150 ml of the same buffer containing 0.5 $\underline{M}$ KCl. The
0.5 $\underline{M}$ KCl eluate, which contained over 90% of the amidase activity
of the urine, as determined with BPNA, was dialyzed exhaustively
against distilled water and lyophilized. Two such batches were
combined, dissolved in 5.0 ml of 0.1 $\underline{M}$ NH$_4$OAc containing 0.2 $\underline{M}$ NaCl,
pH 7.0, and applied to a 2.5 x 90 cm column of Sephacryl S-200, at
5°, equilibrated and eluted with the same buffer. The effluent
was monitored for amidase activity with BPNA and the contents of
the tubes containing the first peak of amidase activity were combined,
dialyzed against distilled water and frozen in small aliquots.
Polyacrylamide gel electrophoresis of this enzyme in Tris-glycine,
pH 8.5, showed the coomassie blue one major band with a minor band
preceding and following. All three bands were stained yellow upon
incubation with BPNA, and probably represent kallikrein variants
containing different amounts of carbohydrate. No kininase activity
could be demonstrated by incubation of the purified enzyme with
kallidin, followed by bioassay. Amidase activity was monitored
during enzyme purification by incubation of fractions with the
chromogenic substrate BPNA at pH 7.85; liberated p-nitroaniline
was read at 405 nm.

Rates of hydrolysis of substrates by RUK were monitored with
fluorescamine, which reacts with amino groups to yield a fluorescent
product. Purified RUK was preincubated for 20 min in 0.1 $\underline{M}$ tricine

buffer, pH 8.2, at 37°; appropriate amounts of solutions of substrates KS-1 or KS-3 were added and the incubation continued at
37°. Aliquots (8μl) of the reaction mixture were removed at
selected times, diluted with 30 volumes of 0.1 M tricine, pH 8.2,
and mixed vigorously while 6 volumes of a 1 mg/ml solution of
fluorescamine (Fluram[R], Roche) in spectro grade acetone was added.
The solution was transferred to the fluorometer (Gilson, model
3301) cuvette and fluorescence read one minute later (excitation
390 nm, emission 475 nm). Appropriate blanks corrected for
fluorescence contributions of the buffer, substrate and enzyme.

High pressure liquid chromatography (HPLC) was used for identification of the products of enzymatic reactions and for purification
of synthetic peptides. Reversed phase partition chromatography was
done on a 1 x 25 cm column of Lichrosorb RP-18, 5 μ particle size,
using methanol-ammonium formate mixtures at pH 5.0. The pump was
an Altex model 100, samples were injected via a Valco loop valve,
and UV absorbance of the effluent was measured with an Altex-
Hitachi monitor. Absorbance was monitored at 210 nm when low
concentrations of formate were used in the buffers; higher formate
concentrations necessitated use of longer wavelengths (215-225 nm)
because of buffer absorbance.

Biologically active kinin liberated from KS-1 by RUK was
assayed on the isolated guinea pig ileum at pH 7.2, 29°, as previously described (Freer and Stewart, 1972).

RESULTS AND DISCUSSION

Purified RUK released biologically active kinin from substrate
KS-1, as shown in Fig. 1. This action was not inhibited by tosyl-
lysine chloromethyl ketone (TLCK), an alkylating inhibitor of
trypsin and plasma kallikrein, but was inhibited by benzamidine.
In this susceptibility to inhibitors the action of RUK on KS-1
parallels the established pattern of action of RUK on natural
protein kininogens. HPLC was used to identify the product of this
reaction. A system was developed which would separate the known
mammalian kinins and resolve them from substrate KS-1 (see Table 1).
As expected, the product of hydrolysis of KS-1 by RUK was found to
be kallidin. Hydrolysis by trypsin yielded bradykinin. This substrate should be a valuable tool for kallikrein research, since it
provides a pure, chemically defined substrate which behaves toward
these enzymes as does the normal protein substrate, without any of
the uncertainties involved in the use of plasma or its derivatives
as substrates.

All three substrates were hydrolyzed by RUK, as shown by the
fluorescamine assay. Peptide KS-3 was a very good substrate
(K_m=6.7 x 10^{-5}M), while hydrolysis of KS-2 was much slower.

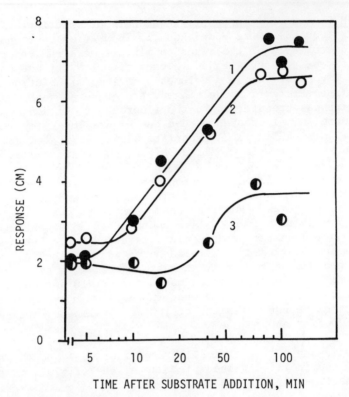

Figure 1.   Release of Kinin from KS-1 by rat urinary kallikrein;
            assay on guinea pig ileum. 1. Kallikrein + KS-1;
            2. Kallikrein + TLCK + KS-1; 3. Kallikrein + Benzamidine
            + KS-1.

With KS-1 the rate-limiting hydrolytic step was similar in velocity
to hydrolysis of KS-2, and probably represents cleavage at the
analogous site in KS-1. Preliminary analysis of the hydrolysis of
KS-2 yielded the data shown in Fig. 2; the k_m thus determined is
similar to that of small molecule substrates for RUK (Silva et al.,
1974). Hydrolysis of KS-2 appears to be accelerated at high substrate concentrations, as has previously been found for other
substrates.

BPNA was found to be a good substrate for RUK (K_m=8.8 x 10^{-4}),
despite the earlier report by Amundsen et al., (1977) that it is not
cleaved by glandular kallikreins such as bovine pancreatic kallikrein; hydrolysis of this substrate was also accelerated at high
substrate concentrations. Hence it does not appear that this substrate will be useful for unequivocal distinction of plasma kalli-

krein from all glandular kallikreins. Carbobenzoxy-L-arginine-p-nitroanilide was also hydrolyzed by RUK, although at a slower rate than was BPNA, whereas Amundsen stated that benzoyl-L-arginine-p-nitroanilide was not hydrolyzed by glandular kallikrein.

TABLE 1.   SEPARATION OF KININS BY HPLC

Peptide	Emergence Time
Bradykinin	3.0 min
Met-Lys-Bradykinin	3.7
Lys-Bradykinin	4.4
Kallikrein Substrate KS-1	2.6

Column: Lichrosorb RP-18 5μ, 1x25 cm
Buffer: Methanol-0.25 $\underline{M}$ Ammonium Formate (9:1), pH 5.0

This system of substrates is being used to develop specific inhibitors for urinary kallikrein, and if such inhibitors are found to be selective for inhibiting cleavage of the substrate at one site, valuable information may be obtained about the catalytic mechanism of these puzzling enzymes.

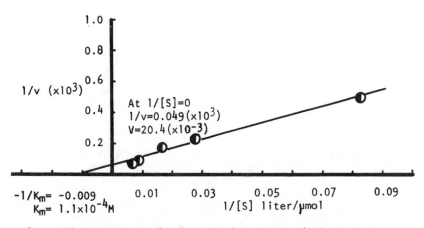

Figure 2.   Lineweaver–Burk plot to determine (K_m) KS-2 for purified rat urinary kallikrein. The line shown and values
derived for K_m and V are based on a linear regression
analysis of primary data.

ACKNOWLEDGEMENTS

The authors thank Renee McIntosh and Virginia Sweeney for technical assistance. This work was supported by contract NO1-HV-72946 from the USPHS.

REFERENCES

Amundsen, E., L. Svendsen, A.M. Vennerod and K. Laake, 1976. Determination of Plasma Kallikrein with a new Chromogenic Tripeptide Derivative, in: Chemistry and Biology of the Kallikrein-Kinin System in Health and Disease, ed. J.J. Pisano (US Government Printing Office Publication (NIH)76-791) p.215.

Freer, R.J., and J.M. Stewart, 1972. Alkylating Analogs of Peptide Hormones. I. Synthesis and Properties of Chlorambucil Derivatives of Bradykinin and Bradykinin Potentiating Factor. J. Med. Chem. 15: 1.

Kato, H., Y.N. Han and S. Iwanaga, 1977. Primary Structure of Bovine Plasma Low-Molecular Weight Kininogen, J. Biochem. (Tokyo) 82: 377.

Morris, D.H., and J.M. Stewart, 1979. A New Assay for Urinary Kallikrein, in: Current Concepts in Kinin Research, ed. G.L. Haberland (Pergamon, Oxford) in press.

Nustad, K., and J.V. Pierce, 1974. Purification of Rat Urinary Kallikreins and Their Specific Antibody, Biochemistry 13: 2312.

Silva, E., C.R. Diniz and M. Mares-Guia, 1974. Rat Urinary Kallikrein: Purification and Properties, Biochemistry 13: 4304.

Biochemical Characterization of
Components of the Plasma and
Tissue Kallikrein-Kinin System

CHEMICAL RELATIONS BETWEEN RENAL AND URINARY KALLIKREIN OF RAT

G. Porcelli, G.B. Marini-Bettòlo, H.R. Croxatto,
M. Di Jorio

Istituto di Chimica, Fac.Med., Università Cattolica,
Rome, Centro Chimica Recettori e delle Molecole Biolo-
gicamente Attive del C.N.R., Rome, Laboratorio di
Fisiologia, Universidad Cattolica, Santiago de Chile,
Chile

ABSTRACT

The ratio in μ-Moles between each aminoacid residue of both
hydrolized renal and urinary kallikrein of rat, is about 1.00 ± 0.3.
Except for Glu, His and Glucosamine a good proportion between all
residues of both enzymes was obtained. It is probable that the different molecular weight, respectively 40,000 for the renal kallikrein and 32,000 for the urinary enzyme, is an artefact of the
different procedures used for the purification of rat kallikrein.

INTRODUCTION

During the last four years we have introduced the chemical a-
nalysis of purified renal and urinary kallikrein of a same animal
species, as a parameter to compare the chemical composition of both
enzymes and to define the renal origin of the urinary kallikrein.

The importance of the latter enzyme, in fact, is related to its
significant decrease in essential hypertensive subjects in comparison with the controls, in hypertensive rats with a ligature in one
kidney and in genetic hypertensive rats in comparison with normal
rats (for references see Porcelli et al. 1978). In that paper we
reported that renal and urinary kallikrein of rat have a different
electrophoretic molecular weight and a different aminoacid com-

221

position. Considering the different procedures used to purify the
kallikreins (affinity chromatography only for the renal enzyme), we
decided to prepare three samples of each enzyme and to compare the
hydrolyzed purified proteins.

MATERIALS AND METHODS

The materials obtained from commercial sources were: DE-32 from
Whatman; Bio-Gel P-200 from Bio-Rad; Sephadex G-100 from Pharmacia;
Trypsin X 2 crystllized and Lysozyme crystallized from Sigma; Bovine
albumin and Egg albumin from Nutritional Biochem.Corp.; N-Benzoyl-
L-arginine ethyl-ester (BAEE) from Cyclo Chemical; Aprotinin
(Trasylol) from Bayer; Dialysing tubing from A.H. Thomas. Other
chemicals used were reagent grade.

For purification procedures of rat kallikreins see Porcelli et
al. (1974) and Porcelli et al. (1978).

Protein was measured either by the method of Lowry et al. (1951)
or by the optical adsorption method in a Beckman spectrophotometer,
model ACTA III C at 280 nm. The purified enzyme proteins were
hydrolyzed with 6N HCl at 137°C for 20 hours in an oil bath under a
current of nitrogen. The molecular weight of kallikrein isolated
from rat kidneys and from rat urines was measured by electrophoresis
on 1% SDS - Cyanogum gel, as described by Weber and Osborn (1969).
The esterase activity and the kinin releasing of urinary and renal
kallikrein were determined by the methods already described (Porcelli
et al. (1975).

RESULTS

At the last step of both procedures used to purify urinary and
renal kallikrein of rat, an isolated urinary enzyme and a 90% purified renal kallikrein were obtained. The purified proteins confirm
the very high esterase and kininogenase activity already described
(Porcelli et al. 1974; Porcelli et al. 1978). A 40,000 m.w. for
renal kallikrein and a 32,000 m.w. for urinary kallikrein was also
confirmed by the Weber and Osborn method, using bovine serum albumine, ovoalbumin, trypsin and lysozyme as marker proteins. Bio-
Rad-P-200-Trasylol, used to purify rat urinary kallikrein, when applied to renal kallikrein was without success. The results of the
aminoacid analysis of urinary and renal kallikrein are shown in
table 1. In that table the mean ratio in μ-Moles for each residue,
obtained after hydrolysis of three different amounts of protein (respectively of renal and urinary enzymes) was reported. That ratio,
mean of three, obtained by dividing each by a whole number which de-

Table 1

Renal kallikrein (R)	Urinary kallikrein (U)
40,000 M.W.	32,000 M.W.

R/U Mean ratio (in μ-Moles)

Asp	1,00
Thr	1,08
Ser	1,02
Glu	1,51 +
Pro	0,88
Gly	0,96
Ala	1,06
1/2 Cys	undetectable
val	1,16
Met	1,00
Ile	0,85
Leu	0,78
Tyr	0,95
Phe	1,03
Lys	1,15
His	0,50 +
Arg	1,07
Glycosamine	1,45 +

+ Different values than 1,00 ± 0,3

pends on the amount of the hydrolyzed protein, is expressed in μ-
Moles of residues.

DISCUSSION

The isolation steps of urinary kallikrein were described
(Porcelli et al. 1974) and the purification steps of renal kallikrein were described too (Porcelli et al. 1978).

It is important to note that from rat urine the most abundant kallikrein was isolated by the Trasylol-affinity chromatography
system, whereas Bio-Gel-P-200-Trasylol when applied to purify renal
kallikrein was without success. The consistent differences between
renal and urinary kallikrein obtained comparing their aminoacid
composition and already described (Porcelli et al. 1978), when we
consider the ratio in μ-Moles between the aminoacid residue of each
hydrolyzed enzyme, are equal to 1.00 ± 0.3, except for Glu, His and
Glutamine. Nevertheless, the molecular weight differences between
renal and urinary kallikrein of rat, respectively 40,000 and 32,000
are consistent. Therefore the question now is whether the protein
of the renal enzyme is a result of a greater number of protein units
than that of the urinary kallikrein, or an effect of the different
purification procedures used for both enzymes.

REFERENCES

1) Lowry O.H., Rosbrough N.J., Farr A.L., Randall R.J.(1951),
   Protein measurement with the folin phenol reagent; J.Biol.Chem.,
   193, 265
2) Porcelli G., Bianchi G., Croxatto H.R. (1975),
   Urinary kallikrein excretion in a spontaneously hypertensive
   strain of rats; Proc.Soc.Exp.Biol.Med. 149, 983
3) Porcelli G., Marini-Bettòlo G.B., Croxatto H.R., Di Jorio M.
   (1974), Purification and chemical studies on rat urinary kallikrein, Ital.J.Biochem., 24, 175
4) Porcelli G., Marini-Bettòlo G.B., Croxatto H.R., Di Jorio M.,
   Micotti G. (1978), Purification of renal rat kallikrein and
   chemical relations with urinary rat kallikrein, Ital. J. Biochem.,
   27, 201
5) Weber K., Osborn M. (1969), The reliability of molecular weight
   determinations by dedecyl-sulfate-poly-acrylamide gel electrophoresis; J.Biol.Chem. 244, 4406

RADIOIMMUNOASSAY OF RAT SUBMANDIBULAR GLAND KALLIKREIN AND THE DETECTION OF IMMUNOREACTIVE ANTIGEN IN BLOOD

Kjell Nustad, Kåre Gautvik and Torill Ørstavik

Dept. of Clin. Chem., The Norwegian Radium Hospital
(K.N., K.G.); Inst. of Physiol., Med. Fac. (K.G.); and
Inst. of Physiol. and Biochem., Dent. Fac., University
of Oslo, (T.Ø.), Oslo, Norway.

INTRODUCTION

Glandular kallikreins are a group of related kinin-forming
enzymes (EC 3.4.21.8) present in the major exocrine glands and in
the kidney. They are found in the ductal cells of the salivary
glands, in the distal tubular cells of the kidney and in the acini
of the pancreas (Nustad et al., 1978b). After activation of the
glands, kallikrein is found in the secreted fluids such as saliva,
pancreatic juice and distal tubular urine. However, evidence indicate that glandular kallikreins may be released to blood during
salivary gland stimulation (Nustad et al., 1978b). The substrate
for glandular kallikreins is present mainly in blood and formation
of the active product lysyl-bradykinin implies that enzyme and substrate combines in the intercellular space or in blood. However,
so far glandular kallikreins have not been detected in blood except
during acute pancreatitis where an inhibitor-pancreatic kallikrein
complex was found (Ofstad, 1970). The establishment of a sensitive
radioimmunoassay for glandular kallikreins has allowed us to explore
the possible occurrence of glandular kallikreins in blood. Employing
antiserum raised against purified rat submandibular gland kallikrein,
we demonstrate the presence of immunological crossreacting material(s)
in plasma. A preliminary report was presented at the Nordic Microcirculation group (Nustad et al., 1978a; Ørstavik et al., 1978).

MATERIALS AND METHODS

Radioimmunoassay of Rat Submandibular Kallikrein (RSK). Antibodies to RSK was obtained in rabbits after multiple intracutaneous
injections of pure RSK (Brandtzaeg et al., 1976). Each rabbit
received 150 µg protein each time and was boostered every 14th day
and bled 10 days after each injection. The first four injections
were in complete Freund adjuvant, later incomplete adjuvant was
used. Antiserum from the best rabbit could be used in a final
dilution of 1 to 80,000 using bleeding five to eleven.

^{125}I-RSK was prepared using hypochlorit as oxidizing agent.
The reagents were added with Hamilton syringes through the rubber
membrane of the iodine-container, which was kept sealed until the
reduction was finished. 1 mCi ^{125}I (The Radiochemical Center,
Amersham, England), was buffered with 25 µl 0.5 M Na-phosphate
(pH 7.5) before adding 10 µg RSK in 10 µl 0.15 M NaCl - 0.1 M Na-
phosphate (pH 7.5). The oxidation was started by adding 10 µl of
freshly prepared 1.2 mM NaClO in 0.05 M Na-phosphate (pH 7.5) and
terminated 30 s later with 50 µl of 0.05 M $Na_2S_2O_5$ in 0.05 M Na-
phosphate-0.6 M KI-0.2% bovine serum albumin (BSA) (pH 7.5). ^{125}I-
RSK was separated from free iodine by gel filtration on a BioGel
P-150 column (Bio Rad, USA) 0.6x10 cm in 1 M NaCl - 0.1% BSA - 0.01%
NaN_3 - 0.01 M Na-phosphate (pH 7.5) using a flow rate of 8 ml/hr and
collecting 0.4 ml fractions with a LKB fraction collector at 4°C.
When the ^{125}I-RSK was used for diffusion studies the BSA and 1 M
NaCl was not used in the gel filtration described above. Fifty to
eighty percent of the iodine was incorporated into RSK. The specific
activity in the best experiments was calculated to be about 74 mCi/mg
assuming 75% recovery of the protein giving about one molecule of
^{125}I per RSK molecule.

Standards of RSK from 0.1 to 20 ng per tube were prepared by
serial dilutions of pure RSK in 0.05 M barbital buffer - 0.1% BSA -
0.01% merthiolate (pH 8.6). The protein concentration of the RSK
was determined by the method of Lowry et al. (1951) using BSA as
standard.

The absorbance of a 0.1% solution at 280 nm of the RSK standard
was 2.28. Samples to be tested were diluted in the same buffer as
the standards.

The assay was run with standards in triplicate and unknowns in
duplicate. The incubate in 0.05 M barbital buffer - 0.1% BSA - 0.01%
merthiolate (pH 8.6) contained 100 µl ^{125}I-RSK (20,000 cpm, 0.2 ng),
100 µl antiserum (1:80,000 final dilution) and 200 µl sample. Antiserum was omitted from the blanks, and the totals contained only
^{125}I-RSK. The tubes were incubated at room temperature overnight
before adding 1.0 ml double antibody solid phase (DASP, Organon, Oss,

Holland) diluted 1:20 in the assay buffer. In most experiments the tubes were rotated for 2 hr and centrifuged (3000 g for 10 min) before decantation and counting. However, later studies showed that rotation with DASP was unnecessary. Decantation was performed simultaneously for all tubes by placing them in a polyethylene tube holder. Counting of ^{125}I was performed in a CG 4000 gammacounter (Intertechnique, France) equipped with a computer which transformed the standard curve into a hyperbola from which the unknowns were calculated.

Diffusion of ^{125}I-RSK from the Rat Submandibular Gland to Blood
^{125}I-RSK (40 µl, 1-3·10^6 cpm) was injected gently into the cannulated main duct or intraglandularly in anaesthetized, heparinized adult rats. Radioactivity was traced in the venous blood continuously and samples were obtained from the anterior facial vein after ligation of the tonsillar vein. Heparinized blood substitution was given during the experimental period through a catheter in the femoral vein.

RESULTS

Evaluation of the Radioimmunoassay for RSK

The radio-labelling procedure for RSK gave no change in esterase activity. When applied to a DEAE-Sephadex A-50 column, one peak of radiolabelled material appeared eluting at a slightly higher salt concentration than native RSK (Brandtzaeg et al., 1976). This change in chromatographic behaviour was probably due to the negatively charged iodine molecule introduced. ^{125}I-RSK could be stored at -20°C for at least 10 weeks without apparent change in immunoreactivity.

Figure 1 shows the standard curve for RSK. Incubation at 4°C rather than at room temperature had little effect on the profile of the standard curve. The sensitivity of the assay was 0.25 ng per tube (8 fmol) or 1 ng/ml. The intraassay coefficient of variance (VC) in the low standard region was 4.2% (n =10) whereas the interassay VC in the same standard region was 11.7% (n =10).

Serial dilution of rat urinary kallikrein (Nustad and Pierce, 1974) gave a standard curve parallel to that of RSK. The same results were obtained with rat pancreatic kallikrein and pro-pancreatic kalli-krein, whereas rat pancreatic trypsin showed no cross reactivity (Proud et al., 1977).

To our surprise rat serum contained immunoreactive material (Fig. 1). The standard curve obtained by diluting rat serum was similar to that obtained by RSK when high dilutions of rat serum was used, but a distinct non-parallel curve was obtained with larger amounts

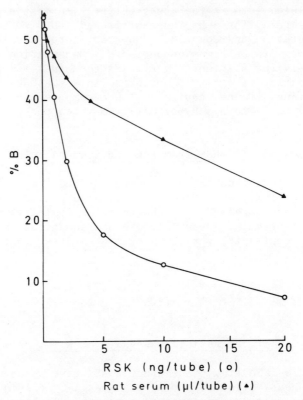

Figure 1. Standard curve for RSK–RIA using RSK and rat serum in
           increasing amounts along the abscissa. Ordinate: per
           cent of total radioactivity bound corrected for non
           specific binding (% B).

of serum in the assay (Fig. 1).

The concentration of immunoreactive material in serum is
difficult to estimate due to the composite and partly non-parallel
behaviour of the curves. A minimal concentration of 150 ng/ml was
calculated from the results with 10 to 20 μl serum in the assay.

Characterization of the Immunoreactive Material in Blood

^{125}I-RSK was added to rat serum and gel filtered on an Ultragel AcA 22 column (LKB, Sweden). The results were very different
from that of ^{125}I-RSK in buffer (Fig. 2). Most of the labelled
kallikrein in serum eluted just ahead of the albumin peak and

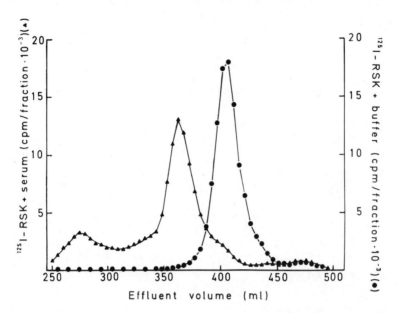

Figure 2. Gel filtration on Ultragel AcA 22 in 0.01 M Na-phosphate
0.10 M NaCl (pH 6.0). Column 2.6x90 cm, flow rate
14 ml/hr, fraction volume 5 ml, 4°C (▲——▲) 5 ml rat
serum + ^{125}I-RSK (140,000 cpm), (●——●) 5 ml buffer +
^{125}I-RSK.

represented probably a RSK-α_1-antitrypsin complex. A small but
distinct peak was excluded from the column presumably representing
^{125}I-RSK complexed to α_2-macroglobulin. However, when the RSK-RIA
was used to assay the eluted endogenous immunoreactivity a third
pattern emerged (Fig. 3). The main immunoreactive peak was excluded
from the column and two incompletely separated peaks were eluted
before and after the albumin peak. The excluded fractions from the
Ultragel AcA22 was further purified on a DEAE cellulose column.
^{125}I-RSK was then eluted as a position clearly different from the
immunoreactive peak (Fig. 4). Both ^{125}I-RSK and the immunoreactive
peak was probably associated with α_2-macroblobulin as judged by the
behaviour of the single protein band in the combined concentrated
fractions on agarose electrophoresis (data not shown).

    The possibility that the immunoreactivity in blood represents
plasma kallikrein could not be tested since no pure rat plasma
kallikrein was available. However, one would expect a rather different elution profile from the Ultrogel AcA 22 column. Furthermore,
immunoreactive material was also found in human serum, and no cross

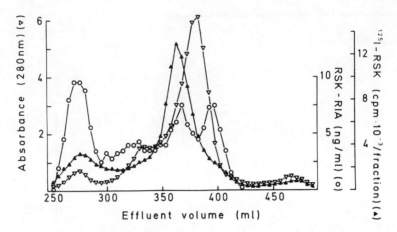

Figure 3.   Gel filtration on Ultragel AcA 22.   Identical to run
            with rat serum in Fig. 2, but with additional assay
            with RSK-RIA (O———O) and absorbance at 280 nm (∇———∇)

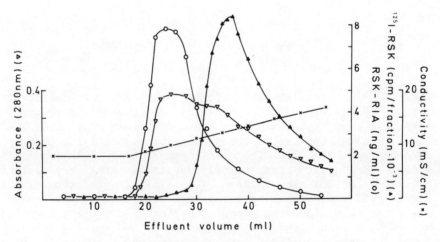

Figure 4.   DEAE-cellulose chromatography with gradient from 0.1 M
            to 0.4 M ammoniumacetate pH 6.0.   Column 0.9x28 cm,
            flow rate 4 ml/hr, fraction volume 1 ml, 4°C.   Sample:
            excluded fractions from Ultragel AcA 22 in the equili-
            bration buffer with ^{125}I-RSK added (200,000 cpm).
            Absorbance 280 nm (∇———∇), RSK-RIA (O———O), ^{125}I-RSK
            (▲———▲) and conductivity (x———x).

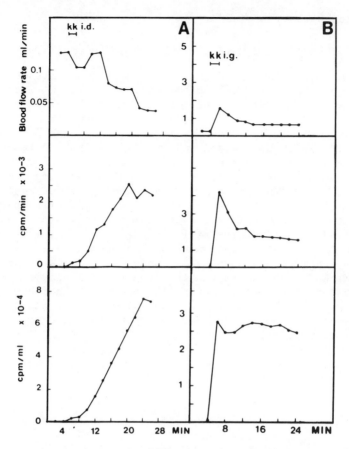

Figure 5.   Administration of ^{125}I-RSK into the resting submandibular
            gland. After intraductal administration (A), maximum
            concentration of ^{125}I-RSK in venous blood is reached
            after about 20 min. After intraglandular (interstitial)
            administration (B), the concentration of ^{125}I-RSK in
            venous blood increased rapidly, reaching a plateau after
            about 2-4 min. Thus, the main permeation barrier in the
            salivary gland seemed to be the duct epithelium.

reactivity was found when pure human plasma kallikrein (150 μg) was
tested in the RSK-RIA (Gallimore et al., 1978). Gel filtration of
human serum with added ^{125}I-RSK gave one broad peak of immunoreactive
material just ahead of the albumin peak and this coincided with the

main elution peak of ^{125}I-RSK.

Passage of ^{125}I-RSK from the Submandibular Gland to Blood

The submandibular gland is far the most abundant source for
glandular kallikrein in the rat (Ørstavik, 1978). We therefore
studied the possible passage of ^{125}I-RSK from the gland to blood
by injection of labelled enzyme into the salivary main duct and
intraglandularly as described in Methods. ^{125}I-RSK permeated
readily from the duct to blood and the duct epithelim represented
the main permeability barrier (Fig. 5). The labelled material in
blood was excluded from a Sephadex G-75 column and no free iodine
was found. The permeation of ^{125}I-RSK across the duct epithelium
was apparently not due to destruction of the epithelial barrier
caused by the experimental procedure for the following reasons:
1. The gland responded with saliva secretion and alteration in
blood flow in a regular fashion when subjected to stimulation.
2. Alteration in gland morphology could not be detected by histochemical methods. 3. Parasympathetic nerve stimulation in rats
given ^{125}I-RSK albumin intraarterially showed no increase in
salivary radioactivity, after intraductal or intraglandular
injections of buffered saline (Ørstavik, Gautvik and Nustad, manuscript in preparation).

DISCUSSION

The radioimmunological determination of glandular kallikrein
in salt solutions represents no difficulty. The same has been
found with assay of rat urinary kallikrein (Oza, 1977; Carretero
et al., 1978) and pig pancreatic kallikrein (Fink et al., 1978).
The composite curve obtained when rat serum was added to the RSK-
RIA may in general be due to the presence of non-identical cross-
reacting immunological material. However, the curve may also be
characteristic of a heteregenous group of material with different
immunological cross-reacting affinities. The immunoreactive material
we demonstrate in blood represents most probably glandular kallikrein inhibitor complexes. The distribution of immunoreactive
material is most complex in rat serum, whereas human and pig serum
have antigen bound mainly to one inhibitor. However, the endogenous
immunoreactive material in blood does not behave like labelled RSK
added to the serum in vitro. This may be explained by stereo-
chemical changes in the RSK introduced during iodination. In addition,
the source for the immunoreactive material in blood is probably both
the salivary glands, the pancreas and the kidney giving rise to a
heterogenous group of related antigens which bind to the natural
occurring inhibitors. Only purification of relatively large quantities
of immunoreactive material from blood and separation of the antigen
from the inhibitor will allow the positive identification of the anti-

gens as intact glandular kallikreins. To obtain this we have coupled our antiserum to Sepharose 4B. This immunosorbent is excellent for a one-step purification procedure of glandular kallikrein from gland homogenates (Gautvik, Svindahl, Nustad and Ørstavik, manuscript submitted for publication), and we intended to use the same method for the purification of the blood antigens.

Diffusion studies of glandular kallikrein across the inter-stitial wall (Moriwaki et al., 1974; Fink et al., 1978) and on studies in the salivary gland also lend support to the conclusion that glandular kallikrein can indeed pass from lumen into blood. This passage of glandular kallikrein from its site of production to blood has important implications for its possible function as a mediator of local vasodilatation.

ACKNOWLEDGEMENTS

We wish to thank Dr. Gallimore for the generous gift of pure human plasma kallikrein, Kirsten Svindahl and Vigdis Teig for excellent technical assistance, and the Norwegian Cancer Society for economical support.

REFERENCES

Brandtzaeg, P., K.M. Gautvik, K. Nustad and J.V. Pierce, 1976. Rat submandibular gland kallikreins: Purification and cellular localization. Br. J. Pharmacol. 56: 155.

Carretero, O.A., V.M. Amin, T. Ocholik, A.G. Scicli and J. Koch, 1978. Urinary kallikrein in rats bred for their susceptibility and resistance to the hypertensive effect of salt. A new radio-immunoassay for its direct determination. Circ. Res. 42: 727.

Fink, E., J. Seifert and C. Güttel, 1978. Development of a radio-immunoassay for pig pancreatic kallikrein and its application in physiological studies. Fresenius Z. Anal. Chem. 290: 183.

Gallimore, M.J., E. Fareid and H. Stormorken, 1978. The purification of plasma kallikrein with weak plasminogen activation activity. Thromb. Res. 12: 409.

Lowry, O.H., N.J. Rosebrough, A.L. Farr, and R.J. Randall, 1951. Protein measurement with the folin phenol reagent. J. Biol. Chem. 193: 265.

Moriwaki, C., K. Yamaguchi and H. Moriya, 1974. Studies on kalli-kreins. III. Intra-intestinal administration of hog pancreatic kallikrein and its appearance in the perfusate from the mesen-teric vein. Chem. Pharm. Bull. (Tokyo), 22: 1975.

Nustad, K. and J.V. Pierce, 1974. Purification of rat urinary
    kallikrein and their specific antibody. Biochemistry 13: 2312.
Nustad, K., T.B. Ørstavik and K.M. Gautvik, 1978a. Radioimmuno-
    logical measurements of rat submandibular gland kallikrein (RSK)
    in tissues and serum. Microvasc. Res. 15: 115.
Nustad, K., T.B. Ørstavik, K.M. Gautvik and J.V. Pierce, 1978b.
    Glandular kallikreins. Gen. Pharmacol. 9: 1.
Ofstd, E., 1970. Formation and destruction of plasma kinins during
    experimental acute hemorrhagic pancreatis in dogs. Scand. J.
    Gastroenterol. 5: suppl. 5.
Oza, N.B., 1977. A direct assay for urinary kallikrein. Biochem.
    J. 167: 305.
Proud, D., G.S. Bailey, K Nustad and K.M. Gautvik, 1977. The
    immunological similarity of rat glandular kallikreins.
    Biochem. J. 167: 835.
Ørstavik, T.Z., 1978. The distribution and secretion of kallikrein
    in some exocrine organs of the rat. Acta physiol. scand.
    in press.
Ørstavik, T.B., K.M. Gautvik, K. Nustad and J. Hedemark-Poulsen,
    1978. Diffusion of ^{125}I-labeled glandular kallikrein after
    local administration in the rat submandibular gland. Microvasc.
    Res. 15: 115.

HUMAN URINARY KALLIKREIN - BIOCHEMICAL AND PHYSIOLOGICAL ASPECTS

R. Geiger, U. Stuckstedte, B. Förg-Brey and E. Fink

Abteilung für Klinische Chemie und Klinische Biochemie

in der Chirurgischen Klinik der Universität München

Nussbaumstrasse 20, D-8000 München 2, Germany

The history of kallikrein begins with the discovery of urinary kallikrein more than fifty years ago. The renal origin of urinary kallikrein, though not finally proved, is largely accepted. A possible role of kallikrein in the regulation of kidney function and blood pressure has been debated for a long time (Pisano and Auster, 1976). However, neither the question for its origin, nor for its physiological role is finally settled.

Isolation and Characterization

As a first step in the development of a radioimmunoassay and of enzymatic assays for human urinary kallikrein an isolation method for the enzyme was set up (Geiger et al. 1977). The method is summarized in Table 1 (a slightly different method was reported earlier, Mann and Geiger, 1977).

Preparations of human urinary kallikrein obtained from different urine pools were subjected to polyacrylamide gel electrophoresis at pH 6 and 8. Two different patterns of protein bands were obtained. For some preparations only one band was visible after staining, whereas other preparations were resolved into three bands as described also by Matsuda et al. (1976). All bands contained active kallikrein as was demonstrated by active enzyme staining using Z-Ser-Pro-Phe-Arg-MNA and coupling with Fast Blue B Salt (Smith et al. 1975). After incubation with Trasylol, however, only a single band of lower electrophoretic mobility was detected (Fig. 1) for all preparations.

Table 1.

                    Isolation of human urinary kallikrein

          Steps   Purification

Collection of human male urine   -
Dialysis   -
Lyophilization   -
Extraction of the crude urine powder   -
Sephacryl S-200   1
Trasylol Sepharose   89
DEAE-Sepharose   240

        Amino acid analyses of the human urinary kallikrein were
done by common methods, carbohydrate content was determined as
described by Krystal and Graham (1976). The results are shown in
Table 2 and 3. According to our preliminary results, the amino
acid compositions of human urinary kallikrein is very similar to
that of pig pancreatic β-kallikrein. The values for Ser, Gly,
Ala, Cys and Met are identical, whereas minor differences exist for
the other amino acids. Some differences also exist in the amino
acid compositions of preparations isolated from different urine
pools.

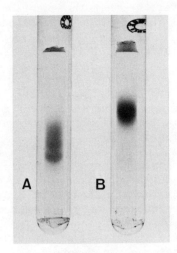

Fig. 1.   Acrylamide gel electrophoresis (7.58% gel, pH 8) of
           human kallikrein.
           A: purified enzyme   B: purified enzyme
                                           complexed with Trasylol

Table 2.

Amino acid composition of kallikreins from human
urine and porcine pancreas.

Tryptophan was not determined, cystein after performic acid oxidation (Hirs 1976).

	Human urinary kallikrein	Porcine pancreatic β-kallikrein (Fiedler et al. 1977)
Asp	20–23	28
Thr	14	15
Ser	14	14
Glu	28–30	23
Pro	14	16
Gly	22	22
Ala	12–14	13
Cys	10	10
Val	13–16	10
Met	4	4
Ile	8–9	12
Leu	18	20
Tyr	9	7
Phe	8–12	10
Lys	8–12	10
His	8–9	8
Arg	6	3
Trp	?	7

Table 3.

Carbohydrate content of human urinary kallikrein
and porcine pancreatic kallikrein

Kallikrein from	Carbohydrate content g/100 g protein	
Porcine pancreas		(Fiedler et al. 1975)
form A	5.6	
form B.	11.5	
Human urine	10.5 – 15.6	

The differences in both amino acid composition and electrophoretic patterns suggest that our preparations of human urinary
kallikrein contain multiple forms as a result of limited proteolysis. Limited proteolytic attack causes cleavages within a
protein chain, eventually resulting in the release of single amino
acids or peptides. These cleavages and the loss of parts of the
protein molecule can give rise to changes in electrophoretic
mobility and amino acid composition. Multiple forms caused by
limited proteolysis have also been observed for pig pancreatic
kallikrein (Fiedler et al. 1977).

Assay Methods

It has been observed in our laboratory that Ac-Phe-ArgOMe is
a much better substrate for porcine pancreatic (Fiedler 1976),
submandibular and urinary kallikreins (Fritz et al. 1977) than α-
N-acetylated arginine esters. The corresponding ethyl ester, Ac-
Phe-ArgOEt , is the most rapidly hydrolyzed substrate for human
urinary kallikrein described as yet (Fiedler et al. 1978). Therefore, a highly sensitive assay for human urinary kallikrein could
be developed employing Ac-Phe-ArgOEt as substrate. The assay
(Table 4) is analogous to that with Bz-ArgOEt developed by
Trauschold and Werle (1961). The reaction sequence is shown in
Fig. 2. The sensitivities of this and other assays for human
urinary kallikrein are compiled in Table 5. The sensitivity of
the assay allows the convenient measurement of the esterase
activity of human urine. Urine samples 20 20 - 100 µl cause a
linear absorbance increase of 0.04 to 0.2 per 10 min. Known
amounts of human urinary kallikrein added to urine samples raised
the esterase activity to the expected extent. If the urine samples
contain ethanol it has to be removed by dialysis. Therefore,
ethanol intake should be avoided during the urine collection period.

Table 4.
              Assay of human urinary kallikrein using the substrate
              Ac-Phe-ArgOEt

2.00 ml	0.15 M sodium diphosphate buffer, pH 8.7 containing 0.15 M semicarbazidium chloride and 0.0375 M glycine
0.10 ml	0.03 M NAD
0.10 ml	0.015 M AcPheArgOEt acetate
0.02 ml	alcohol dehydrogenase (100 mg/3.4 ml)
(0.28+x) ml	water

5 min preincubation at 25°C

(0.5-x) ml	enzyme solution
Final volume:	3 ml

The change in absorbance is monitored for 10 min. at 366 nm.

$$Ac\text{-}Phe\text{-}ArgOEt \xrightarrow{\text{KALLIKREIN}} Ac\text{-}Phe\text{-}Arg + C_2H_5OH$$

$$C_2H_5OH + NAD \xrightarrow[(\longleftarrow)]{\text{ALKOHOLDEHYDROGENASE}} CH_3 - C \underset{H}{\overset{O}{\lessgtr}} + NADH_2$$

Fig. 2.   Reaction scheme of kallikrein assay using Ac-Phe-ArgOEt
          as substrate.

A number of experiments were undertaken to verify that the
esterase activity reflects the kallikrein content of urine.   Trasylol completely inhibited the esterase activity.   Dialysed urine
samples of 10 different persons were assayed.   The results were
compared with those obtained by the dog blood pressure assay, by
a radioimmunoassay for human urinary kallikrein (Mann and Geiger
1977) and by the assay with D-Val-Leu-ArgNHNp as substrate (Fig.
3).   Though the correlation coefficient of the results of the
Ac-Phe-ArgOEt assay and the dog blood pressure assay (Fig. 3a)

Table 5.   Absorbance changes in assays of human urinary
           kallikrein with various substrates.

(Reaction volume 3 ml, cuvette light path 1 cm)

	BLANK $(\Delta A \cdot 10^3 \times \text{MIN}^{-1})$	REACTION $(\Delta A \cdot 10^3 \times \text{MIN}^{-1} \times U^{-1})$	RELATIVE SENSITIVITIES
Ac-Phe-ArgOEt	0.6	1 100	46
D-Val-Leu-ArgOEt	0.6	430	20
B$_z$-ArgOEt	0.5	24	1
Z-TyrONp	15	460	19
D-Val-Leu-Arg-p-nitranilide	0.0	29	1.2
D-Pro-Phe-Arg-p- "		3	
Tos-Gly-Pro-Arg-p- "		1	
Bz-Phe-Val-Arg-p- "		0.3	
Glu-Gly-Arg-p- "		0.3	

is rather close to 1, a considerable scattering of the data is observed.   This is not too surprising, since the coefficient of variation of the blood pressure assay for kallikrein amounts to 20% (Arens and Haberland 1973).   The correlation between the Ac-Phe-ArgOEt assay and both the radioimmunoassay (Fig. 3b) and the D-Val-Leu-Arg-p-nitroanilide assay is even more satisfactory. The excellent correlation between the two enzymatic assays (Fig. 3c) strongly suggests that in both assays the same enzyme is determined.   For a mixture of enzymes a similarly good correlation would only be expected if these enzymes were always excreted in identical ratios.

D-Val-Leu-Arg-p-nitroanilide has been suggested quite recently by KABI (Amundsen et al. 1978) as a substrate for the determination

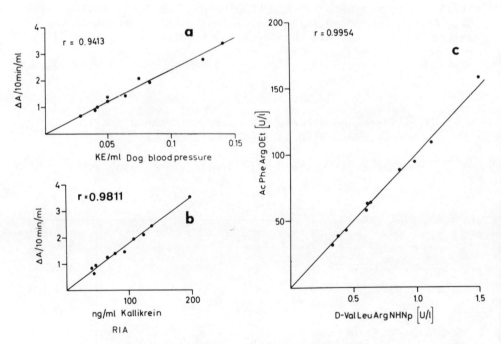

Fig. 3.   Comparision of the Ac-Phe-ArgOEt assay for human urinary kallikrein with the blood pressure assay (a), the radio-immunoassay (b) and the D-Val-Leu-ArgNHNp assay (c).

10 samples of human urine were measured.

of human urinary kallikrein. Hydrolysis of p-nitroanilides can
be monitored at 405 nm. Negligible spontaneous hydrolysis of
these compounds allows working at 37°C. To obtain abosrbance
changes of sufficient magnitude, an incubation time of 30 min was
necessary for urine samples of 50 to 500 µl. This long incubation
time precluded continuous monitoring of the reaction. The results
had to be corrected for the inherent absorbance of the urine
samples that was determined in parallel (blanks contain water
instead of substrate). The reaction conditions are given in
Table 6.

Evidently, both Ac-Phe-ArgOEt and D-Val-Leu-ArgNHNp are useful
substrates for kallikrein determination in human urine. The
advantage of the Ac-Phe-ArgOEt assay is the possibility of continuous monitoring during the test, a drawback is the alcohol
sensitivity of the reaction. This is not found in the assay with
D-Val-Leu-ArgNHNp, but due to its low sensitivity, this method
suffers from the disadvantages of a two point assay.

The radioimmunoassay for human urinary kallikrein was also
applied to clarify, whether endogenous glandular kallikrein is
present in the blood. We found glandular kallikrein in human
serum in concentrations of 10-15 ng/ml. In order to ascertain
that the radioimmunoassayable substance was not a low molecular
degradation product, serum samples were subjected to gel filtration
and the fractions tested by radioimmunoassay (Fig. 4). After gel
filtration one peak was detected in the position of a molecular
weight of about 80,000 whereas our kallikrein preparation was
eluted in the position of about 50,000. The exact origin of the
glandular kallikrein in blood is unknown, a discrimination by
radioimmunoassay is impossible because of the immunological cross-

Table 6.
            Assay of human urinary kallikrein using the substrate
                        D-Val-Leu-ArgNHNp

        0.4 ml   0.4 M TRIS/HCl, pH 8.2
          x ml   urine
    (0.5-x) ml   water

                      5 min preincubation at 37°C

        0.1 ml   0.001 M D-Val-Leu-ArgNHNp

                      Incubation at 37°C

    The absorbance increase (405 nm) after 30 min. is read.

reactivity of the various tissue kallikreins. The presence of glandular kallikrein in blood leads to the assumption that renal filtration might contribute to some extent to the amount of kallikrein found in urine.

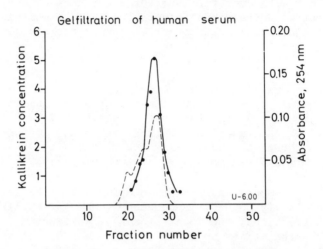

Fig. 4. Gel filtration of human serum through Sephacryl S-200.

The fractions were assayed by a radioimmunoassay for human urinary kallikrein.

ABBREVIATIONS

Bz-ArgOEt: N^{α}-Benzoyl-arginine ethyl ester, Z-TyrONp: Carbobenzoxytyrosine nitrophenyl ester, Ac-Phe-ArgOMe: Acetyl-phenylalanyl-arginine methyl ester, Ac-Phe-ArgOEt: Acetyl-phenylalanyl-arginine ethyl ester, Z-Ser-Pro-Phe-Arg-MNA: Carbobenzoxy-seryl-prolyl-phenylalanyl-arginine-p-nitroanilide, D-Val-Leu-ArgOEt: D-valyl-leucyl-arginine ethyl ester.

ACKNOWLEDGEMENT

This work was supported by Deutsche Forschungsgemeinschaft, Sonderforschungsbereich 51, Munchen. We are indebted to Dr. C. Kutzbach, Bayer AG, for providing preprocessed starting material for the isolation of human urinary kallikrein. We thank very much Prof. H. Fritz for his interest in this work and his stimulating discussions and comments.

REFERENCES

Amundsen, E., J. Püttner, P. Friberger, M. Knös, M. Larsbråten, and G. Claeson (1978). Methods for the Determination of Glandular Kallikreins by Means of a Chromogenic Tripeptide Substrate. In press.

Arens, A., and G.L. Haberland (1973). Determination of Kallikrein Activity in Animal Tissue Using Biochemical Methods. In: G.L. Haberland, and J.W. Rohen (Eds.) Kininogenases - Kallikrein 1, F.K. Schattauer Verlag, Stuttgart, pp. 43-53.

Fiedler, F., C. Hirschauer, and E. Werle (1975). Characterization of pancreatic kallikreins A and B. Hoppe Seylers Z. Physiol. Chem. 356, 1879-1891.

Fiedler, R. (1976). Pig Pancreatic Kallikrein: Structure and Catalytic Properties. In: J.J. Pisano and K.F. Austen (Eds.) Chemistry and Biology of the Kallikrein-Kinin System in Health and Disease, DHEW Publ. No. (NIH) 76-791, pp. 93-95.

Fiedler, F., W. Ehret, G. Godec, C. Hirschauer, C. Kutzbach, G. Schmidt-Kastner, and H. Tschesche (1977). The Primary Structure of Pig Pancreatic Kallikrein B. In: G.L. Haberland, J.W. Rohen, and T. Suzuki (Eds.) Kininogenases - Kallikrein 4, F.K. Schattauer Verlag, Stuttgart, pp. 7-14.

Fiedler, F., R. Geiger, C. Hirschauer, and G. Leysath (1978). Peptide esters and nitroanilides as substrates for the assay of human urinary kallikrein. Hoppe Seylers Z. Physiol. Chem., in press.

Fritz, H., F. Fiedler, T. Dietl, M. Warwas, E. Truscheit, H.J. Kolb, G. Mair, and H. Tschesche (1977). On the Relationship between Porcine Pancreatic, Submandibular, and Urinary Kallikreins. In: G.L. Haberland, J.W. Rohen, and T. Suzuki (Eds.) Kininogenases - Kallikrein 4, F.K. Schattauer Verlag, Stuttgart, pp. 15-28.

Geiger, R., K. Mann, and T. Bettels (1977). Isolation of Human Urinary Kallikrein by Affinity Chromatography. J. Clin. Chem. Clin. Biochem. 15, 479-483.

Hirs, C.H.W. (1976). Methods Enzymol. 11, 197-199.

Krystal, G., and A.F. Graham (1976). A sensitive method for estimating the carbohydrate content of glycoproteins. Anal. Biochem. 70, 336-345.

Mann, K., and R. Geiger (1977). Radioimmunoassay of Human Urinary Kallikrein. In: G.L. Haberland, J.W. Rohen, and T. Suzuki (Eds.) Kininogenases - Kallikrein 4, F.K. Schattauer Verlag, Stuttgart, pp. 55-61.

Matsuda, Y., K. Miyazaki, H. Moriya, Y. Fujimoto, Y. Hojima, and C. Moriwaki (1976). Studies on Urinary Kallikrein, I. Purification and Characterization of Human Urinary Kallikrein. J. Biochem. 80, 671-679.

Pisano, J.J., and K.F. Austen (1976). Chemistry and Biology of the Kallikrein-Kinin-System in Health and Disease. DHEW Publication No. (NIH) 76-791.

Smith, R.E., and R.M. Van Frank (1975). The use of amino acid
    derivatives of 4-methoxy-β-naphtylamine for the assay and
    subcellular localization of tissue proteinases. In: A.
    Neuberger and E.L. Tatum (Eds.) Frontiers of Biology 43,
    North-Holland Publishing Co., Incl., New York, 193-249.
Trautschold, I., and E. Werle (1961). Spektrometrische Bestimmung
    des Kallikreins und seiner Inaktivatoren. Hoppe Seylers Z.
    Physiol. Chem. 325, 48-59.

THE PRIMARY STRUCTURE OF PORCINE GLANDULAR KALLIKREINS

Harald Tschesche, Gerhard Mair and Gudrun Godec
Department of Biochemistry, University Bielefeld
D-4800 Bielefeld 1, GFR
Franz Fiedler, Werner Ehret and Christa Hirschauer
Marius Lemon and Hans Fritz
Department of Clinical Chemistry and Clinical Bio-
chemistry, University Munish, D-8000 Munich 1, GFR
Gunther Schmidt-Kastner and Carl Kutzbach
Bayer AG, D-5600 Wuppertal 1, GFR

ABSTRACT

The amino acid sequence of the A- and B-chains of porcine
pancreatic kallikrein B is presented and compared to that of porcine
trypsin. The overall homology between both enzymes is 37% identical
residues in corresponding position and 51% chemically similar
residues. Comparison of the sequences with the crystal structure
of bovine trypsin reveals that the trypsin "autolysis loop" is enlarged in kallikrein by two residues but lacks the basic residue
at the cleavage site. Substitutions at the calcium-binding site
of trypsin which include Arg 70 for Glu 70 possibly interfere with
ion binding. Insertions between trypsin residues 95 and 96
obviously form a new kallikrein "autolysis loop" containing the
site of cleavage between the A- and B-chains. One carbohydrate
moiety is attached to this surface loop at Asn 95, the second to
Asn 239 at the same edge of the globular molecule. The residues
at the surface of the substrate binding site are substituted to
an extent of 85% while the residues forming contacts to the trypsin
inhibitor (Kunitz) are highly preserved. Immunodiffusion studies
as well as identity of the N-terminal sequences of pancreatic,
submandibular and urinary kallikrein reveal the same genetic origin
of the three glandular kallikreins.

INTRODUCTION

Kallikrein$^{(R)}$ (Ec 3.4.21.8) denotes those serine proteinases
which liberate kinins from kininogens by limited proteolysis. The
proteinases are highly specific and have no or little proteolytic
activity on other proteins (Habermann, 1962). Their pharmacological
effects became known already in the late twenties (Kraut et al.,
1930).

Two types of kallikreins have so far been detected in mammals:
plasma kallikrein and different species of glandular kallikreins
which have been found in exocrine glands and their secretions.
Both types differ in (a) physicochemical properties, (b) enzyme
kinetics of kinin release from kininogen and (c) rates of reaction
with synthetic substrates or pseudosubstrates, e.g. inhibitors
(Pisano, 1975).

It was the aim of the present investigations to determine the
first amino acid sequence of a glandular kallikrein isolated from
porcine pancreas and to compare the data obtained with sequences
of kallikreins isolated from other secretions. The results are
due to concerted efforts of Kutzbach and Schmidt-Kastner in pancreas
kallikrein isolation, Ehret and Fiedler in peptide preparations and
purification, and my group in peptide sequence determinations.
Submandibular kallikrein was isolated by Lemon and Fritz and urinary
kallikrein by Mair, Tschesche and Fritz.

Properties of Pancreatic Kallikrein

Porcine pancreatic kallikrein isolated from autolyzed pancreas
shows multiple forms at least in part due to varying carbohydrate
content and could be resolved upon gel electrophoresis at pH 8 and
9 into the components A and B (Habermann, 1962). Preparative isolation of both components was achieved by chromatography on DEAE-
ion exchangers (Fiedler and Werle, 1967; Kutzbach and Schmidt-Kastner,
1972). The only difference between kallikreins A and B was found
in the carbohydrate content (Fiedler, 1976). Kallikrein B has
about 11.5% carbohydrate which is about twice as high as in kallikrein A (Fiedler et al., 1975). No differences in enzymic properties
have so far been detected between kallikreins A and B against natural
and synthetic substrates (Fiedler, 1976). Kallikreins A and B have
identical amino acid compositions and contain 232 amino acid residues
(protein part MW. 25,600) but differ in carbohydrate compositions
(Fiedler et al., 1977). The molecule of kallikrein (form B, MW.
28,9000 without sialic acid content; Fiedler et al., 1977) contains
5 disulfide bridges and no free cysteine (Zuber and Sache, 1974).

It is still an open question whether kallikreins A and B are
of biological significance and are distinct products of separate
biosynthetic pathways or whether kallikrein A is an intermediate

in synthesis or degradation of kallikrein B. However, two prekalli-
kreins have been identified in pancreatic extracts (Fiedler et al.,
1970).

Primary Structure

Kallikreins A and B are obviously constructed from two peptide
chains interlocked by disulfide bridges. After reduction of the
disulfide links both chains were separated by gel electrophoresis
or gel filtration on Sephadex G-75 in 0.1 M ammonium bicarbonate,
pH 7 (Tschesche et al., 1976). The A-chains of kallikrein A and B
both contain isoleucine as amino terminal residue and about half a
residue of leucine and serine as carboxy-terminal residues (Fiedler
et al., 1975). Both B-chains contain alanine at their amino terminus
and proline at their carboxyl terminal end (Fiedler et al., 1975).

Kallikrein B (266 U/mg protein, measured with Bz-Arg-OEt (Fiedler, 1976) was treated with neuraminidase to remove sialic acid
residues and to eliminate charge differences in the carbohydrate-
containing peptides. The reduced and carboxymethylated A- and B-
chains of the enzyme were subjected to selective cleavages by
cyanogen bromide and trypsin (Tschesche et al., 1976). The amino
acid sequence of the peptides was determined by means of an automatic Edman Sequencer (model Beckman 890 B) making use of the Beckman DMAA-program or a modified program with 0.25 M DMBA (Hermodson
et al., 1972). The amino acid phenylthiohydantoins from Edman
degradations were identified by either mass spectrometry and/or by
amino acid analysis after back hydrolysis with hydrogen iodide as
described previously (Tschesche and Wachter, 1970; Tschesche and
Dietl, 1975).

The previously reported partial sequence (Tschesche et al., 1976;
Fiedler et al., 1977) has been completed by determination of the
amino acid sequence of a 41 residue peptide (residue 127-165*),
Fig. 1b. This peptide was obtained in about 30% yield from selective
tryptophan cleavage at residue 141 of the cyanogen bromide peptide
(residues 105 to 180) from the kallikrein B-chain. The cleavage was
performed by making use of the BNPS-skatol reagent (Fontana et al.,
1973). The amino acid composition and integral values of the
isolated 41 residue peptide is given in Table 1.

The almost completed data of the A- and B-chains of the kallikrein B sequence from porcine pancreas is presented in Fig. 1a,b.
The peptides were ordered into the sequence of kallikrein B on the
basis of information obtained during stepwise degradation and using
selective cleavages of the isolated A- and B-chains (Tschesche et
al., 1976). Only the sequence of residues 170 to 174 shown in

---

*Chymotrypsinogen numbering (Hartley, 1964).

Table 1.   Amino acid composition of the 41-residue peptide
             from cleavage at Trp 141 in the cyanogen bromide
             fragment (residues 105-180) after 24 h hydrolysis
             in 6 N HCl at 100°C.

AMINO ACID	NO. 142-180	
	Moles AA/mole Peptide	
CARBOXYMETHYL-CYSTEINE	1.27	2
ASPARTIC ACID	5.87	6
THREONINE	2.95	3
SERINE	2.16	2
GLUTAMIC ACID	7.28	7
PROLINE	3.92	4
GLYCINE	2.22	2
ALANINE	2.07	2
VALINE	1.79	2
ISOLEUCINE	1.94	2
LEUCINE	3.04	3
PHENYLALANINE	2.80	3
HISTIDINE	1.03	1
LYSINE	0.95	1
HOMOSERINE	0.91	1
TOTAL		41

brackets is tentative and subject to error and needs reconfirmation
as well as a few of the amino acid amides, i.e. residues 148A, 153
and 240.

Homology To Other Serine Proteinases

The amino acid sequence of porcine pancreatic kallikrein B
is compared to that of porcine trypsin as determined by the group
of Neurath (Hermodson et al., 1973), Fig. 1a,b. The A-chain
represents the amino terminal part of the sequence and is clearly
homologous to trypsin as is the B-chain. Maximal homology is
obtained between both enzymes with only one insertion in the A-
chain, i.e. Gln 41A after position 41. Maximal homology of the B-
chain of kallikrein is obtained with insertion of only 3 residues
in the sequence of kallikrein B, i.e. residues Pro 145A, Gly 145B
and Thr 218. Thr 218 corresponds to Ser 218 in bovine chymotrypsin
A and B (Hartley, 1964). The alignment given in Fig. 1a,b is
restricted to a comparison with porcine trypsin only due to limited

```
                    16          20      22       25
    Kallikrein  Ile-Ile-Gly-Gly-Arg-Glu-Cys-Glu-Lys-Asn-Ser-His-
    Trypsin     Ile-Val-Gly-Gly-Tyr-Thr-Cys-Ala-Ala-Asn-Ser-Val-

                        30                  40          42
    K.      -Pro-Trp-Gln-Val-Ala-Ile-Tyr-His-Tyr-Ser-Ser-Phe-Gln-Cys-
    T.      -Pro-Tyr-Gln-Val-Ser-Leu-Asn-Ser-Gly-Ser-His-Phe———Cys-

                    45                  50                  55
    K.      -Gly-Gly-Val-Leu-Val-Asn-Pro-Lys-Trp-Val-Leu-Thr-Ala-Ala-
    T.      -Gly-Gly-Ser-Leu-Ile-Asn-Ser-Gln-Trp-Val-Val-Ser-Ala-Ala-

            57  58      60                  65                  70
    K.      -His-Cys-Lys-Asn-Asp-Asn-Tyr-Glu-Val-Gly-Trp-Leu-Arg-His-
    T.      -His-Cys-Tyr-Lys-Ser-Arg-Ile-Gln-Val-Arg-Leu-Gly-Glu-His-

                        75                  80                  85
    K.      -Asn-Leu-Phe-Glu-Asn-Glu-Asn-Thr-Ala-Gln-Phe-Phe-Gly-Val-
    T.      -Asn-Ile-Asp-Val-Leu-Glu-Gly-Asn-Glu-Gln-Phe-Ile-Asn-Ala-

                            90              CHO
    K.      -Thr-Ala-Asp-Phe-Pro-His-Pro-Gly-Phe-Asn-Leu-[Ser]
    T.      -Ala-Lys-Ile-Ile-Thr-His-Pro-Asn-Phe-Asn-
```
                                                                    a)

```
                                            99          102         105
Kallikrein, B-chain             Ala-Asp-Gly-Lys-Asp-Tyr-Ser-His-Asp-Leu-Met-Leu
Porcine Trypsin                 Gly-Asn-Thr-Leu-Asp-Asn-Asp-Ile-Met-Leu

                110             115             120             125
K.  -Leu-Arg-Leu-Gln-Ser-Pro-Ala-Lys-Ile-Thr-Asp-Ala-Val-Lys-Val-Leu-Glu-Leu-Pro-Thr-
T.  -Ile-Lys-Leu-Ser-Ser-Pro-Ala-Thr-Leu-Asn-Ser-Arg-Val-Ala-Thr-Val-Ser-Leu-Pro-Arg-

            130             136         140
K.  -Gln-Glu-Pro-Glu-Leu-Gly-Ser-Thr-Cys-Glu-Ala-Ser-Gly-Trp-Gly-Ser-Ile-Glu-Pro-Gly-
T.  -Ser-Cys-Ala-Ala-Ala-Gly-Thr-Glu-Cys-Leu-Ile-Ser-Gly-Trp-Gly-Asn-Thr-Lys————

            150                 157
K.  -Pro-Asp-(Asp)-Phe-Glu-Phe-Pro-Asp-Glu-Ile-Gln-Cys-Val-Gln-Leu-Thr-Leu-Leu-Gln-Asn-
T.  -Ser-Ser- Gly -Ser-Ser-Tyr-Pro-Ser-Leu-Leu-Gln-Cys-Leu-Lys-Ala-Pro-Val-Leu-Ser-Asp-

            168             175             180     182
K.  -Thr-Phe-Cys-(Ala-His-Ala-Asx-Pro-Asx)-Lys-Val-Thr-Glu-Ser-Met-Leu-Cys-Ala-Gly-Tyr-
T.  -Ser-Ser-Cys- Lys-Ser-Ala-Tyr-Pro-Gly -Gln-Ile-Thr-Gly-Asn-Met-Ile-Cys-Val-Gly-Phe-

    185             189     191 192     194 195                     201
K.  -Leu-Pro-Gly-Gly-Lys-Asp-Thr-Cys-Met-Gly-Asp-Ser-Gly-Gly-Pro-Leu-Ile-Cys-Asn-Gly-
T.  -Leu-Glu-Gly-Gly-Lys-Asp-Ser-Cys-Gln-Gly-Asp-Ser-Gly-Gly-Pro-Val-Val-Cys-Asn-Gly-

            210             215             220                 225
K.  -Met-Trp-Gln-Gly-Ile-Thr-Ser-Trp-Gly-His-Thr-Pro-Cys-Gly-Ser-Ala-Asn-Lys-Pro-Ser-
T.  -Gln-Leu-Gln-Gly-Ile-Val-Ser-Trp-Gly-Tyr————Gly-Cys-Ala-Gln-Lys-Asn-Lys-Pro-Gly-

            230             235         CHO 240                 245
K.  -Ile-Tyr-Thr-Lys-Leu-Ile-Phe-Tyr-Leu-Asp-Trp-Ile-(Asx)(Asx)-Thr-Ile-Thr-Glu-Asn-Pro
T.  -Val-Tyr-Thr-Lys-Val-Cys-Asn-Tyr-Val-Asn-Trp-Ile- Gln -Gln -Thr-Ile-Ala-Ala-Asn
```
                                                                    b)

Fig. 1a,b. Amino acid sequence of the A-chain (a, above) and the
            B-chain (b, below) of porcine pancreatic kallikrein B.
            For details see text.

space. The alignment reveals an extended loop between residues
Asn 95 and Gly 96 in kallikrein. The residues Asn 95 and Gly 96 in
trypsin are linked directly. All half-cystine residues 22, 42, 58,
136, 157, 168, 182, 191 and 226 are then in equivalent positions in
kallikrein B and trypsin. On disulfide bridge linking positions 22
and 157 is unique for trypsins and is not present in chymotrypsin,
elastase and thrombin (Hartley and Shotton, 1971). The A-chain
contains half-cystine residue 157. Obviously, this bridge is present
in kallikrein B as well. This documents the close relationship
between the enzyme families of trypsin and kallikrein. However,
the second cystine bridge 128-232 unique to trypsin is not present
in kallikrein, underlining that kallikreins are a family of serine
proteinases of its own.

The overall homologies between kallikrein and other mammalian
serine proteinases are compared in Table 2. A close relationship
between kallikrein and trypsin with 37% identical residues and 51%
chemically similar residues (acc. to Hartley and Shotton, 1971)

Table 2. Overall homologies between mammalian serine proteinases

ENZYME	KALLIKREIN B	(%) PERCENT IDENTITY (OR CHEMICAL SIMILARITY[a]) WITH[b]				CHAIN LENGTH
		TRYPSIN	CHYMOTRYPSIN B	ELASTASE	THROMBIN	NO. OF RESIDUES
KALLIKREIN B[c]	–	37 (51)	30 (44)	31 (42)	29 (39)	232
TRYPSIN[c]		–	38 (49)	35 (48)	32 (38)	
CHYMOTRYPSIN A[d]		43 (53)	78 (85)	39 (51)	32 (39)	230
CHYMOTRYPSIN B[d]			–	38 (47)	31 (38)	230
ELASTASE[c]				–	27 (39)	240
THROMBIN[e]					–	265

[a]Chemical similarities are defined as Arg = Lys, Asp = Asn, Glu = Gln,
Asp = Glu, Asn = Gln, Ser = Thr, Val = Ile, Ile = Leu, Tyr = Phe =
Trp, in addition to identities

[b]Calculated as percent of the minimum length required to accomodate
the sequences being compared when aligned as in Fig. 1a,b, discoun-
ting deletions or insertions.

[c]From porcine pancreas

[d]From bovine pancreas, based on residues 16-245 only (Chymotrypsin
numbering, acc. to Hartley, Nature 201, 1284 (1964).)

[e]bovine

in both enzymes is obvious. Thus, the homology between trypsin
and kallikrein is as close as between porcine trypsin or elastase
compared to bovine chymotrypsin B. Comparison with chymotrypsin
reveals lack of the chymotryptic residues No. 35, 36, 67, 68, 99A
and 99B, 126, 131, 205 and 206 in kallikrein and trypsin, indicating
a close relationship between the latter two enzymes. This is
documented as well by the similar substrate specificity for basic
residues for which Asp 189 in the specificity binding pocket is
responsible in kallikrein and trypsin. Further homologies include
such important residues as (a) the amino-terminal Ile 16 and Asp
194 forming an ion pair in activated serine proteinases (b), the
basic Arg 107 residue arresting the carboxylat at the carboxy
terminus by a salt bridge and (c) the reactive site residues of the
charge relais-system of serine proteinases, His 57, Asp 102 and
Ser 195 (Stroud et al., 1971; Bode and Schwager, 1975a; Kossiakoff
et al., 1977). Comparison of the kallikrein sequence with bovine
chymotrypsin A and B, however, reveals a number of similarities
between both enzymes, which are unique to chymotrypsins, e.g. Met
192 and Ser 218. Methionine 192 closes the binding site in chymotrypsinogen. Its side-chain is turned to the outside surface in
the activated enzyme and lines up at the substrate binding site
(Freer et al., 1969).

Comparison to the Crystal Structure of Trypsin

In the crystal structure of trypsin, Fig. 2, residues 92-100
located on the surface of the molecule (Stroud et al., 1971). The
additional residues 95A-95Z in the sequence form a unique "kallikrein autolysis loop" not present in other serine proteinases of
pancreas nor present in bovine thrombin (Hartley and Shotton, 1971).
This loop contains the site of cleavage between the A- and B-chains
of kallikrein. The split obviously is the result of proteolytic
attack during isolation of kallikrein from autolyzed pancreas,
during which part of the newly formed carboxy-terminal Ser is
cleaved from the A-chain. This has been discussed previously
(Tschesche et al., 1976; Fiedler et al., 1977) and is supported by
the finding that porcine submaxillary and urinary kallikreins are
single-chain molecules. Preliminary and indirect evidence for the
loss of as many as three residues from this loop of the A-chain was
obtained (Fritz et al., 1977).

The extended "kallikrein autolysis loop" contains the attachment site of one of the carbohydrate moieties at Asn 95 in the
sequence Asn-Leu-Ser 97. A second carbohydrate moiety is obviously
attached to the carboxy terminal end of the B-chain on Asn 239 in
the sequence Asx-Asc-Thr. Indirect evidence came from complete
lack of a phenylthiohydantoin recovery at position 95 and 239
during sequence determinations. Both carbohydrate moieties are thus
located at the same edge of the globular molecule as indicated in

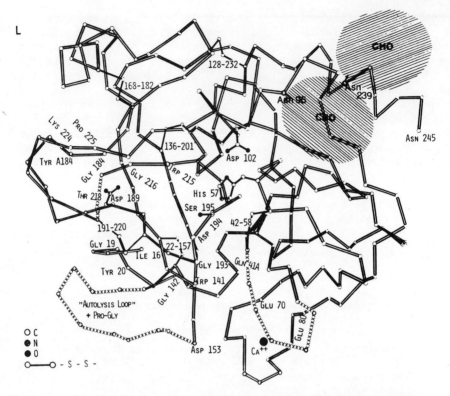

Fig. 2.   α-Carbon drawing of the complete polypeptide chain of
refined bovine β-trypsin (Bode and Schwager, 1975).
The broken lines indicate sites carrying insertions
in kallikrein, i.e. residues Gln 41A, Gly 145A–Pro 145B,
and Thr 218. The "kallikrein autolysis loop" residues
95A–96Z is not indicated, but the carbohydrate attachment
site (CHO in hatched areas) in kallikrein Asn 95 and
Asn 239 are illustrated.

Fig. 2.   They could perhaps serve to cover hydrophobic clusters in
the regions of residues 88–94 and 114–123 remote from the reactive
site cleft.

        In the drawing of the globular structure of bovine trypsin
(Fehlhammer et al., 1977), Fig. 2, those main chain segments of
trypsin are indicated which carry insertions in kallikrein. These
regions are necessarily subject to major differences in their atom
positions. Mainly concerned are (a) the "autolysis loop" of trypsin
and chymotrypsin (Blow et al., 1969 with Lys (or Arg) 145 in the
sequence Gly 142 to Pro 152, furthermore (b) the calcium binding

site (Bode and Schwager, 1975) containing the loop or residues Arg 70 to Ala 80 and (c) the specificity binding pocket with residues Gly 216 to Cys 220, where Thr 218 is inserted.

The "trypsin autolysis loop" is enlarged in kallikrein by insertion of two residues; Fig. 1a,b. It is, however, not subject to autolytic cleavage, since the basic residue Lys or Arg in trypsin, chymotrypsin or elastase is substituted by Pro 145 in kallikrein.

Substitution of Arg 117 in porcine and bovine trypsin by Ala 117 in kallikrein eliminates a second preferred splitting site at another external loop (Bode and Schwager, 1975). However, Lys 188A is present in kallikrein as well as in both trypsins. This potential tryptic splitting site which leads to pseudotrypsin is preserved in porcine kallikrein (Smith and Shaw, 1968).

The calcium ion is complexed by six different ligands positioned at the edges of an almost regular octahedron (Bode and Schwager, 1975). Two ligands are the carbonyl oxygens of Asn 72 and Val 75, two are water molecules, close to the carboxylic group of Glu 77 and the side chain of Glu 70. The residual two ligands are the side chains of Glu 70 and Glu 80 in porcine trypsin. In kallikrein Asn 72 is preserved; the other residues are substituted by Arg 70, Glu 75 and Glu 80 in porcine kallikrein. Besides changes in the atom positions of the calcium-binding loop, substitution of the negatively charged Glu 70 by the positively charged Arg 70 would possibly interfere with binding of the positive calcium ion.

In the substrate specificity binding pocket Gly 266 of trypsin is substituted by Ser 226 in kallikrein. However, the pocket is not closed for larger residues as in elastase (Hartley and Shotton, 1971). Except for residues Ser 39 and Asp 189 all other amino acids are in the surface of the substrate binding region in porcine kallikrein are changed when compared to porcine trypsin, Table 3. Thus, the degree of 85% accepted mutations affecting the surface in the binding site of kallikrein is by far higher than is the overall number of 37% substitutions in the entire chain. A detailed explanation of the restricted specificity has therefore to await the elucidation of the x-ray crystallographic structure of kallikrein B. A discussion of the restricted specificity of kallikrein on the basis of new experimental data from investigations of various substrates is given by Fiedler and Leysath (this volume).

In this regard it is striking that 57% of the residues mediating the contact in the complex of trypsin-kallikrein inhibitor (Kunitz) and either kallikrein of trypsin are preserved in both enzymes, Table 4. Especially important, residues forming more than just one interaction with the inhibitor remained unchanged in kallikrein. From the numerous interactions listed (Huber et al., 1974) on

Table 3. Amino acids in the surface of the substrate binding region
          (acc. to Hartley and Shotton, 1971)

RESIDUE NO.	PORCINE KALLIKREIN	PORCINE TRYPSIN	BOVINE TRYPSIN	BOVINE CHYMOTRYPSIN
39	SER	SER	TYR	PHE
97	LYS	ASN	ASN	LEU
99	TYR	LEU	LEU	ILE
143	SER	ASN	ASN	LEU
149	PHE	SER	THR	ALA
150	GLU	SER	SER	ASN
151	PHE	TYR	TYR	THR
172	ASX	TYR	TYR	TRP
189	ASP	ASP	ASP	SER
192	MET	GLU	GLU	MET
217	HIS	TYR	SER	SER
218	THR	-	-	SER
219	PRO	GLY	GLY	THR

the basis of the amino acid sequence about 70% seem to be possible
in kallikrein, especially the contacts around the reactive site
Lys 15-Ala 16 of the inhibitor.

Relationships Between Glandular Kallikreins

The isolation, purification and partial characterization of
porcine submandibular (Lemon et al., 1976) and porcine urinary
(Tschesche et al., 1976) kallikrein have been reported previously.
A high degree of similarity between submandibular and urinary
kallikreins and to some extent with porcine pancreatic kallikrein
was revealed from identical or respectively similar kinetic behaviour
from SDS gel electrophoretic and chromatographic separation into
A- and B-forms of all three kallikreins, as well as from similar
amino acid compositions (Fritz et al., 1977). New values of the
amino acid composition of urinary kallikrein were obtained from a
time-release plot of the acid hydrolysis, Table 5, and are
compared to the compositions of submandibular and pancreatic kallikrein. All three compositions indicate a close relationship of
the protein part of the enzymes. Pancreatic kallikrein is a two
chain molecule with some distinctly different properties, while
submandibular and urinary kallikrein are single chain enzymes (Fritz
et al., 1977). The difference seems to result from cleavage of the
kallikrein autolysis loop in the pancreatic enzyme and is reflected

Table 4. Interactions of Kunitz inhibitor (Trasylol) and trypsin
(Huber et al., 1974) compared to the corresponding
kallikrein residues

Inhibitor		TKI	Thr	Gly	Pro	Cys	Lys	Ala	Arg	Ile	Val	Tyr	Gly	Gly	Cys	Arg	
Trypsin			11	12	13	14	15	16	17	18	34	35	36	37	38	39	Kallikrein
Porcine	Bovine																Porcine
Ser	Tyr 39							V									Ser
	His 40							H									Ser
	Phe 41						V	H,V	V								Phe
	Cys 42						V										Cys
	His 57				V	V	V					V	V	V			His
	Cys 58						V										Cys
	Tyr 59																Lys
	Lys 60								V								Asn
	Asn 97														H,V		Lys
	Thr 98														V		Asp
	Leu 99				V									V	V		Tyr
	Tyr 151								V,CT	V							Phe
	Gln 175														H		Lys
	Asp 189						S										Asp
	Ser 190						H,V										Thr
	Cys 191						V										Cys
	Gln 192	H?	H?,V		H		V	V									Met
	Gly 193						H,V	V	V								Gly
	Asp 194																Asp
	Ser 195					V	C,HV,V										Ser
	Ser 214						H										Ser
	Tyr 215				V	V	V							V			Trp
	Gly 216					H,V											Gly

Phe = Tyr = Trp and Thr = Ser,   C covalent, H hydrogen bond, V Van der Waals
interaction, CT charge transfer, S salt bridge

in the amino acid composition with three additional residues present
in submandibular or urinary kallikrein. Additional differences
between the enzymes derive from differences in the carbohydrate
content which is higher in submandibular and urinary kallikrein
than in the pancreatic enzyme.

Data on the inhibition properties of all three glandular
kallikreins with synthetic and with naturally occurring inhibitors
have been published recently (Fritz et al., 1977).

The close structural relationship of all three glandular
enzymes becomes clearly evident from immunological cross-reactivities
in the immunodiffusion using the OUCHTERLONY test. The precipitin
lines show a pattern of identity after diffusion of the three
kallikreins against rabbit α-globulins directed against either

Table 5.   Amino acid compositions of porcine glandular
           kallikreins (integral values).

AMINO ACID	KALLIKREIN PANCREATIC	KALLIKREIN SUBMANDIBULAR	KALLIKREIN URINARY
	MOLES AMINO ACID PER MOLE PROTEIN		
ASPARTIC ACID	28	28	28
THREONINE	15	16	15-16
SERINE	14	14	14
GLUTAMIC ACID	23	23	23
PROLINE	16	15-16	16
GLYCINE	22	22	22
ALANINE	13	13	13
HALF-CYSTINE	10	10	10
VALINE	10	10	10
METHIONINE	4	4	4
ISOLEUCINE	12	11	11
LEUCINE	20	21	20
TYROSINE	7	7	7
PHENYLALANINE	10	10	9
LYSINE	10	11	10
HISTIDINE	8	9	9
ARGININE	3	3	3
TRYPTOPHAN	7	7	N.D.
TOTAL	232	234-235	

kallikrein, Fig. 3. However, immunelectrophoretic studies with
all three glandular kallikreins reveal minor differences in mobility
between pancreatic and even submandibular and urinary kallikrein
(Fritz et al., 1977). The experiments indicate complete immunological identity of all three glandular kallikreins and the various
forms of pancreatic kallikrein as well.

    Clear evidence for identity of the primary structure of all
three proteins was obtained from the amino-terminal sequences.
Automatic Edman-degradation of carboxymethylated submandibular
kallikrein and of the A-chain of carboxymethylated pancreatic
kallikrein revealed identity of the first 28 residues (Fritz et al.,
1977). Edman-degradation of porcine urinary kallikrein resulted
in an N-terminal sequence identical in the first ten residues to
that of sumbandibular and pancreatic kallikrein, Fig. 4.

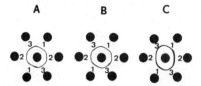

Fig. 3. Immunodiffusion of the three porcine glandular kallikreins against purified rabbit α-globulins directed against other kallikrein. 1=pancreatic, 2=urinary, 3=submandibular kallikrein. A=urinary, B=pancreatic, C=submandibular kallikrein-directed α-globulins (Fritz et al., 1977).
0.25 µg of each kallikrein dissolved in 5 µl sodium barbital buffer pH 8.2 were applied in the outer wells, 5 µl of the corresponding α-globulin solution (1%, w/v) in the central well. After diffusion (48 hours at 20°C), the precipitate was stained with Coomassie Brilliant blue.

All evidence accumulated from biophysical studies, from immunological and from N-terminal sequence investigations point to a common genetic origin of all three glandular kallikreins. The three enzymes are structurally homologous proteins. Existing differences obviously originate from differences in the carbohydrate part and different stages of limited proteolytic degradations, as e.g. in the β-, α- and π-trypsin series (Smith and Shaw, 1968).

Pancreatic B   Ile-Ile-Gly-Gly-Arg-Glu-Cys-Glu-Lys-Asn-Ser-His-Pro-Trp
                                                                    10

Submandibular   Ile-Ile-Gly-Gly-Arg-Glu-Cys-Glu-Lys-Asn-Ser-His-Pro-Trp
                                                                    10

Urinary   Ile-Ile-Gly-Gly-Arg-Glu-Cys-[Glx-Lys]-Asn-[Ser]- X -Pro-
                                                                    10

Fig. 4. Amino terminal amino acid sequences of glandular kallikreins.

ACKNOWLEDGEMENT

The authors are grateful to the Sonderforschungsbereich 51, Munich, for financial support (projects B-2, B-3, B-17). We are indebted to the Stiftung Volkswagenwerk, Hannover, for providing a Beckman Sequencer, model 890 B. The financial aid of the Fonds der Chemischen Industrie, Frankfurt, is gratefully acknowledged. We wish to thank Prof. R. Huber and Dr. W. Bode for helpful discussions on the x-ray crystallographic structure of bovine β-trypsin and their generous help in building a structural model of the enzyme.

REFERENCES

Blow, D.M., J.J. Birktoft and B.S. Hartley, 1969. Role of a buried acid group in the mechanism of action of chymotryspin, Nature (London 221: 337.

Bode, W. and P. Schwager, 1975. The single calcium-binding site of crystalline bovine β-trypsin, FEBS letters 56: 139.

Bode, W. and P. Schwager, 1975a. The refined crystal structure of bovine β-trypsin at 1.8 A resolution, J. Mol. Biol. 98: 693.

Flhlhammer, H., W. Bode and R. Huber, 1977. Crystal structure of bovine trypsinogen at 1.8 A resulution, J. Mol. Biol. 111: 415.

Fiedler, F., C. Hirschauer and E. Werle, 1970. Anreicherung von Prakallikrein B aus Schweinepankreas und Eigenschaften verschieder Formen des Pankreaskallikreins, Hoppe-Seyler's Z. Physiol. Chem. 351: 225.

Fiedler, F., C. Hirschauer and E. Werle, 1975. Characterization of pig pancreatic kallikreins A and B, Hoppe-Seyler's Z. Physiol. Chem. 356: 1879.

Fiedler, F., 1976. Pig pancreatic kallikreins A and B, in: Methods in Enzymology 45: 289.

Fiedler, F., W. Ehret, G. Godec, C. Hirschauer, C. Kutzbach, G. Schmidt-Kastner and H. Tschesche, 1977. The primary structure of pig pancreatic kallikrein B, in: Kininogenases-Kallikrein 4, eds. G. Haberland, J.W. Rohen and T. Suzuki (Schattauer-Stuttgart), p. 7.

Fontana, A., C. Vita and C. Toniolo, 1973. Selective cleavage of the single tryptophanyl peptide bond in horse heart cytochrome C, FEBS letters 32: 139.

Freer, S.T., J. Kraut, J.D. Robertus, H.T. Wright, and N.H. Xuong, 1970. Chymotrypsinogen: 2.5 A crystal structure, comparison with α-chymotrypsinogen, and implication for zymogen activation, Biochemistry 9: 1977.

Fritz, H., F. Fiedler, T. Dietl, M. Warwas, E. Truscheit, H.J. Kolb, G. Mair and H. Tschesche, 1977. On the relationship between porcine pancreatic, submandibular, and urinary kallikrein, in:

Kininogenases-Kallikrein 4, eds. G. Haberland, J.W. Rohen and
   T. Suzuki (Schattauer-Stuttgart), p. 15.

Habermann, E., 1962. Trennung und Reinigung von Pankreaskallikrein,
   Hoppe-Seyler's Z. Physiol. Chem. 328: 15.

Hartley, B.S. and Shotton, D.M., 1971. Pancreatic elastase, in:
   The Enzymes, ed. P.D. Boyer (Academic Press-New York) p. 323.

Hermodson, M.A., L.H. Ericsson, K. Titani, H. Neurath and K.A.
   Walsh, 1972. Application of sequenator analysis to the study
   of proteins, Biochemistry 11: 4493.

Hermodson, M.A., L.H. Ericsson, H. Neurath and K.A. Walsh, 1973.
   Determination of the amino acid sequence of porcine trypsin
   by sequenator analysis, Biochemistry 12: 3146.

Huber, R., D. Kukla, W. Steigemann, J. Deisenhofer and T.A. Jones,
   1974. in: Proteinase Inhibitors - Bayer Symposium V, eds.
   H. Fritz, H. Tschesche, L.J. Green and E. Truscheit (Springer-
   Berlin), p. 497.

Kossiakoff, A.A., J.L. Chambers, L.M. Kay and R.M. Stroud, 1977.
   Structure of bovine chymotrypsinogen at 1.9 A resolution,
   Biochemistry 16: 654.

Kraut, H., E.K. Frey and E. Werle, 1930. Der Nachweis eines
   Kreislaufhormons in der Pankreasdruse, Hoppe-Seyler's Z.
   Physiol. Chem. 189: 97.

Kutzbach, C. and G. Schmidt-Kastner, 1972. Kallikrein from pig
   pancreas. Purification, separation of components A and B,
   and crystallization. Hoppe-Seyler's Z. Physiol. Chem. 353: 1099.

Lemon, M., B. Forg-Grey and H. Fritz, 1976. Isolation of porcine
   submaxillary kallikrein, in: Kinins-pharmacodynamics and biological roles, eds. F. Sicuteri, N. Back and G.L. Haberland
   (Plenum-New York) p. 209.

Pisano, J.J., 1975, Chemistry and biology of the kallikrein-kinin
   system, in: Proteases in Biological Control, eds. E. Reich,
   D.B. Rifkin and E. Shaw (Cold Spring Harbor Laboratory - Cold
   Spring Harbor) p. 199.

Smith, R.L. and E. Shaw, 1968. Pseudotrypsin, J. Biol. Chem. 244:
   4704.

Stroud, R.M., L.M. Kay and R.E. Dickerson, 1971. The crystal and
   molecular structure of DIP-inhibited bovine trypsin at 2.7 A
   resolution, Cold Spring Harbor Symposium Quant. Biol. 36: 125.

Stroud, R.M., L.M. Kay and R.E. Dickerson, 1974. The structure of
   bovine trypsin: Electron density maps of the inhibited enzyme
   at 5 A and 2.5 A resolution, J. Mol. Biol. 83: 185.

Tschesche, H. and E. Wachter, 1970. The structure of the porcine
   pancreatic secretory trypsin inhibitor I. A sequence determination by Edman degradation and mass spectral identification
   of the p-bromophenyl-thiohydantoins, Eur. J. Biochem. 16: 187.

Tschesche, H. and T. Dietl, 1975. The amino acid sequence of iso-
   inhibitor K from snails (Helix pomatia) Eur. J. Biochem. 58:
   439.

Tschesche, H., W. Ehret, G. Godec, C. Hirschauer, C. Kutzbah, G.
    Schmidt-Kastner and F. Fiedler, 1976. The primary structure of
    pig pancreatic kallikrein B, in: Kinins-pharmacodynamics and
    biological roles, eds. F. Sicuteri, N. Back and G.L. Haberland
    (Plenum-New York) p. 123.
Tschesche, H., G. Mair, B. Forg-Brey and H. Fritz, 1976a. Isolation
    of urinary kallikrein, in: Kinins-pharmacodynamics and biologi-
    cal roles, eds. F. Sicuteri, N. Back and G.L. Haberland (Plenum
    New York) p. 119.
Zuber, M. and E. Sache, 1974. Isolation and characterization of
    porcine pancreatic kallikrein, Biochemistry 13: 3098.

SUBSTRATE SPECIFICITY OF PORCINE PANCREATIC KALLIKREIN

Franz Fiedler and Gisela Leysath

Abteilung für Klinische Chemie und Klinische Biochemie

der Chirurgischen Klinik der Universität München

Nussbaumstr. 20, D-8000 Muenchen 2, W. Germany

INTRODUCTION

The glandular kallikreins (EC 3.4.21.8) of the pig have revealed themselves as members of the family of pancreatic serine
proteinases that includes the digestive enzymes trypsin (EC 3.4.
21.4), chymotrypsin (EC 3.4.21.1), and elastase (EC 3.4.21.11)
(Tschesche et al., this volume). Outstanding in this family of
proteinases is the narrow and seemingly inconsistent specificity
of porcine pancreatic kallikrein. A protein as casein is hydrolyzed at least 200 times slower than it is by trypsin (Habermann
1962), though the rate of cleavage of certain specific peptide
bonds may reach about 10% of the rate of tryptic attack (see
below). Porcine pancreatic kallikrein contains in its sequence
the same aspartic acid residue that is responsible for the specificity of trypsin for basic amino acids (Tschesche et al., this
volume). Nevertheless, this kallikrein – as well as the other
glandular kallikreins studied so far – exhibits the strange
property of cleaving in kininogen a bond involving a neutral amino
acid, methionine, with formation of kallidin. Moreover, this bond
is located just adjacent to a basic lysine residue, that is readily accessible to trypsin that liberates bradykinin. In contrast,
the cleavage of the second bond linking the kinin part to kininogen,
an arginyl bond, conforms to the primary specificity for basic
amino acids of both enzymes (Fig. 1).

These peculiar features of kallikrein prompted us to a study
of the hydrolysis of kininogen model peptides and peptide esters

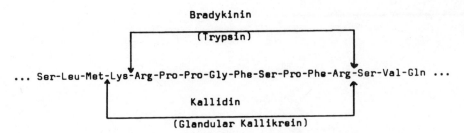

Fig. 1.   Partial amino acid sequence of bovine kininogen (Haber-
          mann 1966; Han et al. 1976) and sites of attack by
          trypsin and by glandular kallikreins.

by porcine pancreatic kallikrein in an attempt to pinpoint those
structural elements of kininogen essential in the interaction with
kallikrein. For comparison, the digestive enzyme trypsin was
included in the investigations.

MATERIALS AND METHODS

Initial rates of the hydrolysis of synthetic substrates at
several concentrations by neuraminidase-treated porcine pancreatic
kallikrein B (mainly the two-chain β-form, Fiedler et al. 1977a)
or bovine β-trypsin (Schroeder and Shaw 1968) were followed in
0.1 M NaCl, 0.1 mM thioglycolic acid or EDTA (to counteract a
possible inhibition by heavy metal ions) at pH 9.0, 25°C, in a
Radiometer Autotitrator. Where appropriate, the necessary small
corrections for ionization of the α-amino groups of substrates and
products were applied. Cleavage sites in peptides were identified
by thin-layer chromatography of the mixture of products with
appropriate reference compounds and were always found to involve
only the arginyl bond. Some differences in kinetic constants
reported here to previous preliminary values (Fiedler 1976) are
due to repetition of the measurements with a larger number of
experimental points and to more elaborate evaluation of the data.

RESULTS AND DISCUSSION

Peptide Models for the Cleavage of the Bond at the C-Terminus of
                        Kinin in Kininogen

We have shown previously (Werle et al. 1973) that among a
number of arginine-containing peptides most were hydrolyzed by
porcine pancreatic kallikrein at a rate lower than 0.05 sec^{-1},

with the exception of two peptides comprising part of the C-terminal
sequence of kinin and some further residues of kininogen. Valid
models for the events taking place at this site in kallikrein-
catalyzed cleavage of kininogen must display maximal turnover
rates k_{cat} and specificity constants (Bender and Kézdy 1965)
k_{cat}/K_m not less favourable than those for kinin release. The
rate of kallidin liberation by porcine pancreatic kallikrein from
highly purified bovine HMW kininogen at 8 µM concentration has
been determined as 0.94 sec^{-1} by Dittmann and Wimmer (1978; pH 8,
37°C). A lower limit of 120 mM^{-1} sec^{-1} follows from these data
for the specificity constant. k_{cat} for the kallikrein-catalyzed
hydrolysis of the peptide Pro-Phe-Arg-Ser-Val-Gln, comprising
six amino acid residues of the kininogen sequence, is well above
the lower limit of the same constant for the cleavage of the
corresponding Arg-Ser bond in kininogen (Table 1). Also, k_{cat}/K_m
approaches the lower limit of this constant for the cleavage of
kallidin from kininogen. The interactions of this hexapeptide
with kallikrein appear thus to comprise the interactions essential
for the kallikrein-catalyzed release of the C-terminus of kinin
in kininogen.

Now, which structural elements of the hexapeptide are involved
in essential interaction with kallikrein? We have shown previously
that elongation of the peptide at the amino terminus beyond the
proline residue up to completion of the sequence of bradykinin
does not significantly influence the substrate properties (Fiedler
1976). A favourable effect on binding of the substrate is exerted
by the proline residue in position P_3 (according to the nomenclature of Schechter and Berger 1967) as follows from a comparison
of the kinetic constants with those of the corresponding Phe-Arg-
and Ac-Phe-Arg-peptides (Table 1). At the carboxy terminus of the
peptides, substitution of the glutamine residue in P_3' by an amino
group even notably favours hydrolysis by kallikrein, while all the
other modifications in the sequence of the hexapeptide-kininogen-
fragment tried so far proved detrimental. If the valine residue
in P_2' is also removed, a comparably poor kallikrein substrate
results. Substitution of the serine residue in P_1' by an isosteric
α-aminobutyryl residue significantly impairs the substrate properties (Table 1). The β-hydroxy amino acid serine appears to be
much better a leaving group.

In the interaction of these peptide substrates with bovine
trypsin, K_m is - with a single exception - remarkably similar
(within a factor of two or less) to the corresponding figures for
kallikrein (Table 1). k_{cat} values for kallikrein are generally
significantly lower than those for trypsin. They still can attain
9 and 17% of the rates of tryptic turnover. Changes made in

Table 1. Kinetic constants (pH 9, 25°C) for the hydrolysis of peptides and peptide esters by porcine pancreatic β-kallikrein B and by bovine β-trypsin.

P_3 P_2 P_1 / P_1' P_2' P_3'	Kallikrein			Trypsin		
	K_m (mM)	k_{cat} (sec^{-1})	k_{cat}/K_m ($mM^{-1}sec^{-1}$)	K_m (mM)	k_{cat} (sec^{-1})	k_{cat}/K_m ($mM^{-1}sec^{-1}$)
Bovine HMW kininogen[+]	0.057	0.94[++]	120[+++]			
Pro-Phe-Arg-Ser-Val-Gln		5.7	100	0.063	33	520
Phe-Arg-Ser-Val-Gln	2.2	2.8	1.3	0.33	7.5	23
Ac-Phe-Arg-Ser-Val-Gln	0.31	6.8	22	0.15	55	370
Ac-Phe-Arg-Ser-Val-NH$_2$	0.040	11.6	290	0.082	130	1600
Ac-Phe-Arg-Ser-NH$_2$	0.21	2.1	10	0.32	81	250
Ac-Phe-Arg-Abut-Val-NH$_2$	0.073	4.2	58	0.18	100	560
Ac-Gly-Arg-Ser-Val-Gln	26	0.77	0.030	0.35	87	250
Z-Gly-Arg-Ser-Gly			5×10^{-5}[+++]	0.28	30	110
Ac-Phe-ArgOMe	0.030	920	31000	0.019	94	4900
Ac-Gly-ArgOMe	1.4	350	250	0.063	230	3700

+ Dittmann and Wimmer (1978)   ++ $\dfrac{v}{[E]_o}$ +++ $\dfrac{v}{[E]_o \cdot [S]}$

positions P_3 and P_1' to P_3' tend to affect hydrolysis by both enzymes in a similar way, though quantitatively much less so in the case of trypsin: k_{cat}/K_m value for all peptides with six residues (counting also acyl and C-terminal amide groups) differ by a factor of 13 in kallikrein-catalyzed, but only by a factor of three in tryptic hydrolyses. Evidently, the active sites of both kallikrein and trypsin can interact with at least six consecutive positions of peptide substrates.

In addition to these minor quantitative differences in specificities of the various subsites in kallikrein and trypsin, there is one very conspicuous difference as regards subsite S_2. Ac-Gly-Arg-Ser-Val-Gln displays a nearly tenfold reduction of k_{cat} in the kallikrein-catalyzed reaction, and K_m is raised to a still much larger amount. The combined effects reduce the specificity constant as much as 700-fold in comparison to the corresponding peptide carrying a bulky phenylalanine residue instead of the small glycine residue in position P_2 (Table 1). With trypsin, the minor rise of K_m is even partially compensated by an increase of k_{cat}, resulting in only 30% decrease of the sepcificity constant. Some additional minor modifications in the peptide structure leading to Z-Gly-Arg-Ser-Gly nearly abolish hydrolysis by kallikrein, while the substrate properties for trypsin are only little impaired.

The same phenomenon is observed with the corresponding peptide esters (Table 1). Ac-Phe-ArgOMe is 120-fold better a kallikrein substrate in terms of k_{cat}/K_m than is Ac-Gly-ArgOMe, while trypsin hardly differentiates between the two compounds. The pronounced secondary substrate specificity for a phenylalanine residue in P_2 exhibited by porcine pancreatic kallikrein is thus practically non-existent in bovine trypsin. Incidentally, in the related serine proteinase chymotrypsin, there has also been observed secondary specificity for bulky side chains in P_2 (Kurachi et al. 1973 and further references therein), though the effect appears not so pronounced as in kallikrein. Possibly, these differences can be attributed to interaction with residue 99 in serine proteinases, that is leucine in trypsin, isoleucine in chymotrypsin, and tyrosine in kallikrein.

That it is the bulk of the amino acid side chain in P_2 that is the crucial feature in interactions with kallikrein is demonstrated by two further aminoacyl arginine esters (Table 2). A bulky leucyl or methionyl residue in this position also leads to very good kallikrein substrates, though they are distinctly inferior to the ester carrying the still more voluminous phynylalanine residue.

At least one of the main reasons for the narrow substrate

specificity of porcine pancreatic kallikrein is thus evidently the
high selectivity for the Phe-Arg sequence as it occurs in kininogen.
It is interesting to note that Suzuki and coworkers observed two
additional bonds involving basic amino acid residues in bovine HMW
kininogen to be cleaved to a minor extent by pancreatic kallikrein,
located in a His-Arg(or Lys)-Ser and in a Trp-Arg-Thr sequence
(Iwanaga et al. 1977; Kato et al. 1977). Both sequences comprise
the features of a bulky amino acid residue in P_2 and a good β-
hydroxy amino acid leaving group, though the reasons for the relatively slow rate of hydrolysis have still to be elucidated.

The pronounced secondary specificity for a bulky amino acid
residue in P_2 might well be a general characteristic of the whole
group of glandular kallikreins. Ac-Phe-ArgOMe is a much better
substrate than Bz-ArgOEt not only for porcine β-pancreatic, but
also for single-chain submandibular and urinary kallikreins (Fritz
et al. 1977; Lemon et al.) and for human urinary kallikrein that
also exhibits a much slower hydrolysis of Ac-Gly-ArgOMe (Fiedler
et al. 1978). The three porcine glandular kallikreins also showed
an increase rate of inhibition by peptide chloromethyl ketones
with increasing size of the residue in P_2 (Fiedler et al. 1977b).

Peptide Ester Models for the Cleavage of the Bond at the N-Terminus
of Kinin in Kininogen

As to the strange cleavage by glandular kallikreins of the
methionyl bond in kininogen at the aminoterminal end of kallidin
one might suppose that this reaction is directed by a specific conformation of the kininogen molecule. Recently, however, Iwanaga
et al. (1977) reported that a small kininogen fragment of the
sequence shown in Figure 1 is also cleaved by porcine pancreatic
kallikrein at the methionyl bond, with formation of kallidin.

Interestingly, in position P_2 to this bond there is also
located a bulky residue, leucine, that conceivably might determine
the site of attack by kallikrein. We therefore synthesized Ac-Leu-
MetOMe as a model compound and were somewhat disappointed to learn
that this ester was a very poor kallikrein substrate in comparison
not only with the corresponding arginine ester (Table 2) but also
with kininogen (Table 1) where a peptide bond of much lower inherent reactivity than the ester bond has to be cleaved.

The leucine residue in P_2 is not without influence, though.
The increase in hydrolytic efficiency as compared to Bz-DL-MetOMe
is quite drastic, as it is in the arginine ester series (Table 2).
An analogous effect is observed also with other unspecific ester
substrates of kallikrein. A phenylalanine residue in P_2 of Ac-
Phe-PheOMe substantially promotes hydrolysis when compared to the

Table 2.   Preliminary specificity constants (pH 9, 25°C) for the hydrolysis of peptide esters by porcine pancreatic ß-kallikrein B.

$P_3 \quad P_2 \quad P_1$	k_{cat}/K_m $(mM^{-1}sec^{-1})$
Ac–Phe–ArgOMe	31 000
Ac–Leu–ArgOMe	15 000
Ac–Met–ArgOMe	6 000
Ac–Gly–ArgOMe	250
Bz–ArgOMe[+]	1 230
Z–Pro–Phe–ArgOMe	35 000
Ac–Leu–Met–ArgOMe	3 000
Ac–Leu–Met–LysOMe	120
Ac–TyrOEt[+]	0.22
Ac–Phe–PheOMe	48
Bz–DL–MetOMe[++]	0.07
Ac–Leu–MetOMe	3
Z–Ser–Leu–MetOMe	6

[+] Fiedler et al. 1973 (pH 8)

[++] Fiedler 1968 (pH 8)

related Ac-TyrOEt, and the specificity constant of this compound
even is notably higher than that of the methionine esters comprising
more features of kininogen (Table 2). Nevertheless, none of these
compounds can be regarded as a valid kininogen model. Ester substrates modelling the structure of the C-terminal part of kinin
exhibit specificity constants three to four orders of magnitude
more favourable (Table 2).

The same is true for the methionine ester Z-Ser-Leu-MetOMe
(Table 2) containing all the amino acid residues of the N-terminal
part of the kininogen fragment studied by Iwanaga et al. (1977).
An unfavourable influence of the carbobenzoxy group in P_4 is ruled
out by the example of Z-Pro-Phe-ArgOMe that is not worse a kallikrein substrate than Ac-Phe-ArgOMe (Table 2)(though this argument
is weakened by possibly altered steric relationships at the proline
residue). Unfortunately, no data were available for a comparison
with the kinetic constants of the kallikrein-catalyzed hydrolysis
of the kininogen fragment. Possibly, as well as the methionine
esters studied, this peptide is also a kallikrein substrate inferior to kininogen because of the lack of some further N-terminal
amino acid residues. On the other hand, three amino acid residues
of kininogen in an equivalent position relative to the site of
cleavage are sufficient to yield an optimal model peptide for the
region at the C-terminus of kinin, though this might reflect again
the influence of the terminal proline residue in P_3.

Another strange fact that has to be explained is the lack of
cleavage by kallikrein of the lysyl bond in the immediate vicinity
of the methionine residue in kininogen, though this bond is readily
accessible to trypsin and esters of lysine are the second best
substrates next to those of arginine for porcine pancreatic kallikrein (Fiedler et al. 1973). One might suppose that the subsite
S_3 of kallikrein is unable to accomodate a bulky leucine residue.
A minor negative effect is indeed seen in comparing Ac-Leu-Met-
ArgOMe with Ac-Met-ArgOMe hydrolysis (Table 2), but it is much too
small to suggest an important steering action of the leucine
residue. The corresponding lysine ester Ac-Leu-Met-LysOMe comprising main features of the kininogen fragment is 20-fold better
a substrate than the best methionine ester of equal length (Table
2). Incidentally, with the more extended peptide esters one
observes the same strong discrimination by porcine pancreatic
kallikrein between arginine and lysine as found previously for the
benzoylated amino acid esters (Fiedler et al. 1973).

From the results of the present studies, one would expect
practically exclusive hydrolysis of the lysyl instead of the
methionyl bond in the kininogen fragment by porcine pancreatic
kallikrein. A result not in accordance with this prediction as
obtained by Iwanaga et al. (1977) can only be explained by the

really important interactions with kallikrein taking place in that
part of the peptide extending from the site of cleavage towards the
C-terminal end.

SUMMARY

The primary specificity of porcine pancreatic kallikrein is
directed predominantly against arginyl and much less so against
lysyl bonds. In addition, the enzyme exhibits pronounced secondary
specificity for a bulky residue, preferentially phenylalanine, in
position P_2 of substrates. This feature is found also in porcine
submandibular and urinary and in human urinary kallikrein, but
not in bovine trypsin. Residues in P_3 and P_1' to P_3' also affect
hydrolysis by pancreatic kallikrein distinctly more than tryptic
hydrolysis. The hexapeptide Pro-Phe-Arg-Ser-Val-Gln with the
sequence of bovine kininogen around the C-terminus of kinin
contains all the structural elements essential for the interaction
with kallikrein, and even glutamine appears dispensable. In
contrast to ester models for this site, peptidyl methionine esters
with the structure of kininogen towards the N-terminus of kinin,
notably bulky leucine in P_2, are very poor kallikrein substrates,
and appear to be of no value as models for the cleavage of kininogen under formation of kallidin.

ACKNOWLEDGEMENT

Our thanks are due to DRs. E. Wünsch and G. Wendlberger, Max-
Planck-Institut für Eiweiß- und Lederforschung, München, for the
synthesis of several of the peptides and to Drs. C. Kutzbach and
G. Schmidt-Kastner, Bayer AG, Werk Elberfeld, for providing us
with purified preparations for the isolation of porcine pancreatic
kallikrein B. This work was sponsored by Deutsche Forschungsgemeinschaft, Sonderforschungsbereich 51.

REFERENCES

Bender, M.L. and F.J. Kézdy, 1965, Mechanism of action of proteo-
    lytic enzymes, Ann. Rev. Biochem. 34, 49.
Dittmann, B. and R. Wimmer, 1978, Comparison of kinin release and
    blood pressure activity of porcine pancreatic, submandibular,
    and urinary kallikrein. In: Current Concepts in Kinin Research,
    eds. G.L. Haberland and U. Hamberg (Pergamon Press, Oxford)
    in press.
Fiedler, F., 1968, Heterogenität und enzymatische Eigenschaften
    von Pankreaskallikrein, Hoppe-Seylers Z. Physiol. Chem. 349,
    926.
Fiedler, F., 1976, Pig pancreatic kallikrein: structure and cataly-
    tic properties. In: Chemistry and Biology of the Kallikrein-

Kinin-System in Health and Disease, eds. J.J. Pisano and K.F. Austen
    (US Government Printing Office, Washington) p. 93.
Fiedler, F., G. Leysath and E. Werle, 1973, Hydrolysis of amino-
    acid esters by pig-pancreatic kallikrein, Eur. J. Biochem.
    36, 152.
Fiedler, F., W. Ehret, G. Godec, C. Hirschauer, C. Kutzbach, G.
    Schmidt-Kastner and H. Tschesche, 1977a, The primary structure
    of pig pancreatic kallikrein B. In: Kininogenases - Kallikrein,
    Vo. 4, eds. G.L. Haberland, J.W. Rhen and T. Suzuki (F.K.
    Schattauer, Stuttgart, New York) p. 7.
Fiedler, F., C. Hirschauer and H. Fritz, 1966b, Inhibition of three
    porcine glandular kallikreins by chloromethyl ketones, Hoppe-
    Seylers Z. Physiol. Chem. 358, 447.
Fiedler, F., R. Geiger, C. Hirschauer and G. Leysath, 1978, Peptide
    esters and nitroanilides as substrates for the assay of human
    urinary kallikrein, Hoppe-Seylers Z. Physiol. Chem., in press.
Fritz, H., F. Fiedler, T. Dietl, M. Warwas, E. Truscheit, H.J.
    Kolb, G. Mair and H. Tschesche, 1977- On the relationship
    between porcine pancreatic, submandibular, and urinary kalli-
    kreins. In: Kininogenases - Kallikrein, Vol. 4, eds. G.L.
    Haberland, J.W. Rohen and T. Suzuki (F.K. Schattauer, Stuttgart
    New York) p. 15.
Habermann, E., 1962, Trennung und Reinigung von Pankreaskallikrein,
    Hoppe-Seylers Z. Physiol. Chem. 328, 15.
Habermann, E., 1966, Strukturaufklärung kininliefernder Peptide
    aus Rinderserum-Kininogen, Arch. exp. Path. Pharmak. 253, 474.
Han, Y.N., H. Kato and S. Iwanaga, 1976, Identification of Ser-Leu-
    Met-Lys-bradykinin isolated from chemically modified high-
    moleculr-weight bovine kininogen, FEBS Lett. 71, 45.
Iwanaga, S., Y.N. Han, H. Kato and T. Suzuki, 1977, Actions of
    various kallikreins on HMW kininogen and its derivatives. In:
    Kininogenases - Kallikrein, Vol. 4, eds. G.L. Haberland,
    J.W. Rohen and T. Suzuki (F.K. Schattauer, Stuttgart, New
    York) p. 79.
Kato, H., Y.N. Han, S. Iwanaga, N. Hashimoto, T. Sugo, S. Fuji and
    T. Suzuki, 1977, Mammalian plasma kininogens: their structures
    and functions. In: Kininogenases - Kallikrein, Vol. 4, eds.
    G.L. Haberland, J.W. Rohen and T. Suzuki (F.K. Schattauer,
    Stuttgart, New York) p. 63.
Kurachi, K., J.C. Powers and P.E. Wilcox, 1973, Kinetics of the
    reaction of chymotrypsin Aα with peptide chloromethyl ketones
    in relation to its subsite specificity, Biochemistry 12, 771.
Lemon, M., F. Fiedler, B. Förg-Brey, C. Hischauer, G. Leysath and
    H. Fritz, The isolation and properties of porcine submandibular
    kallikrein, Biochem. J., in press.
Schechter, I. and A. Berger, 1967, On the size of the active site
    in proteases: I. Papain, Biochem. Biophys. Res. Commun. 27,
    157.

Schroeder, D.D. and E. Shaw, 1968, Chromatography of trypsin and
    its derivatives. Characterization of a new active form of
    bovine trypsin, J. Biol. Chem. 243, 2943.
Werle, E., F. Fiedler and H. Fritz, 1973, Recent studies on kalli-
    kreins and kallikrein inhibitors. In: Pharmacology and the
    Future of Man, Vol. 5 (S. Karger, Basel) p. 284.

PURIFICATION AND CHARACTERIZATION OF HOG PANCREATIC KALLIKREIN I, II AND III

Heizo Kira, Seiji Hiraku and Hiroshi Terashima

Research Institute, Ono Pharmaceutical Co., Ltd.

Sakurai, Shimamoto-cho, Mishima-gun, Osaka 618, Japan

Three forms of kallikrein [EC 3.4.4.21] were purified from hog pancreas powder by affinity chromatography on bovine lung trypsin inhibitor-Sepharose column and DEAE-Sephadex A-50 column chromatography. Each form of kallikrein was tentatively named II, III and I, in the order of elution on DEAE-Sephadex A-50 column. Final yields of I, II and III, per kg of the starting material, were 6.7, 7.6 and 1.9 mg, respectively. Kallikrein I and II were crystallized.

Kinin forming activities of the three kallikreins were 324(I), 280 (II) and 206 (III)(μg bradykinin eq/mg/min, 30°C, pH 8.0). The vasodilator activities were 2,390 (I), 2,180 (II) and 1,500 (III)(kallikrien units (KU)/mg), and esterolytic activities towards N-α-benzoyl-L-arginine ethyl ester were 167 (I), 157 (II) and 118 (III)(μmoles/mg/min, 25°C, pH 8.0). The molecular weights of I,II and III were estimated to be 28,300, 32,000 and 28,300, respectively, by Sephadex G-100 gel filtration.

Kallikrein I and II were comparable with kallikrein A and B, respectively, reported by Fiedler (1976, in: Methods in Enzymology, Vol. 45, p. 389), while kallikrein III differed from them.

INTRODUCTION

During a last few years, detailed studies about hog pancreatic kallikrein [EC 3.4.4.21] were reported by several investigators (Kutzbach et al, 1972; Zuber et al, 1974; Fiedler et al, 1975). All of them confirmed two principal components named as kallikrein A and B, or kallikrein d_1 and d_2. However, some discrepancies between authors are observed in enzymatic and physicochemecal pro-

perties of kallikreins obtained by them. Moreover, any methods
reported until now need complicated procedures to obtain purified
kallikrein, and yields are low.

    This report deals with the purification of hog pancreatic kal-
likrein from pancreas powder by affinity chromatography on bovine
lung trypsin inhibitor-Sepharose and DEAE-Sephadex A-50 chromatography, and also with the characterization of three kallikreins
obtained.

MATERIALS AND METHODS

Materials

    N-α-bebzoyl-L-lysine methyl ester, acetyl glycine methyl ester
and benzoyl methionine methyl ester were obtained from Vega Biochemicals; other synthetic ester substrates and casein (Hammarsten)
from Sigma and E. Merck AG, respectively; limabean trypsin inhibitor,
ovomucoid trypsin inhibitor, beef pancreas inhibitor, N-α-p-tosyl-
L-lysine chloromethyl ketone (TLCK) and diisopropylfluorophosphate
(DFP) from Sigma; soybean trypsin inhibitor (SBTI, No. 37329) and
N-α-tosyl-L-phenylalanine chloromethyl ketone (TPCK) from Serva
and Seikagaku Kogyo Co., respectively; bovine serum albumin and
ovalbumin from Sigma and Nutritional Biochemicals Corp., respectively; pepsin (No. P7012) and trypsin (Type I) from Sigma; alcohol
dehydrogenase (yeast) and cytochrome c from Boehringer; Sepharose
4B, DEAE-Sephadex A-50, blue dextran (2000) and Sephadex G-100 from
Pharmacia Fine Chemicals; carrier ampholite from LKB Produkter AB.
Standard kallikrein (hog pancreatic, No. 751-M, 26.67 KU/mg) for
vasodilator activity determinatin was supplied by Science University
of Tokyo. Bovine lung trypsin inhibitor was prepared from lung by
the extraction as described by Kassell (1970) and by affinity chromatography using trypsin-Sepharose. Trypsin-Sepharose, bovine lung
trypsin inhibitor-Sepharose and soybean trypsin inhibitor-Sepharose
were prepared by coupling each protein to Sepharose 4B activated by
CNBr as described by Cuatrecasas (1970), and these coupling reactions were resulted in 30, 7.7 and 8.0 g protein per 1 of Sepharose
bed, respectively.

Methods

    Enzyme assay. Kinin forming activity was determined by the
method of Moriwaki et al (1974), using rat uterus instead of guinea
pig ileum. Partially purified bovine kininogen (Seikagaku Kogyo)

Abbreviations used: BAEE, N-α-benzoyl-L-arginine ethyl ester;
TAME, N-α-tosyl-L-arginine methyl ester; SBTI, soybean trypsin
inhibitor; BLTI, bovine lung trypsin inhibitor; SDS, sodium dodecyl
sulfate.

was used as a substrate, and the activity was expressed in terms of
μg of synthetic bradykinin eq per min at 30°C, pH 8.0.

Vasodilator activity was determined by measuring the increase
of blood flow in the dog femoral artery as described by Moriwaki et
al (1974). Standard kallikrein (No. 751-M) was used as the standard.

Esterolytic activity was measured by the formation of hydro-
xamic acid-ferric complex from the residual substrate. 0.5 ml of
30 mM substrate in 0.2 M Tris-HCl buffer (pH 8.0) and 0.5 ml of
sample in 0.01 M Tris-HCl buffer (pH 8.0) were mixed and incubated
at 25°C for 30 min. 3 ml of the stop solution (mixture of equal
volume of 3.5 M NaOH and 2 M NH_2OH-HCl) was added to the enzyme
reaction mixture, and kept at 25°C for 20 min. Then, 2 ml of 4 N
HCl, 2 ml of 18 % trichloroacetic acid and 2 ml of 10 % $FeCl_3$ (in
0.1 N HCl) were added and kept at 25°C for 20 min. After filtration
to remove the insoluble precipitate, the formed ferric complex was
determined colorimetrically at 530 nm. Esterolytic activities were
expressed in terms of units; one unit is defined as the amount of
enzyme which hydrolyzes 1 μmol of substrate per min.

Caseinolytic activity was determined at 37°C, pH 8.0 by the
method of Kunitz (1947).

Protein concentrations were estimated as described by Lowry
(1951), with bovine serum albumin as the standard.

Disc electrophoresis was carried out in 7.5 % polyacrylamide
gel(0.5 x 7 cm) at pH 8.0 gel (Williams et al, 1964).

Isoelectric focusing fractionation was carried out in the LKB
Ampholine column (110 ml capacity) with a pH range of 3.5 - 5.0 at
1 % ampholine solution (Vesterberg et al, 1966). Electrophoresis
was carried out for 50 hr at 4°C, 500 - 800 V. Afterwards, fractions of 2.1 ml were collected and examined for absorbance at 280
nm, pH and enzyme activity.

Molecular weight. The molecular weights of kallikreins were
estimated by the two methods, i.e. gel filtration on Sephadex G-100
column (Andrews, 1964) and SDS-polyacrylamide gel electrophoresis
(Weber et al, 1969).

A Sephadex G-100 column (1.8 x 90 cm) was equilibrated with
0.05 M Tris-HCl buffer (pH 8.0) containing 0.1 M NaCl. Blue dextran
for the determination of the void volume, bovine serum albumin,
ovalbumin, soybean trypsin inhibitor and cytochrome c were used as
the markers. 2 mg of each protein in 1 ml was applied to the column.
The elution was performed at a flow rate of 15.6 ml per hr, and
fractions of 2.6 ml were collected. The elution volumes of the
proteins and blue dextran were determined from the absorbance at
280 nm and 610 nm, respectively.

For SDS-electophoresis, the samples were incubated for 15 hr at
37°C with 25 % glycerol, 1% SDS and 1 % β-mercaptoethanol. Urea
treatment of the kallikreins was performed by the incubation with
8 M urea, 25 % glycerol, 1 % SDS and 4 % β-mercaptoethanol for 15
hr at 37°C (pH 7.0). Electrophoresis was performed in 10 % acrylamide gel containing 0.1 % SDS. Bovine serum albumin, ovalbumin,
pepsin and cytochrome c were used as protein standards.

Amino acid analysis. Sample (0.5 mg) was hydrolyzed in twice distilled constant-boiling HCl at 110°C for 24, 48 and 72 hr in an evacuated sealed tube, and the hydrolysate was analyzed according to Spackman et al (1958) with a Hitachi KLA-5 amino acid analyzer. The sample was oxidized by the method of Moore (1963) and hydrolyzed for 24 hr at 110°C for determination of cysteine and methionine. Tryptophan was determined by a spectrophotometric method (Edelhoch, 1967).

Carbohydrate analysis. For the determination of hexosamine, the sample (10 mg) was hydrolyzed in 2 ml of 4 N HCl at 100°C for 4 hr in a N_2-replaced sealed tube. The hydrolysate was evaporated to dryness, dissolved in water and applied on a Dowex 50-X-8 column (1 x 1.6 cm). The column was washed with distilled water and eluted with 0.5 N HCl. The hexosamine content in the eluate was determined colorimetrically at 535 nm by the method of Blix (1948).

Neutral sugar content in the sample (1 mg/ml) was determined by the phenol and sulfuric acid method of Dubois et al (1956).

RESULTS

Enzyme Purification

All purification steps were performed at 4°C unless otherwise noted.

Step 1. Extraction. 3 kg of the defatted acetone powder from hog pancreas was suspended in 35 l of distilled water (4°C) and stirred for 30 min at pH 4.1 (adjusted with about 400 ml of conc. acetic acid) at room temperature. The suspension was centrifuged to remove insoluble material. The supernatant adjusted to pH 8.0 with 8 N NaOH was centrifuged again to remove the precipitate formed.

Step 2. First affinity chromatography. The extract was diluted with equal volume of 0.1 M Tris-HCl buffer (pH 8.0) and applied to the connected affinity columns, SBTI-Sepharose (upper, ϕ20 x 22 cm) and BLTI-Sepharose (lower, ϕ25 x 6 cm), both equilibrated with 0.1 M Tris-HCl buffer (pH 8.0). After washing the columns with 20 l of the equilibration buffer, the lower column was washed with 50 l of 0.1 M acetate buffer (pH 5.3) to remove chymotrypsin-like enzyme, and the kallikrein was eluted with 0.1 M acetic acid at a flow rate of 30 l per hr. The eluate was collected into the vessel containing 1 ℓ of 2 M Tris-HCl buffer (pH 9.0) with stirring, to avoid the inactivation of kallikrein. Upper and lower columns were regenerated separately with 0.1 N HCl to remove proteins still adsorbed on them (upper, trypsin and chymotrypsin; lower, trypsin) (Table 1). Steps 1 and 2 were repeated 7 times.

Step 3. Second affinity chromatography. The combined eluates (equivalent to 21 kg pancreas powder) from step 2 were adjusted to pH 8.0 with 8 N NaOH and applied to the affinity columns equilibrated with 0.1 M Tris-HCl (pH 8.0). In the second chromatography, a column ϕ25 x 3 cm was used for lower one. After washing the columns

Table 1. First affinity chromatography of hog pancreatic kallikrein. Extract from 3 kg pancreas powder was applied to connected affinity columns, SBTI-Sepharose 4B (upper, ϕ20 x 22 cm) and BLTI-Sephadex 4B (lower, ϕ25 x 6 cm), both equilibrated with 0.1 M Tris-HCl buffer (pH 8.0). BLTI-Sepharose separated was washed with 0.1 M acetate buffer (pH 5.3), and elution was carried out stepwise. BAEE hydrolyzing activity was measured in the presence of SBTI. The values were expressed in averages of 7 times experiments.

Fraction	Volume (ℓ)	Protein (A 280) $\times 10^4$	Activity BAEE (Units) $\times 10^4$	S.A (U/A 280)	Esterase TAME (Units) $\times 10^4$	Activity ATEE (Units) $\times 10^4$
Extract	29	191	4.96	0.026	1,404	880
Passed Through	76	144	0.14	0.001	55.6	62.9
BLTI-Sepharose						
pH 5.3 Washed	50	20.5	0.11	0.005	82.2	175
0.1M AcOH Eluted	20	1.4	3.62	2.58	7.0	20.2
0.1N HCl Washed	30	0.8	0		346	8.1
SBTI-Sepharose						
0.1N HCl Washed	60	29.4	0		698	528

Table 2. Second affinity chromatography of hog pancreatic kallikrein. The combined eluates of 7 times chromatography from step 2 were applied to connected columns, SBTI-Sepharose 4B (ϕ20 x 22 cm) and BLTI-Sepharose 4B (ϕ25 x 3 cm), equilibrated with 0.1 M Tris-HCl buffer (pH 8.0). Elution was carried out stepwise. BAEE activity was determined in the presence of SBTI.

Fraction	Volume (ℓ)	Protein (A 280) $\times 10^4$	Activity BAEE (Units) $\times 10^4$	S.A (U/A 280)	Esterase TAME (Units) $\times 10^4$	Activity ATEE (Units) $\times 10^4$
1st Step Eluates	140	9.8	25.3	2.58	49.1	141
Passed Through	160	5.2	0	0	0	0
BLTI-Sepharose						
pH 4.5 Washed	10	1.54	0.76	0.49	0	5.8
0.1M AcOH Eluted	10	0.92	17.7	19.2	1.80	0.92
0.1N HCl Washed	15	0.092	0		2.50	0
SBTI-Sepharose						
0.1N HCl Washed	60	1.75	0		42.3	131

with 20 1 of the equilibration buffer, the lower column was washed
with 10 1 of 0.1 M acetate buffer (pH 4.5) and the kallikrein was
eluted with 0.1 M acetic acid into the vessel containing 500 ml of
2 M Tris-HCl buffer (pH 9.0). The recovery of the kallikrein activity (BAEE hydrolysis) in the above two affinity chromatographies
resulted in 51 %, and those of TAME activity (trypsin) and ATEE
(chymotrypsin) were 0.018 and 0.014 %, respectively (Table 2).

Step 4. First DEAE-Sephadex A-50 chromatography. Ethanol was
added to the eluate obtained from the step 3 to make 75 % concentration. The precipitate formed was collected by centrifugation,
dissolved in 0.3 M ammonium acetate buffer (pH 6.0) and dialyzed
against the same buffer. The dialysate (204 ml) was applied to a
DEAE-Sephadex A-50 column (4.6 x 65 cm) equilibrated with the above
buffer and the kallikrein was eluted with a linear gradient elution
system from 0.3 to 0.7 M ammonium acetate buffer (pH 6.0), according
to the method of Takami (1969 a). Three active components (two
peaks and one shoulder) were eluted and named kallikrein II, III and
I in the order of the elution (Fig. 1).

Step 5. Second DEAE-Sephadex A-50 chromatography. Three
active components obtained from the step 4 were individually precipitated by adding ethanol, and the precipitate was collected by centrifugation, dissolved and dialyzed as in the step 4. The dialysate
(50 ml) was rechromatographed on DEAE-Sephadex A-50 column (4.6 x
43 cm) as in the step 4 (Fig. 2).

The active fractions eluted were divided into three parts
(main and others), taking into account the specific activities of
TAME and BAEE activities. The main parts were homogeneous,except
kallikrein III having a slow migrating component (Fig. 3).

The main parts were lyophilized after precipitation by ethanol
and dialysis against distilled water, and used in the following experiments as kallikrein I, II and III.

Results of the individual purification steps are summarized in
Table 3. From the initial extract, about 1,700- to 2,500-fold purification was achieved with 15.3 % recovery of the total activity.

Enzyme Properties

Various activities. Table 4 shows the vasodilator, kinin forming, esterolytic and caseinolytic activities of the three kallikreins obtained.

Substrate specificities. The activities of the kallikreins
towards synthetic ester substrates are shown in Table 5. The kallikreins readily hydrolyzed benzoyl arginine methyl ester and BAEE.
Kallikrein III hydrolyzed TAME at a faster rate than I and II.

Effects of various inhibitors and reagents. The effects on
esterolytic activity towards BAEE are shown in Table 6. Only beef
pancreas trypsin inhibitor (Kunits inhibitor) inhibited the kallikreins completely. DFP weakly inhibited the kallikreins.

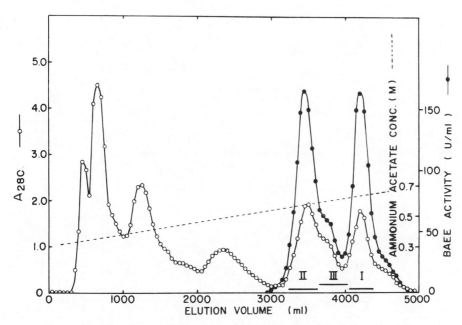

Fig. 1.   Chromatographic separation of hog pancreatic kallikrein on
DEAE-Sephadex A-50.   Material from step 3 was applied to the column
(4.6 x 65 cm)equilibrated with 0.3 M ammonium acetate buffer (pH 6.0).
Elution was carried out in linear gradient system with 5.0 1 of 0.3 -
0.7 M ammonium acetate buffer (pH 6.0).

Effects of metal ions.   The effects on esterolytic activity
towards BAEE are shown in Table 7. Zn^{2+} and Hg^{2+} showed a particularly strong inhibitory effect. Cu^{2+} showed not so strong inhibition.
On the other hand, in the experiments of preincubation with these

metal ions, only Hg^{2+} had an inhibitory effect, and Zn^{2+} had no
effect (Table 7)

Effects of pH and temperature on stability.   0.1 ml of each kallikrein (about 0.1 mg/ml) was incubated with 0.1 ml of Walpole buffer (pH 1 - 4), McIlvaine buffer (pH 3 - 8) and Kolthoff buffer

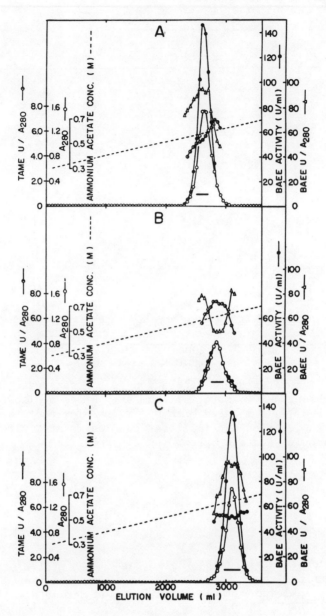

Fig. 2. DEAE-Sephadex A-50 rechromatography of hog pancreatic
kallikrein. Each kallikrein from the step 4 was applied to the
column (4.6 x 43 cm) equilibrated with 0.3 M ammonium acetate
buffer (pH 6.0). Elution was carried out in linear gradient with
3.6 l of 0.3 - 0.7 M ammonium acetate buffer (pH 6.0). A, B and C
show the rechromato-patterns of kallikrein II, III and I, respectively.

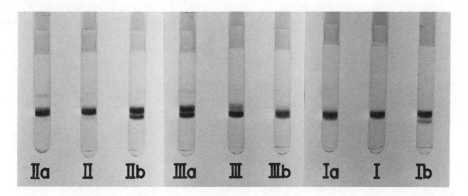

Fig. 3 Disc electrophoretic patterns of hog pancreatic kallikreins obtained from DEAE-Sephadex A-50 rechromatograpy. II, III and I are the main parts of elutions; IIa, IIIa and Ia, ascending limb; IIb, IIIb and Ib, descending limb.

Table 3. Summary of purification for hog pancreatic kallikrein I, II and III, from 21 kg pancreas powder.

Step	Total Protein (g)	Total Act. (BAEE U)	S.A (U/mg protein)	Recovery (%)
Extract	6,085	347,200	0.057	100
1 st Affinitychromato	44.6	253,200	5.68	72.9
2 nd Affinitychromato	5.64	177,000	31.4	51.0
1 st DEAE-Sephadex A-50				
Kallikrein I	0.317	42,780	135	12.3
Kallikrein II	0.363	49,370	136	14.2
Kallikrein III	0.137	14,770	108	4.25
2 nd DEAE-Sephadex A-50				
Kallikrein I	0.168	23,350	139	6.73
Kallikrein II	0.176	25,170	143	7.24
Kallikrein III	0.048	4,720	98.3	1.36

Table 4. Various activities of hog pancreatic kallikrein I, II and
III. Vasodilator activities were expressed in terms of KU per mg;
kinin forming activities, µg of released kinin eq to synthetic bradykinin per min per mg at 30°C (pH 8.0); ester hydrolyzing activities,
unit (µmol substrate hydrolyzed per min at 25°C, pH 8.0) per mg;
caseinolytic activities, Kunitz U/mg. The ratio of BAEE hydrolyzing
activity to TAME hydrolyzing activity is shown as BAEE/TAME.

	I	II	III
Vasodilator Activity KU/mg	2,390	2,180	1,500
Kinin Forming Activity µg BK eq/mg	324	280	206
BAEE Hydrolyzing Activity U/mg	167	157	118
BAEE/TAME	15.4	15.7	8.69
Caseinolytic Activity Kunitz U/mg	0.0042	0.0005	0.0053

Table 5. Hydrolysis of synthetic substrates by hog pancreatic
kallikrein I, II and III. Each relative activity was expressed as
per cent of BAEE activity in 0.1 M Tris-HCl buffer (pH 8.0) and 15
mM substrate at 25°C for 30 min.

Substrate	Relative Activity (%)		
	I	II	III
Bz-Arg-OEt	100	100	100
Tos-Arg-OMe	6.49	6.39	11.5
Bz-Arg-OMe	158	162	151
Arg-OMe	8.88	9.09	11.6
Bz-Lys-OMe	16.2	15.8	14.1
Tos-Lys-OMe	3.05	3.17	4.37
Lys-OMe	0	0	0
Ac-Tyr-OEt	3.10	3.08	2.92
Ac-Phe-OEt	3.80	3.81	3.28
Ac-Gly-OMe	0	0	0
Bz-Met-OMe[*]	0	0	0

*   Methanol concentration in assay was 25 %

Abbreviation: Bz, benzoyl; Tos, tosyl; Ac, acetyl;
OEt, ethyl ester; OMe, methyl ester.

Table 6. Effects of various inhibitors and reagents on the activity of hog pancreatic kallikrein I, II and III. Each enzyme (about 0.1 µM) was incubated with various inhibitors and reagents at 25°C pH 8.0 for the time indicated and then the remaining activity towards BAEE was assayed by the standard assay method.

Reagent	Final Conc. (% or mM)	Time of Incubation (min)	Remaining Activity (%)		
			I	II	III
Soybean Trypsin Inhibitor	0.075 %	10	101.5	102.1	98.2
Limabean Trypsin Inhibitor	0.075	10	99.9	97.9	102.1
Ovomucoid Trypsin Inhibitor	0.075	10	97.1	97.9	102.1
Beef Pancreas Trypsin Inhibitor	0.01	10	0	0	0
EDTA	5.0 mM	60	100.0	99.9	99.9
MIA	5.0	60	98.2	96.3	96.3
PCMB	2.5	60	81.5	79.9	81.2
DFP	2.5	60	23.6	28.9	22.8
TPCK	5.0	60	96.8	99.0	95.5
TLCK	5.0	60	103.9	97.6	100.0
2-Mercaptoethanol	5.0	60	100.3	97.7	100.6
Cysteine	5.0	60	100.0	99.9	100.4
Thioglycollic Acid	5.0	60	103.0	104.5	94.6
Potassium Cyanide	5.0	60	96.7	101.2	94.7

(pH 7 - 12) at 37°C for 3 hr. After 25-fold dilution with 0.1 M Tris-HCl buffer (pH 8.0), the remaining esterolytic activity (BAEE) was determined by the standard assay method. Between pH 5 - 10, the three kallikreins showed more than 80 % residual activity, and kallikrein II was slightly more stable at basic pH range.

Each kallikrein (about 0.005 mg/ml) in 0.01 M Tris-HCl buffer (pH 8.0) was heated at various temperatures (40 - 98°C) for 15 min and quickly chilled in ice bath for 5 min, and remaining BAEE activity was assayed. Differences of stability among these three kallikreins were not observed. They were stable at 40 - 50°C, and 50 % inactivation was observed at 90°C. They still retained about 30 % of the initial activities at 98°C.

Effects of pH and temperature on activity. The optimun pH was measured by the incubation of 0.5 ml of each kallikrein (about 0.005 mg in water for BAEE activity and about 0.06 mg in water for TAME

activity) with 0.5 ml of 30 mM substrate in 0.2 M Tris-HCl buffer
(pH 6.5 - 9.5) at 25°C for 30 min. Spontaneous hydrolysis of substrate at each pH was also measured. These three kallikreins, I, II
and III, exhibited almost the same pH-activity curves, and the
optimum pH towards BAEE and TAME were 8.5 - 9.0 and 7.50 - 7.75,
respectively.

BAEE hydrolyzing activity was measured at 30 - 70°C for 30 min
in 0.1 M Tris-HCl buffer (pH 8.0). Almost the same temperature-
activity curves for thr three kallikreins were shown with maximum
activity at 55°C.

Disc electrophoresis. As shown in Fig. 4, kallikrein I migrated
faster than II, while kallikrein III, which was eluted close to II
and far from I on DEAE-Sephadex chromatography(Fig.1), migrated to
the same distance as I.

Isoelectric focusings. Each kallikrein was resolved into
several active fractions. The pI values of fractions from kallikrein I was 3.75, 3.92 (major) and 4.04; from II 3.67, 3.83 (major)
and 4.03; from III 3.83 and 3.94 (major). (Table 8).

Molecular weights. By Sephadex G-100 gel filtration, the
molecular weights of kallikrein I, II and III were estimated to be
28,300, 32,000 and 28,300, respectively (Table 8).

By SDS-electrophoresis, the molecular weights of kallikrein I,
II and III were estimated to be 25,000, 30,300 and 25,000, respectively. As shown in Fig. 5, by the treatment with 8 M urea, each
kallikrein exhibited apparently two major bands, and the molecular
weights of these bands were estimated to be 16,300 and 12,600 from
kallikrein I, 19,000 and 12,800 from II and 20,000 and 9,700 from
III. The sums of them, 28,900 from kallikrein I, 31,800 from II and
29,700 from III were nearly consistent with the molecular weights
estimated by SDS-electrophoresis without 8 M urea treatment.

Carbohydrate analyses. Hexosamine contents of kallikrein I,
II and III were estimated to be 2.00, 4.95 and 3.31 %, respectively,
as glucosamine eq. Neutral sugar contents of kallikrein I, II and
III were estimated to 3.50, 5.95 and 3.60 %, respectively, as
glucose eq. (Table 8).

Amino acid compositions. As shown in Table 9, the kallikreins
were found to have similar amino acid composition each other.
Kallikrein I, II and III were composed of 223, 231 and 216 amino
acid residues, respectively, on a basis of molecular weights of
28,300, 32,000 and 28,300, respectively. From the amino acid compositions, the molecular weights of the protein moieties of kallikrein
I, II and III were calculated as 24,600, 25,500 and 23,800, respectively.

Crystallization of kallikrein I and II. 50 mg of each kallikrein I and II was dissolved in 2 ml of 0.1 M Tris-HCl buffer (pH 8.0),
to which a saturated ammonium sulfate solution was added to make
45 % saturation by micropipette, and allowed to stand at 23°C.
The crystals of kallikrein I appeared after 2 days, and 55 % of the
initial protein was crystallized after 22 days. On the other hand,
the crystals of kallikrein II appeared after 20 days, and 63 % was

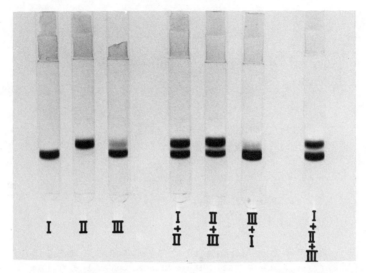

Fig. 4.   Disc electrophoresis of hog pancreatic kallikrein I, II
and III.   Electrophoresis was carried out in 7.5% gel (0.5 x 7 cm)
at pH 8.0 gle, 2.5 mA/tube for 70 min.   25 µg of each kallikrein
was applied.

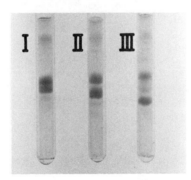

Fig. 5.   SDS- electrophoresis of hog pancreatic kallikrein I, II
and III, treated with 8 M urea.   Urea treatment was in 8 M urea,
25% glycerol, 1% SDS and 4% β-mercaptoethanol at 37°C (pH 7.0)
for 15 hr; electrophoresis, in 10% gel (0.5 x 8 cm) with 0.1% SDS
at pH 7.0, 8 mA/tube for 150 min, 34 µg protein/tube.

crystallized after 35 days.   Each crystals of kallikrein I and II
collected by centrifugation had the same specific activities (vasodilator and BAEE activities) as the initial preparations.   As
shown in Fig. 6, the crystal form of kallikrein I was columnar,
while that of II was needle-like.

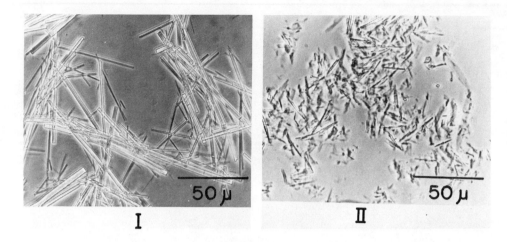

Fig. 6.   Crystals of hog pancreatic kallikrein I and II.   Condition
of crystallization ; 45 % saturated ammonium salfate (pH 8.0).

Table 7.   Effects of metal ions on the activity and stability of hog
pancreatic kallikrein I, II and III.   Effects on activity were determined in final concentration of 1 mM metal ion (chloride), 15 mM
BAEE, 0.1 M Tris-HCl buffer (pH 8.0) and about 0.1 μM enzyme at 25°C
for 30 min.   Effects on stability were determined as follows: The
mixture of 2 mM metal ion (chloride), 0.1 M Tris-HCl buffer (pH 8.0)
and about 20 μM enzyme was preincubated at 25°C for 60 min, and
remaining BAEE activity was assayed after 100-fold dilution.

	on activity				on stability		
	Remaining Activity (%)				Remaining Activity (%)		
Ion	I	II	III	Ion	I	II	III
Cu^{++}	93.0	90.1	85.2	Cu^{++}	96.1	93.1	100
Zn^{++}	37.1	27.8	23.4	Zn^{++}	96.5	91.3	100
Mn^{++}	93.8	93.2	80.3	Mn^{++}	96.4	93.4	96.4
Co^{++}	96.0	82.9	80.4	Co^{++}	92.7	91.7	96.2
Cd^{++}	81.0	76.7	66.3	Cd^{++}	100	100	100
Fe^{++}	87.7	81.5	78.6	Fe^{++}	93.6	89.0	92.9
Mg^{++}	100	100	100	Mg^{++}	100	98.1	100
Ca^{++}	100	100	100	Ca^{++}	100	100	100
Hg^{++}	74.9	72.0	50.8	Hg^{++}	45.6	42.4	46.3
Ni^{++}	82.5	82.3	70.4	Ni^{++}	97.6	100	100

Table 8. Various analytical data of hog pancreatic kallikrein I, II and III.

	I	II	III
Extinction Coefficient $E_{280nm}^{1\%}$ pH 8.0	17.5	16.1	17.5
Neutral Sugar Content Glucose eq %	3.50	5.95	3.60
Amino Sugar Content Glucosamine eq %	2.00	4.95	3.31
Total Sugar Content	5.50	10.90	6.91
Protein Content mg BSA/mg	1.20	1.10	1.20
Isoelectric Point	3.75 3.92 4.04	3.67 3.83 4.03	3.83 3.94
Molecular Weight			
SDS Electrophoresis	25,000	30,300	25,000
Sephadex G-100 Gelfiltration	28,300	32,000	28,300

Table 9. Amino acid compositions of hog pancreatic kallikrein I, II and III. The values were obtained from 24, 48 and 72 hr hydrolysates. Values of threonine and serine were obtained by extrapolation to zero time of hydrolysis. Cystine(1/2) and methionine were determined after 24 hr hydrolysis of performic acid oxidized protein. Tryptophan was determined spectrophotometrically.

Amino Acid	Nearest Integer for Residues per Mol Protein			
	I	II	III	Kallikrein A and B[*]
Lys	10	10	9	10
His	7	8	7	8
(NH₃)	(35)	(43)	(35)	
Arg	3	3	3	3
Asp	27	27	25	27
Thr	14	15	15	14
Ser	12	13	12	14
Glu	22	23	22	23
Pro	16	16	15	16
Gly	21	22	20	22
Ala	12	12	12	13
1/2Cys	12	13	12	10
Val	10	10	9	10
Met	4	4	4	4
Ile	11	11	11	12
Leu	19	20	18	19
Tyr	7	7	6	7
Phe	9	10	9	10
Try	7	7	7	7
Total	223	231	216	229
Mol. wt.	24,600	25,500	23,800	25,200

* Fiedler : Method in Enzymology , 45 , 289

DISCUSSION

The weights of kallikrein I, II and III finally obtained from
21 kg pancreas powder were 140, 160 and 40 mg, respectively. The
amount of kallikrein III accounted for 11.8 % of total weight.

In purification procedures, affinity chromatography using the
connected columns of SBTI-Sepharose 4B and BLTI-Sepharose 4B were
particulary effective. By the two consecutive affinity chromatographies, about 700 folds purification was achieved with 51 % yield
of BAEE activity. At this step, trypsin and chymotrypsin contained
in the extract were almost removed and the purity of kallikrein
amounted to about 20 %.

By further purification on DEAE-Sephadex A-50 columns, about
2,500 folds purification for kallikrein I and II, and 1,700 folds
purification for kallikrein III were achieved. Kallikreins I and
II obtained were almost homogeneous at disc electrophoresis.
However, kallikrein III had one additional band as shown in Fig. 3.
This additional band seemed to be contaminated kallikrein II.

Specific activities of kallikrein I, II and III towards BAEE
were 139, 143 and 98.3 U/mg protein, respectively. Specific activities of kallikrein I and II were almost equal, and that of kallikrein III was about 70 % of kallikrein I and II. The vasodilator
and kinin forming activities of these kallikreins were nearly parallel to BAEE activities as shown in Table 4. The relative activities
of kallikrein I and II towards various synthetic substrates were
nearlythe same, but kallikrein III differed from them on the ability of hydrolyzing TAME and tosyl-L-lysine methyl ester. The ratios
of BAEE hydrolyzing activity to TAME hydrolyzing activity of kallikrein I, II and III were 15.4, 15.7 and 8.69, respectively. Since
the TAME activity of kallikrein III was not inhibited by SBTI (not
described in the experimental section), the possibility of trypsin
contamination in kallikrein III preparation was denied. pH-relative
activity curves of the three kallikreins were almost the same.
Thus kallikrein III was characterized as a new type kallikrein
possesing high activity towards TAME and low one towards BAEE.

Zn^{2+} inhibited most strongly the esterase activities. This
results well agreed with the data by Takami (1969 b). On the stability of three kallikreins, Zn^{2+} had no inhibitory effect, while
Hg^{2+} showed inhibition (Table 7). Potentiating effects of SH compound and chelator reported by Fiedler et al (1968) were not
observed (Table 6).

The contents of amino sugar of kallikrein I, II and III were
2.00, 4.95 and 3.31 %, respectively. The values of amino sugar
content were well correlated with the elution order from the DEAE-
Sephadex A-50 column, The total sugar contents of kallikrein I and
II were almost the same as those of kallikrein A and B,respectively
(Fiedler, 1976). All of the three kallikreins were resolved into
two or three enzymically active fractions on electrofocusing at pH
3.5 - 5.0. The pI values of major fractions of each kallikrein

were nearly equal. Although a new active kallikrein named kallikrein B' was isolated by Fiedler et al (1970), kallikrein B' and kallikrein III are probably not related, because kallikrein B' has a pI value of 4.32. Each kallikrein I, II and III treated with 8 M urea was divided into two major bands on SDS-electrophoresis. This result suggests that the three kallikreins consist of two polypeptide chains. Zuber et al (1974) have suggested that kallikrein d_1 and d_2 consist of several polypeptide chains.

Judging from the similarities of amino acid composition, sugar content, molecular weight and the behavior on anion exchanger, kallikrein I and II obtained by us from hog pancreas powder are comparable with kallikrein A and B, respectively, reported by Fiedler (1976).

ACKNOWLEDGEMENTS

We wish to thank Prof. C. Moriwaki, Science University of Tokyo, for his useful advice and suggestion. We are also grateful to our research colleagues, especially to Mr. H. Aishita and Mr. M. Morita for vasodilator activity determinations, and to Mr. M. Katsura for his cooperation during this work.

REFERENCES

Andrews, P., 1964, Estimation of the molecular weights of proteins by Sephadex gel-filtration, Biochem. J., 91, 222.
Blix, G., 1948, The determination of hexosamines according to Elson and Morgan, Acta Chem. Scand., 2, 467.
Cuatrecasas, P., 1970, Protein purification by affinity chromatography, J. Biol. Chem., 245, 3059.
Dubois, M., K. A. Gilles, J. K. Hamilton, P. A. Rebers and F. Smith, 1956, Colorimetric method for determination of sugars and related substances, Anal. Chem., 28, 350.
Edelhoch, H., 1967, Spectroscopic determination of tryptophan and tyrosine in proteins, Biochemistry, 7, 1948.
Fiedler, F., 1976, Pig pancreatic kallikreins A and B, in: Methods in Enzymology, Vol. 45, eds L. Lorand (Academic Press, New York) P. 289.
Fiedler, F. and E. Werle, 1967, Vorkommen zweier Kallikreinogene im Schweinepankreas und Automation der Kallikrein- und Kallikreinogenbestimmung, Hoppe-Seyler's Z. Physiol. Chem., 348, 1087.
Fiedler, F. and E. Werle, 1968, Activation, inhibition, and pH dependence of the hydrolysis of α-N-benzoyl-L-arginine ethyl ester catalyzed by kallikrein from porcine pancreas, Europ. J. Biochem., 7, 27.

Fiedler, F., C. Hirschauer and E. Werle, 1970, Anreicherung von
    Präkallikrein B aus Schweinepankreas und Eigenschften vershie-
    dener Formen des Pankreaskallikreins.
Fiedler, F., C. Hirschauer and E. Werle, 1975, Characterization of
    pig pancreatic kallikrein A and B, Bd. 356, 1879.
Kassell, B., 1970, Bovine trypsin-kallikrein inhibitor, in: Methods
    in Enzymology, Vol. 19, eds G. E. Perlmann and L. Lorand
    (Academic Press, New York) P. 844.
Kunitz, M., 1947, Crystalline soybean trypsin inhibitor. II. General
    properties, J. Gen. Physiol., 30, 291.
Kutzbach, C. and G. Schmidt-Kastner, 1972, Kallikrein from pig pan-
    creas. Purification, separation of components A and B, and
    crystallization, Hoppe-Seyler's Z. Physiol. Chem., 353, 1099.
Lowry, O. H., N. J. Rosebrough, A. L. Farr and R. J. Randall, 1951,
    Protein measurement with the Folin phenol reagent, J. Biol.
    Chem., 193, 265.
Moore, S., 1963, The determination of cystine as cysteic acid, J.
    Biol. Chem., 238, 235.
Moriwaki, C., Y. Hojima and H. Moriya, 1974, A proposal-use of com-
    bined assays of kallikrein activity measurement, Chem. Pharm.
    Bull. (Tokyo), 22, 975.
Spackman, D. H., W. H. Stein and S. Moore, 1958, Anal. Chem.,30, 1190.
Takami, T., 1969 a, Purification of hog pancreatic kallikreins and
    their proteolytic activities, Seikagaku (Tokyo), 41, 777.
Takami, T., 1969 b, Action of hog pancreatic kallikrein on synthetic
    substrates and its some other enzymatic properties, J. Biochem.
    (Tokyo), 66, 651.
Vestererberg, O. and H. Svensson, 1966, Isoelectric fractionation,
    analysis, and characterization of ampholytes in natural pH
    gradients, Acta Chem. Scand., 20 820.
Weber, K. and M. Osborn, 1969, The reliability of molecular weight
    determinations by dodecyl sulfate-polyacrylamide gel electro-
    phoresis, J. Biol. Chem., 244, 4406.
Williams, D. E. and R. A. Reinsfold, 1964, Disk electrophoresis in
    polyacrylamide gels, Ann. N. Y. Acad. Sci., 121, 373.
Zuber, M. and E. Sache, 1974, Isolation and characterization of
    porcine pancreatic kallikrein, Biochemistry, 13, 3098.

RAT STOMACH KALLIKREIN: ITS PURIFICATION AND PROPERTIES

K. Uchida, A. Yokoshima, M. Niinobe, H. Kato and
S. Fujii

Institute for Protein Research, Osaka University
Suita, Osaka 565, Japan

SUMMARY

From rat stomach, kallikrein was purified by chromatographies on columns of p-aminobenzamidine-Sepharose, DEAE-Sephadex
A-50 and Sephadex G-150 and by isoelectric focusing, measuring its
activities to hydrolyse prolylphenylalanyl-arginine-4-methyl-
coumarine amide (Pro-Phe-Arg-MCA) and to release kinin from rat
heated-plasma. The purified stomach kallikrein showed a single
band on Disc electrophoresis at pH 7.0. The molecular weight of
the kallikrein was calculated to be 29,000 by gel-filtration on a
column of Sephadex G-50. The kallikrein was stable between pH 6
and 11 and hydrolysed Pro-Phe-Arg-MCA optimally at pH 11.0. The
Pro-Phe-Arg-MCA hydrolysing activity of rat stomach kallikrein was
inhibited by DFP and Trasylol, but not by trypsin inhibitors from
soyabean, limabean and ovomucoid. These properties of rat stomach
kallikrein was clearly distinguishable from those of partially
purified rat plasma kallikrein, but similar properties to other
glandular kallikreins from other species.
From these results, it was concluded that kallikrein is present in rat stomach, which can be classified into glandular kallikrein.

INTRODUCTION

In the mammalian organisms, kinin-releasing enzymes are found
in plasma and the various tissues such as pancreas (Kraut et al.,
1930), salivary gland (Werle et al., 1936), intestine (Seki et al.,
1972) and kidney (Werle et al., 1955), which can be classified
into two types of enzymes, plasma kallikrein and glandular kalli-

291

krein. It has been suggested that the function of the glandular
kallikrein is closely related with the function of organs containing kallikrein.

For example, excretion of kallikrein in urine reflects renal
kallikrein which has been reported to regulate renal blood flow
cooperating with renin-angiotensin system in kidney, therefore,
taking part in the regulation mechanism of blood pressure (McGiff
et al., 1976). Kallikrein is also present in glands or cells of
the gastrointestinal tract, which has been suggested to influence
transport of glucose and amino acids and absorption of water and
electrolytes in intestine (Moriwaki et al., 1973).

Geiger et al. (Geiger et al., 1977) have recently suggested
that kininogen is present in human gastric mucus, but the presence
of kallikrein in stomach has not been reported. It is very interesting to know whether kallikrein-kinin system would be present in
stomach, since the secretion of gastric mucus is regulated by
gastrin and secretin.

In this paper, we will report on the purification of kallikrein from rat stomach, and present the evidence that rat stomach-
kallikrein shares the properties with other glandular kallikrein.

MATERIALS AND METHODS

The following reagents were obtained commercially: Ovalbumin,
bovine serum albumin and 𝛾-globulin (Nutritional Biochemical Corp-
oration, Cleaveland, Ohio, U.S.A.). DEAE-Sephadex A-50, Sephadex
G-150, Sephadex G-50 and Sepharose 4B (Pharmacia Fine Chemicals Co.,
Uppsalla, Sweden). Soybean trypsin inhibitor, limabean trypsin
inhibitor, ovomucoid trypsin inhibitor and p-aminobenzamidine HCl
(Sigma Chemical Co., U.S.A.). Diisopropylfluorophosphate (Katayama
Chemical Co., Japan). Trasylol (Bayer AG., Germany). Pro-Phe-Arg-
MCA, Z-Phe-Arg-MCA, Boc-Val-Pro-Arg-MCA, Boc-Ile-Glu-Gly-Arg-MCA,
Glutaryl-Gly-Arg-MCA, and Boc-Val-Leu-Lys-MCA (Protein Research
Foundation, Osaka, Japan). p-Chlorobenzylamine-Sepharose 4B was
prepared by coupling ε-aminocaproyl-p-chlorobenzylamine (Protein
Research Foundation, Osaka) with Sepharose 4B by cyanogen bromide.

Activated Factor XII was isolated from bovine plasma, according to the method of Fujikawa et al. (1977). Snake venom kininogenase from the venom of <u>agkistrodon</u> <u>halys</u> <u>blomhoffii</u> was purified
as reported previously (Suzuki et al., 1966). Disc electrophoresis
in polyacrylamide gel at pH 7.0 using diethylbarbituric acid-Tris
buffer was performed according to the method (Williams and
Reisfeld, 1964). Isoelectric focusing was performed with a 110 ml
column (LKB product) using Ampholine of pH range of 2.5-5. pH-
optimum and stability were examined using Britton-Robinson buffer.
<u>Homogenate of rat stomach</u>

Male Wister rat weighing 150-200 g were killed by decapitation
and stomach was washed with ice-cold saline. Tissues collected
from 130 animals were homogenized with Polytron PCU-2-110 in 3

volumes of 10 mM Na-phosphate buffer pH 7.4 at 4°C.

Measurement of amidase activity

Peptidyl-MCA was used for enzyme assay at 37°C in 0.5 ml of 50 mM Na-phosphate buffer, pH 7.4, containing 0.1 mM substrate. Reaction was started by the addition of 20 μl of enzyme and the amounts of AMC liberated after 30 min was measured using a Hitachi fluorescence spectrophotometer, model 650-10 M with excitation at 380 nm and emission at 460 nm as described previously (Morita et al., 1977).

Bioassay of kinin

In 0.15 ml of 50 mM Tris-HCl buffer, pH 9.0, containing 3 mM 0-phenanthroline, 100 μl of heated plasma (60°C, 30 min) was added. Aliquots of enzyme solution was added to the mixture and kinin was measured after the incubation at 37°C. Kinin activity was measured by its ability to cause smooth muscle contraction of isolated rat uterus as described previously (Yano et al., 1971). Standard bradykinin was a product of Sandoz, Co. Ltd.

Preparation of p-aminobenzamidine-Sepharose 4B

ε-Aminohexanoic acid was first coupled to Sepharose 4B by the cyanogen bromide method (Cuatrecassas, 1970). p-Aminobenzamidine was attached to the Sepharose 4B by 1-ethyl-3-(dimethyl-aminopropyl)-carbodiimide according to the method of Holleman et al. (1975).

Preparation of rat plasma kallikrein

From rat plasma, prekallikrein was partially purified by chromatographies on columns of DEAE-Sephadex A-50, p-chlorobenzylamine-Sepharose 4B and Sephadex G-150, and activated by bovine activated Factor XII. Blood was drawn from the inferior caval vein of anesthetized wister strain male rats and anticoagulated with 3.8 % sodium citrate. After centrifugation, plasma (160 ml) was dialysed against 1,500 ml of 0.02 M Tris-HCl buffer, pH 8.0, containing 3 mM EDTA, 0.005 % polybrene and 0.05 % benzamidine, overnight. The dialysate was applied to a column (3.8 x 14 cm) of DEAE-Sephadex which was equilibrated with the same buffer containing 0.02 M NaCl. The nonadsorbed fraction was applied to a column (6.5 x 17 cm) of p-chlorobenzylamine-Sepharose which was equilibrated with the same buffer. After washing with 500 ml of the buffer, elution was made with the buffer containing 25 % dioxane. The eluate was concentrated by ultrafiltration using Diaflow membrane UM-10. The sample was applied on a column (2 x 140 cm) of Sephadex G-150 which was equilibrated with 0.02 M Tris-HCl buffer containing 0.15 M NaCl. Throughout the procedures, prekallikrein was assayed after the activation with the activated bovine Factor XII, using Z-Phe-Arg-MCA as substrate. The partially purified prekallikrein obtained after gel-filtration on a column of Sephadex G-150, was treated with the activated bovine Factor XII and applied to the column of Sephadex G-150.

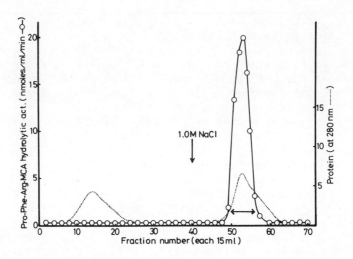

Fig. 1. p-Aminobenzamidine-Agarose Affinity Chromatography of Rat
Stomach Kallikrein.
After ammonium sulfate fractionation of the homogenate of rat
stomach, sample was applied to a column (3.0 x 24 cm) of p-aminobenzamidine agarose equilibrated with 50 mM Na-phosphate buffer,
pH 7.4, containing 0.05 M NaCl. After washing with the buffer,
stepwise elution was performed with the buffer containing 1 M NaCl
at the point indicated by arrow.

RESULTS AND DISCUSSION

Purification of Rat Stomach Kallikrein
        Homogenates of rat stomach prepared from 130 animals as
described in MATERIALS AND METHODS was centrifuged at 105,000 x g
for 60 min. To the supernatant, solid ammonium sulfate was added
with gentle stirring to make 70 % saturation. After 3 hr, the
precipitate was collected by centrifugation at 5,000 r.p.m. for 20
min, and dissolved in 300 ml of cold 50 mM Na-phosphate buffer, pH
7.4, containing 0.05 M NaCl.
        After dialysis against 50 mM Na-phosphate buffer, pH 7.4, con-
taining 0.05 M NaCl, overnight, the sample was applied to a column
(3.0 x 24 cm) of p-aminobenzamidine agarose equilibrated with the
same buffer. After washing with 600 ml of the buffer, stepwise
elution was performed with 50 mM Na-phosphate buffer, pH 7.4, containing 1.0 M NaCl. All the Pro-Phe-Arg-MCA hydrolytic activity was
found in the eluate, as shown in Fig. 1. Each fractions (No. 50-56)
were pooled and subjected to dialysis against 50 mM Na-phosphate
buffer, pH 7.4, containing 0.05 M NaCl, overnight.

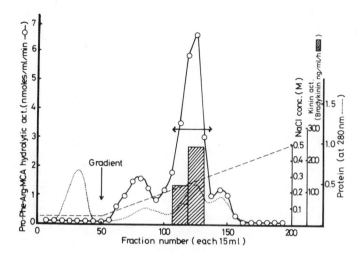

Fig. 2. DEAE-Sephadex A-50 Chromatography of Rat Stomach Kallikrein (Active Fraction from p-Aminobenzamidine-Agarose Affinity Chromato-Graphy)
The kallikrein fraction from p-aminobenzamidine-Sepharose column was applied to a column (3.3 x 14 cm) of DEAE-Sephadex A-50 equilibrated with 50 mM Na-phosphate buffer, pH 7.4, containing 0.05 M NaCl.
Salt gradient elution was performed at the point indicated by arrow, which was formed with each one liter of the buffer containing 0.05 M NaCl and 0.5 M NaCl.

    The sample was applied to a DEAE-Sephadex A-50 column (3.3 x 14 cm) equilibrated with 50 mM Na-phosphate buffer, pH 7.4, containing 0.05 M NaCl. After washing with 750 ml of the buffer gradient elution was performed with 1 l of 50 mM Na-phosphate buffer, pH 7.4, containing 0.05 M NaCl and 1 l of the same buffer containing 0.5 M NaCl. As shown in Fig. 2, three peaks with Pro-Phe-Arg-MCA hydrolytic activity were separated, but the second peak only had the kinin-releasing activity from rat heated-plasma as shown by shaded bar. Each fractions (No. 110-135) were pooled and concentrated to about 9 ml by ultrafiltration using Diaflow membrane UM-10.
    The sample was then applied to a Sephadex G-150 column (3.8 x 130 cm), equilibrated with 50 mM Na-phosphate buffer, pH 7.4, containing 0.15 M NaCl. As shown in Fig. 3, the Pro-Phe-Arg-MCA hydrolytic activity was found in the fractions with the molecular weight of about 29,000 and kinin-releasing activity was associated with the peak. Each fractions (No. 180-220) were collected and subjected to isoelectric focusing using carrier ampholytes of pH 2.5 to pH 5.0. As shown in Fig. 4, the Pro-Phe-Arg-MCA hydrolytic activity

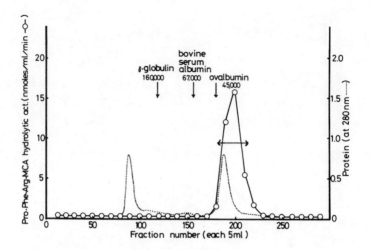

Fig. 3. Gel-filtration of the Kallikrein Fraction from DEAE-
Sephadex A-50 Column.
The kallikrein fraction from DEAE-Sephadex A-50 column was applied
on a column (3.8 x 130 cm) of Sephadex G-150 equilibrated with 50
mM Na-phosphate buffer, pH 7.4 containing 0.75 M NaCl. The elution
positions for r-globulin, bovine serum albumin and ovalbumin are
indicated in the figure.

was focused at pI of 4.05 with a shoulder. Fractions (No. 39-45)
were pooled and the homogeneity was examined by polyacrylamide gel
electrophoresis at pH 7.0. As shown in Fig. 5, a single protein
band was stained with Coomassie Brilliant Blue. Non-stained gel
was sliced into each pieces of 0.28 cm and suspended in 0.2 ml of
50 mM Na-phosphate buffer, pH 7.4. Fig. 5 also shows that Pro-Phe-
Arg-MCA hydrolytic activity corresponds to the protein band.

     Table I summarizes the purification procedures for rat stomach
kallikrein. From 130 animals, 10.2 mg of kallikrein was obtained
with the yield of 13.6 %. About 115-fold purification was achieved
from the supernatant of the homogenate.

     In this purification procedures, the affinity chromatography
on p-aminobenzamidine-Sepharose column was useful very much. However, when sonication was used to homogenate the stomach in the early
stages of this study, the affinity chromatography was found to be
not reproducible, and the Pro-Phe-Arg-MCA hydrolysing activity
sometimes appeared in the nonadsorbed fraction. In such case, the
eluate with 1 M NaCl had the maximum absorbance at 260 nm.   It

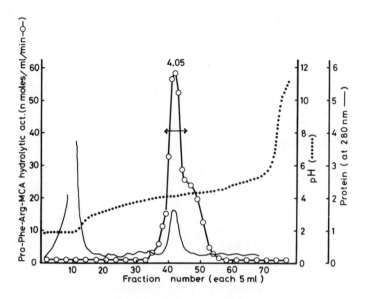

Fig. 4. Isoelectric Focusing Fraction of Rat Stomach Kallikrein.
The kallikrein fraction from gel-filtration was subjected to isoelectric focusing using Ampholine with pH range of 2.5 to 5.0.

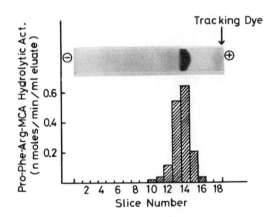

Fig. 5. Disc Gel Electrophoresis of Rat Stomach Kallikrein
Each 10 µg of the purified rat stomach kallikrein was applied to 8
% polyacrylamide gel column and electrophoresis was made at pH 7.0.
The upper half of the figure shows a protein band stained with
Coomassie Brilliant Blue. Non-stained gel was sliced into each
0.28 cm segment and suspended in 50 mM Na-phosphate buffer, pH 7.4.
The Pro-Phe-MCA hydrolysing activity in each segments is shown in
the lower half of the figure.

seemed that sonication solubilized substance which had higher affinity to p-aminobenzamidine-Sepharose. Therefore, we skipped sonication to get higher capacity and reproducibility of the affinity column.

Properties of Rat Stomach Kallikrein

Optimum pH and stability of rat stomach kallikrein ——— When Pro-
Phe-Arg-MCA was used as substrate, optimum pH for rat stomach
kallikrein was found to be apparently at pH 11, as shown in Fig. 6.
Since optimum pH for glandular kallikreins was reported to be
around pH 8.0, using BAEE as substrate, we examined the optimum
pH for hog pancreatic kallikrein and human urinary kallikrein using
Pro-Phe-Arg-MCA as substrate and found that they also showed abnormally alkaline optimum pH at 11. It can not be explained why
rat stomach kallikrein has such abnormal profile of optimum pH,
however, it seems to be common properties for glandular kallikrein.
On the contrary, rat plasma kallikrein showed the optimum pH at
8.0 as shown in Fig. 6. Rat stomach kallikrein was most stable
between pH 6 and 11. As shown in Fig. 6a, rat stomach kallikrein
did not hydrolyse the substrate appreciably above pH 12, which
may be due to the inactivation of the enzyme as shown in Fig. 6b.
    No spontaneous hydrolysis of Pro-Phe-Arg-MCA and no change of
the extinction coefficient of AMC, were observed until pH 13.0
under the conditions used.

Kinin-Releasing Activity and Amidase Activity of Rat Stomach Kallikrein

    As shown in Fig. 7, rat stomach kallikrein released kinin
from rat heated-plasma. The maximum amounts of kinin released by
the enzyme was lower than that by snake venom kininogenase. We
did not yet identify the kinin released by rat stomach kallikrein,
but the above result suggests that it may be kallidin, because it
has been established that snake venom kininogenase released bradykinin and that the contractile activity of kallidin is smaller
than that of bradykinin.
    Rat stomach kallikrein hydrolysed Pro-Phe-Arg-MCA and Z-Pro-
Arg-MCA but did not hydrolyse appreciably Boc-Val-Pro-Arg-MCA, Boc-
Ile-Glu-Gly-Arg-MCA, Glutaryl-Gly-Arg-MCA and Boc-Val-Leu-Lys-MCA
which are specific fluorogenic substrates for thrombin, Factor Xa,
urokinase and plasmin. It has been reported that hog pancreatic
kallikrein and human urinary kallikrein prefer to hydrolyse Pro-
Phe-Arg-MCA to Z-Phe-Arg-MCA, while bovine plasma kallikrein pre-
fers Z-Phe-Arg-MCA. As shown in Table II, among these two substrates for kallikreins, rat stomach kallikrein hydrolysed Pro-Phe-
Arg-MCA better than Z-Phe-Arg-MCA. On the contary, partially purified rat plasma kallikrein hydrolysed Z-Phe-Arg-MCA, better than
Pro-Phe-Arg-MCA. The Pro-Phe-Arg-MCA hydrolytic activity of rat
stomach kallikrein was completely inhibited by DFP and Trasylol
but not by soybean trypsin inhibitor, limabean trypsin inhibitor
and ovomucoid trypsin inhibitor as shown in Table II. Partially
purified rat plasma kallikrein was inhibited by all these inhibi-

TABLE 1.

PURIFICATION OF RAT STOMACH KALLIKREIN

Steps	Total protein (A 280nm)	Total unit (μmoles/min)	Specific act. U/A 280nm(x10^{-4})	Yield (%)
1. Homogenated with 3 volumes of 50mM Na-P.B, pH7.4				
2. Centrifuged at 105,000xG for 60min	8534	6.6	7.7	100
3. Amm. sulfate precipitation(70%)	4027	5.9	14.7	90.0
4. p-Aminobenzamidine agarose affinity chromatography(50mM Na-P.B, pH7.4, 1.0M NaCl stepwise elution)	1576	5.0	32.0	75.4
5. DEAE-Sephadex A-50 column chromatography(50mM Na-P.B, pH7.4, 0.05M-0.5M NaCl linear gradient elution)	198.0	1.7	85.9	25.0
6. Sephadex G-150 gel filtration(50mM Na-P.B, pH7.4, containing 0.15M NaCl)	42.4	1.6	377.0	24.0
7. Isoelectric Focusing Ampholine:pH 2.5-5.0	10.2	0.9	882.3	13.6

TABLE 2.

PROPERTIES OF VARIOUS KALLIKREINS

	Rat stomach	Rat plasma	Rat urinary	Porcine pancreas	Human urinary
Molecular Weight	29,000	98,000	35,300 [a] 33,600 33,100 32,300	33,000 [b]	27,000 [c] 29,000
Inhibitors					
DFP	100%(10^{-3}M)	100%(")	+ [d]	+ [e]	+ [f]
Trasylol	100%(500KIE/ml)	75%(")	+	+	+
Soybean	0%(100ug/ml)	96%(")	−	−	−
Lima bean	0%(100ug/ml)	80%(")		−	−
Ovomucoid	0%(100ug/ml)	57%(")	−	−	−
pI Values	4.05		3.50 [a] 3.68 3.73 3.80	3.64 [g] 3.71 3.85 3.95 4.05	3.9 [c] 4.0 4.2
Optimum pH	11.0	8.0	8.5 [f]	11.0	12.0
Substrate Specificities	(Pro-Phe-Arg-MCA)		(BAEE)	(Pro-Phe-Arg-MCA)	
Pro-Phe-Arg-MCA	1.0	1.0		1.0	
Z-Phe-Arg-MCA	0.23	1.57		0.2	
Fibrin	−	−	−	−	−
Casein	−	−	−	−	−

a) K. Nustad et al., 1974   b) H. Moriya et al., 1963   c) Y. Matsuda et al., 1976
d) K. Nustad, 1970   e) F. Fiedler, 1976   f) H. Moriya, 1959   g) F. Fiedler, 1970

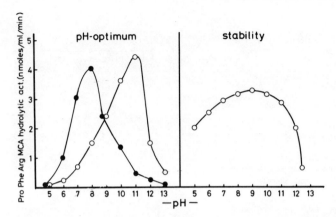

Fig. 6. pH Optimum (a) and Stability (b) for Rat Stomach Kallikrein (-O-) and Rat Plasma Kallikrein (-●-)
Britton-Robinson's wide range buffer (0.04 M) consisting of H_3PO_4-
CH_3COOH-H_3BO_3-NaOH, and Pro-Phe-Arg-MCA as substrate were used.
a) The solution of enzyme in buffer (0.5 ml) was incubated with
10 mM Pro-Phe-Arg-MCA (5 μl) at 37°C for 30 min at the indicated
pH values.
b) The soltuion of enzyme in buffer (20 μl) was preincubated at
37°C for 30 min at the indicated pH values. Then 0.97 ml of 0.1 M
Na-phosphate buffer, pH 7.4, and 10 μl of 20 mM Pro-Phe-MCA were
added, and the incubation was followed at 37°C for 30 min at pH 7.4.

tors. These results strongly indicate that rat stomach kallikrein
purified in this paper, has the similar substrate specificity to
other glandular kallikrein. The susceptibility of rat plasma
kallikrein to these inhibitors is different from those of human
and bovine plasma kallikrein. But it is quite similar to that of
guinea-pig plasma kallikrein, which has been purified recently by
Yamamoto et al.[*]

Molecular Weight of Rat Stomach Kallikrein
      Molecular weight of rat stomach kallikrein was determined by
gel-filtration on a column of Sephadex G-50, and calculated to be
29,000 as shown in Fig. 8a. For comparison, the molecular weight
of the partially purified rat plasma kallikrein was determined by
gel-filtration on a column of Sephadex G-150. As shown in Fig. 8,
the molecular weight of rat stomach kallikrein was clearly different from rat plasma kallikrein.

[*]Personal communication from Dr. T. Yamamoto, Department of Pathophysiology, Toxicology Institute, Kumamoto University Medical
School.

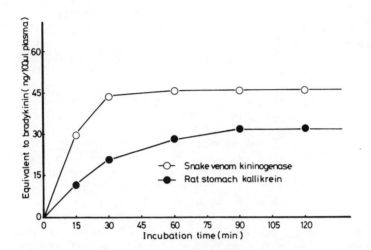

Fig. 7. Liberation of Kinin from Rat Plasma Heated at 60°C for 30 min by Rat Stomach Kallikrein and Snake Venom Kininogenase.
In 0.15 ml of Tris-HCl buffer, pH 9.0, containing 0-phenanthroline (3 mM), 100 µl of heated plasma was added. To the solution, 50 µl of rat stomach kallikrein (A_{280}=1.6) or 50 µl of snake venom kininogenase (A_{280}=1.4) was added, and mixture was incubated at 37°C. Kinin activity was measured by the contaction of rat uterus, using synthetic bradykinin as standard.

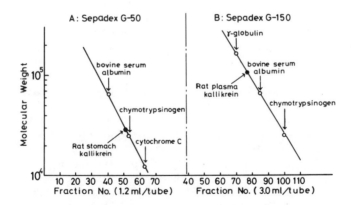

Fig. 8. Determination of molecular weight by gel-filtration on a Sephadex G-50 column (1.6 x 90 cm) and a Sephadex G-150 column (3.8 x 130 cm). The columns were equilibrated with 50 mM Na-phosphate buffer, pH 7.4 containing 0.15 M NaCl.

Table II summarizes the properties of rat stomach kallikrein in comparison with rat plasma kallikrein. They are clearly different molecules in terms of molecular weight, susceptibility to protease inhibitors, optimum pH and substrate specificities. Therefore, these results exclude the possibility that the kallikrein purified in this paper derived from plasma kallikrein. The contamination of plasmin in this preparation also can be excluded, because rat stomach kallikrein did not hydrolyse casein and fibrin.

Table II also shows some properties of glandular kallikrein, rat urinary, porcine pancreas, human urinary kallikreins, which have been reported by other investigators.

The properties of rat stomach kallikrein is very similar to these of glandular kallikrein and it can be concluded that a typical glandular kallikrein is present in rat stomach. We do not know the localization of this enzyme in stomach and the function of the kallikrein remains to be established.

Considering the optimum pH of the kallikrein, it may not be probable that the kallikrein functions on the mucus membrane of the stomach. It is quite interesting to know that the kallikrein regulates the function of stomach responding with gastrin and secretin.

REFERENCES

Cuatrecasas, P., 1970, Protein purification by affinity chromatography. Derivatizations of agarose and polyacrylamide beads. J. Biol. Chem., 245, 3059.

Fiedler, F., C. Hirschauer and E. Werle, 1970, Anreicherung von präkallikrein B aus Schweinepankreas und ligenschaften verschiedener formen des pankreaskallikreins. Hoppe-Seyler's Z. Physiol. Chem., 351, 225.

Fiedler, F., 1976, Methods in Enzymology, ed. by L. Lorand, Academic Press, New York, Vol. 45, p. 287.

Fujikawa, K., K. Kurachi and E. Davie, 1977, Characterization of bovine factor XIIa (activated hageman factor). Biochem., Vol. 16, No. 19.

Geiger, R., G. Feifel and G. L. Haberland, 1977, A precursor of kinins in the human gastric mucus, Kininogenases-Kallikrein, Schattauer, Stuttgart, p. 73-77.

Holleman, W. H., W. W. Andres and L. T. Weiss, 1975, The relation ship between the lysine and the p-aminobenzamidine binding sites on human plasminogen. Thrombosis Research, 7, 683-693.

Kraut, H., E. K. Frey and E. Werle, 1930, Der nachweis lines kreislaufhormons in pankreasdrüse. Z. Physiol. Chem., 189, 97.

Matsuda, Y., K. Miyazaki, H. Moriya, Y. Fujimoto, Y. Hojima and C. Moriwaki, 1976, Studies on urinary kallikreins. J. Biochem., 80, 671-679.

McGiff, J. C., A. Nasjletti, 1976, Kinins, renal function and blood pressure regulation. Fed. Proc., 35, 172.

Morita, T., H. Kato, S. Iwanaga, K. Takada, T. Kimura and S. Sakakibara, 1977, New fluorogenic substrates for α-thrombin, Factor Xa, kallikreins and urokinase. J. Biochem., 82, 1495-1498.

Moriwaki, C., H. Moriya, K. Yamaguchi, K. Kizuki and H. Fujimori, 1973, "Kininogenases", ed. by G. L. Haberland and J. W. Rohen, F. K. Schattauer Verlag·Stuttgart-New York, Vol. 1, p. 57.

Moriya, H., 1959, Chemical studies on kallikrein VIII. Molecular weight of kallikrein and the supplement. J. Pharmacol. Soc. Jap., 79, 1453.

Moriya, H., J. V. Pierce and M. E. Webster, 1963, Purification and some properties of three kallikreins. Ann. N. Y. Acad. Sci., 104, 172.

Nustad, K., 1970, The relationship between kidney and urinary kininogenases. Br. J. Pharmacol., 39, 73-86.

Nustad, K., J. V. Pierce, 1974, Purification of rat urinary kallikreins and their specific antibody. Biochem.,13, No. 11.

Seki, T., T. Nakajima and E. G. Erdös, 1972, Color kallikrein, its relation to the plasma enzyme. Biochem. Pharmacol., 21, 1227.

Suzuki, T., S. Iwanaga, S. Nagasawa and T. Sato, 1966, in Hypotensive Peptide, ed. by E. G. Erdös, N. Back, F. Sicuteri, pp. 149-160, Springer-Verlag, New York.

Werle, E., P. Rodin, 1936, Über das vorkommen des kallikreins in den speicheldrusen und im Mundspeichel. Biochem. Z., 286, 213.

Werle, E., 1955, Polypeptides which stimulated plain muscle, ed. by J. H. Gaddume, p. 20, Livingstone.

Williams, D. E. and R. A. Reisfelf, 1964, Disc electrophoresis in polyacrylamide gels: extension to new conditions of pH and buffer. Ann. N. Y. Acad. Sci., 121, 273.

Yano, M., S. Nagasawa, T. and T. Suzuki, 1971, Partial purification and some properties of high molecular weight kininogen, bovine kininogen-I. J. Biochem., 69, 471-481.

A SIMPLE, LARGE SCALE PROCESS FOR PURIFYING HUMAN URINARY KALLIKREIN,

BASED ON REVERSE OSMOSIS AND AMMONIUM SULFATE PRECIPITATION*

Amintas F.S. Figueiredo and Marcos Mares-Guia

Depto. De Bioquimica, Inst. Cien. Biol. Universidade

Federal De Minas Gerais, CP 2486, 30.000 Belo Horizonte,

Brazil

ABSTRACT

A simple, large scale process for the purification of human urinary kallikrein is described which is based upon concentration by reverse osmosis, ammonium sulfate precipitation, and gel filtration on a column of Sephadex-G-150. The yield in protein is higher than any reported in the literature to this date; the purified enzyme seems to be identical to that reported by Figueiredo and Mares-Guia at the Kinin-Symposium in Paris, 1978, based on the procedure of Hial, et al., (1974).

INTRODUCTION

A simple process has been devised for the purification of human urinary kallikrein that can be applied to large urine samples, provided there is sufficient capacity to perform reverse osmosis.

Filtered, male human urine is subjected to reverse osmosis up to 100-fold concentration, and the concentrate thus obtained is subjected to ammonium sulfate fractionation. An 0.50 saturation cut removes all kininase activity, leaving the kallikrein in the supernatant. A second cut, at 0.75 saturation, precipitates all the kinin-releasing activity. After dialysis and freeze-drying, the material is passed through a Sephadex G-150 column, which results in a final active fraction with properties identical to

---

* This work was supported by FINEP.

the enzyme purified by the scaled-up procedure of Figueiredo and Mares-Guia (1978) based on the work of Hial et al., (1974), but with higher yield.

Although the process to be described is well defined, we are still working on the ammonium sulfate fractionation step, with the goal of preparing the pure enzyme directly from that step.

METHODS

The methods used for determining enzyme activities are cited under Table I. Acrylamide electrophoresis was run at pH 8.3, using 7.5% acrylamide, and applying 200 µg protein to each gel column. Coomassie-blue was used throughout for dyeing, according to Laemmli (1970).

RESULTS

Eighty liters of human urine, collected in the presence of thymol and preserved at 4°C, were filtered and subjected to reverse osmosis using a Millipore Pellicon Cassete System equipped with one pack of membranes. The filtration rate was 3000 ml/hour, and the ultrafiltration was continued to a final volume of 1000 ml.

At this point, the sample was diluted to 10 liters with distilled water, and the solution again subjected to reverse osmosis until a final volume of 850 ml was obtained. Fifty milliliters were removed and subjected to freeze drying, yielding 0.28 g of powder containing 65% protein.

To the remainder 800 ml was added powdered ammonium sulfate to 0.50 saturation, at room temperature. The suspension was left under continuous mixing for 1 hour and was centrifuged at 5000 rpm. always at room temperature (25°C). The precipitate was recovered and stored for further study. Ammonium sulfate was added to the supernatant to give 0.75 saturation, and the resulting suspension was treated as before. After centrifugation, the precipitate was dissolved in the minimum possible volume of distilled water, dialyzed against water for seven days, at 4°C, with daily exchanges of ca. 40 L water. After freeze-drying, each 500 mg of the material were dissolved in 20.0 ml of 0.01 M ammonium acetate buffer, pH 7.0, containing 0.05 M NaCl, yielding a slightly turbid solution. After centrifugation, the clear supernatant was applied to a Sephadex G-150 (super-fine), column 5 x 100 cm, and eluted with the same buffer. Fractions of 10 ml each were collected. The elution profile is shown in Fig. 1. The fractions belonging to the active peak were pooled, dialyzed against water, and freeze-dried.

TABLE I - PURIFICATION OF HUMAN URINARY KALLIKREIN BASED ON REVERSE OSMOSIS AND AMMONIUM SULFATE PRECIPITATION

STEP	PROTEIN[d]		SPECIFIC ACTIVITIES		TOTAL ACTIVITIES			
	Total	REC.	B_z-L-Arg-OEt	KININ-RELEASING	B_z-L-Arg-OEt	REC	KININ-RELEASING	REC
	mg		μmol/(min.mg) KU/mg	μgBK/(min.mg)				
POWDER FROM CONCENTRATED URINE (75L)	3460	100	0.096[b]	0.13[c]	422.2	100	473	100
0.75 SAT. AMMONIUM SULFATE PRECIPITATE	880	25.4	0.121	0.37	107	25.4	325.6	68.8
SEPHADEX G-150	550	15.9	0.141	0.45	77.6	18.4	247	52.2
HUK₁ SCALED-UP BASED ON HIAL et al (1974)			0.113[a]	0.72				

a - data from Figueiredo and Mares-Guia, (1978).

b - at pH 8.0, 25°C, according to Arens and Haberland (1977).

c - determined according to Prado and Prado (1961),but using partially purified human plasma kininogen.

d - protein was determined according to Lowry et al (1951).

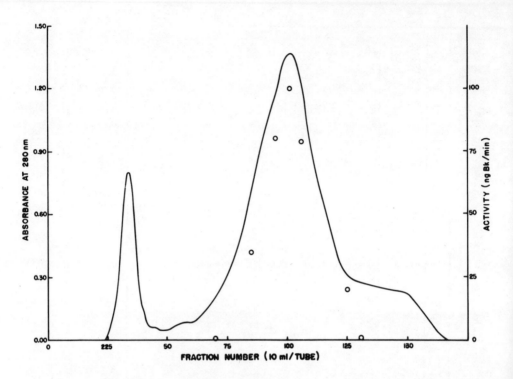

Figure 1. Gel filtration of ammonium sulfate precipitate (0.75 sat)
on Sephadex G-150.

The overall yield of purified enzyme was 550 mg in protein, contained in a total 580 mg of powder; the balance sheet of the
purification process is shown in Table I. For comparison purposes
the enzyme obtained through the above described process will, from
now on, be called HUK-2, whereas the enzyme prepared through the
scaled-up process of Hial et al., (1974), developed by Figueiredo
and Mares-Guia (1978), will now be called HUK-1.

Acrylamide electrophoresis of HUK-2 yielded three bands (Fig.
2), exactly positioned as the three bands, all active, found for
HUK-1 by Figueiredo and Mares-Guia (1978). A sedimentation constant
of S = 3.36 was found which should be compared to S = 3.49 for
HUK-1. Amino acid analysis was performed, and the results are
shown in Table II.

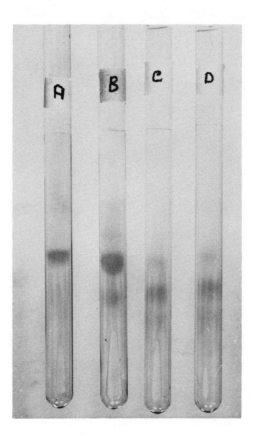

Figure 2.   Acrylamide electrophoresis of concentrated urine,
            ammonium sulfate precipitate (0.75 sat.), HUK-2 e
            HUK-1. Conditions described in the text.

HUK-2 was subjected to preparative electrofocussing with the
purpose of analyzing the behavior of each fraction on acrylamide
electrophoresis. Three major active peaks, with PI values of
3.56, 3.85, and 4.10 were separated, the fractions pooled,
extensively dialyzed against water as described before, and freeze-
dried.

Acrylamide electrophoresis of each electrofocus peak displayed
a common pattern of three components, identical in migration to
those HUK-1 or HUK-2, shown in Fig. 2. Only the proportions of

TABLE II - AMINO ACID ANALYSIS OF HUK-1 AND HUK-2
(HYDROLYSIS - 20.0 Hs)

AMINO ACIDS	HUK-1	HUK-2
Lysine	3.0	3.0
Histidine	1.0	1.0
Arginine	2.0	2.0
Aspartic Acid	5.0	5.0
Threonine	4.0	4.0
Serine	3.0	3.0
Glutamic Acid	7.0	6.0
Proline	2.0	3.0
Glycine	3.0	3.0
Alanine	4.0	4.0
Half Cystine	1.0	3.0
Valine	3.0	3.0
Methionine	1.0	1.0
Isoleucine	1.0	2.0
Leucine	4.0	4.0
Tyrosine	2.0	2.0
Phenylalanine	2.0	2.0

the three acrylamide bands were different from one electrofocus
peak to the other. The constant observation of three components
in acrylamide electrophoresis of HUK leads us to propose that
these active fractions be called HUK A, B, C (Fig. 2), according
to their increasing rate of migration. The electrofocus peaks
are now undergoing chemical study, including amino acid analysis.

DISCUSSION

Preparation of human urinary kallikrein of high degree of purification has been described by Moriya et al., (1963); Hail et al., (1974); Matsuda et al., (1976); Yoi et al., (1977); Geiger et al., (1977); e Narendra et al., (1978).

The procedures are, in general, multi-step and give low yields. The purification procedure described in this paper is sufficiently simple, involving only three steps, and offers a good yield, when contrasted with the above mentioned procedures. HUK-2, purified according to this procedure has properties similar to those of HUK-1, prepared according to Figueiredo and Mares-Guia (1978), using the scaled-up procedure of Hial et al., (1974). Table I shows an esterolytic activity recovery of 18%, whereas recovery of kinin-releasing activity is close to 52%. This clearly shows that, in human urine, there occur other esterolytic activities not related to the kinin-releasing activity. Table I shows, in addition, the very close agreement between specific esterolytic activities of HUK-1 and HUK-2 indicating similar degrees of purity. It is, however, more difficult to compare the two preparations with basis on their kinin-generating activities, given the variations in substrate quality, from batch to batch, mostly related to solubility. The identity between HUK-1 and HUK-2 is further indicated by their acrylamide electrophoretic patterns, both displaying three bands, shown to be all active for HUK-1 (Figueiredo and Mares-Guia, 1978). This identity is further stressed by Table II, where the respective amino acid analyses are shown.

The inherent microheterogeneity of human urinary kallikrein is stressed by the experiments coupling electrofoccus to acrylamide electrophoresis. Through amino acid analysis of the pools obtained from preparative electrofoccussing we hope to gain insight into the causes of microheterogeneity.

ACKNOWLEDGEMENT

The authors are grateful for the help of Drs. Armando Neves and Marcelo Santoro in the experiments at the ultracentrifuge.

REFERENCES

Arens, A., and G.L. Haberland (1977). Determination of kallikrein activity in animal tissue using biochemical methods. In: G.L. Haberland, J.W. Rohen, and T. Suzuki (eds.) Kininogenases. Kallikrein 4. Physiological properties and Pharmacological rationale. F.K. Schattauer Verlag, Stuttgart-New York, pp.43-53.

Figueiredo, A.F.S., and M. Mares-Guia (1978). Some properties of
    human urinary kallikrein obtained through scaled-up purifi-
    cation. In: Current Concepts in Kinin Research. Ed. G.L.
    Haberland. Pergamon Press, 1978. In Press.
Geiger, R., K. Mann, and T. Bettels (1977). Isolation of human
    urinary kallikrein by affinity chromatography. J. Clin. Chem.
    Clin. Biochem. 15: 479-483.
Hial, V., C.R. Diniz, and Mares-Guia (1974). Purification and
    properties of a human urinary kallikrein (kininogenase).
    Biochemistry 13: 4311-4318.
Laemmli, U.K. (1970). Cleavage of structural proteins during the
    assembly of the head of bacteriophage T_4. Nature 227: 680-685.
Lowry, O.H., M.J. Rosenbrough, A.F. Lewis, and R.J. Randall (1951).
    Protein measurement with the folin phenol reagent. J. Biol.
    Chem. 193: 265-275.
Matsuda, Y., K. Miyazaki, H. Moriya, Y. Fujimoto, Y. Hojima, and
    C. Moriwaki (1976). Studies on urinary kallikreins. I.
    Purification and characterization of human urinary kalli-
    kreins. J. Biochem. 80: 671-679.
Moriya, H., J.V. Pierce, and M. Webster (1963). Purification and
    some properties of three kallikreins. Ann. N.Y. Acad. Sci.
    104: 172-185.
Narendra, B.O., and J.W. Ryan (1978). A simple high-yield procedure
    for isolation of human urinary kallikreins. Biochem. J. 171:
    285-288.
Prado, E.S. and J.L. Prado (1961). Partial purification of a plasma
    kinin forming enzyme from horse urine. Experientia (Basel) 17:
    31-33.
Yoi, O.O., K.F. Austen, and J. Spragg (1977). Kinin-generating and
    esterolytic activity of purified human urinary kallikrein
    (urokallikrein). Biochem. Pharmacol. 26: 1893-1900.

COMPONENTS OF THE KALLIKREIN-KININ SYSTEM IN URINE

James W. Ryan, Narendra B. Oza, Larry C. Martin and
Guillermo A. Pena

Department of Medicine, University of Miami School of
Medicine, Miami, Florida 33101, USA

ABSTRACT

The excretion of kallikrein in urine varies, but the
pathophysiologic implications are not clear. To help clarify the
role of the urinary kallikrein-kinin system, we have begun to
define components of the system as they occur in urine. To minimize artifacts which may arise through extensive purification
procedures, we studied urinary protein concentrates prepared by
ultrafiltration. The concentrates were separated by chromatography
on Sephacryl. Urine contains abundant kininase activity, but in
strongly inhibited forms. Kininase II is separable into at least
two forms. Another major kininase can hydrolyze benzoyl-Pro-Phe-
Arg and is inhibited by arginine but not by BPP_{9a} or SQ 14,225.
Its molecular weight is ~63,000. A third kininase, not inhibited
by BPP_{9a}, is excluded from Sephacryl. Human urine appears to contain only one kallikrein-like enzyme (MW 45,000). In addition,
urine contains a protein (MW ~80,000) which reacts with trypsin to
release bradykinin and which inhibits the hydrolysis of Pro-Phe-
Arg-[^{3}H]anilide by urinary kallikrein. Thus, in addition to
kallikrein and kinins, urine contains kininogen and at least three
kininase enzymes. Urinary ultrafiltrate contains an inhibitory
substance (~MW 400).

INTRODUCTION

A number of different groups have adduced evidence to indicate
that the rate of kallikrein excretion in urine varies system-
atically in response to dietary factors (notably salt and H_2O), and
in response to blood levels of mineralocorticoids (for review, see

313

McGiff and Nasjletti, 1976; Mills et al., 1976; Keiser et al., 1976; Margolius et al., 1976; Croxatto et al., 1976). Although there may be racial differences, it appears that unusually small amounts of kallikrein were excreted by patients with essential hypertension (Elliot and Nuzum, 1934; Margolius et al, 1971; Geller et al., 1976). Further, there is growing evidence of interactions between the kallikrein-kinin system and the renin-angiotensin system; some of which are postulated to occur within the kidney. Caldwell et al. (1976) and Ward and colleagues (1975, 1976) have shown that angiotensin converting enzyme (kininase II) occurs in association with brush border of the proximal tubule. Recently, in a collaborative study, we have found that human urinary kallikrein can activate inactive renin (Sealey et al., 1978).

However, further to develop and test hypotheses on the role of the kallikrein-kinin system within the kidney and urinary outflow tract, it will be necessary to know which of the components, in addition to kallikrein, occur in urine. Hial et al. (1976) have shown that urine contains both Lys-bradykinin and bradykinin and have defined conditions under which Met-Lys-bradykinin can be formed by urine in vitro. The de novo synthesis of Met-Lys-bradykinin implies the presence of kininogen (see also Pisano et al., 1978). And the presence of bradykinin implies the action at a kinin converting enzyme (cf. Brandi et al., 1976).

We have found kininase II in urine (e.g., see Ryan et al., 1978b), and Erdös and colleagues (1978) have described a kininase I-like enzyme.   Further to characterize components of the system, we undertook a series of experiments to concentrate and then separate proteins of fresh human and guinea pig urine by means sufficiently mild to allow for quantitative or near-quantitative recoveries.

MATERIALS AND METHODS

Sephacryl-200 was obtained by Pharmacia Fine Chemicals, Inc., and Bio-Gel P-2 and Bio Rex 70 were obtained from BioRad Laboratories, Inc. Kinins were synthesized in this laboratories. The standard human urinary kallikrein used in these studies and its specific antibodies were prepared as described by Oza and Ryan, 1978.

Assays

Kallikrein was assayed as described by Chung et al., (this volume). Angiotensin converting enzyme (kininase II) was assayed by the procedures described by Ryan et al., (1977, 1978b). Other kininase enzymes were measured using [H^3]benzoyl-Pro-Phe-Arg. Protein was

measured by two techniques: 1. The Folin-Lowry method, and 2. By
absorbance at 280 nm. The kinin content of urokininogen was assayed,
after denaturation of proteins followed by incubation with trypsin,
on isolated guinea pig ileum.

RESULTS AND DISCUSSION

Preparation of Urine

Urines of man and guinea pig have been examined. Human urine
was provided by six male volunteers and was collected at room temperature under a thin layer of toluene. Twenty-four hour urines were
collected from 40 female guinea pigs maintained in metabolic cages.
The guinea pig urine was collected under a layer of toluene into a
collection vessel cooled with cracked ice. The latter precaution was
necessary because of the observation that guinea pig urinary kininase
II is highly labile at room temperature (half-life of 2-4 h). However, once partially purified, kininase II is stable for months at
4°C. The results may imply that urine contains other substances,
possibly protease enzymes (cf. Nakahara, 1978, in reactions of plasma kallikrein on kininase II), capable of inactivating or denaturing
kininase II.

The urines were concentrated 50- to 200-fold, at 4°C, using a
Millipore filter apparatus with a membrane (PTGC 142 05) having a
10,000 MW retention limit. The concentrated urinary proteins (~10
ml) were applied to a Sephacryl S-200 column (2.5 x 110 cm), equilibrated with 0.05 M Tris-HCl plus 0.5 M NaCl; all at pH 8.0 (cf. Oza
and Ryan, 1978).

Kallikrein and Kallikrein-like Enzymes

Both human and guinea pig urines contained an enzyme capable of
hydrolyzing Pro-Phe-Arg-[3H]anilide or Pro-Phe-Arg-[3H]benzylamide
(see Chung et al., this volume). The human enzyme behaved as a single
substance having a molecular weight of 45,000. It was inhibited completely by Trasylol at 5µg/ml and was not inhibited by SBTI at 10µg/ml.
The enzyme was inhibited by antibodies to highly purified human urinary kallikrein (cf. Oza and Ryan, 1978).

Similarly, the guinea pig enzyme could not be distinguished from
kallikrein in terms of its response to Trasylol, its ability to bind
to Trasylol-Sepharose, and its pH optimum (pH 9.5) on reaction with
Pro-Phe-Arg-[3H]benzylamide. It was not inhibited by SBTI at 10µg/ml.

A point to be emphasized is that there were no other enzymes of
urine, separable by Sephacryl, capable of hydrolyzing our radio-la-
belled substrates.

Kininogen

Any hypothesis on the role of the kallikrein-kinin system in renal function (or function lower in the urinary outflow tract) requires that conditions must exist in which kinins can be formed and gain access to receptors. Both kallikrein and kinins occur in urine (see references above), and there is abundant evidence to indicate that kinins, if filtered, do not survive passage beyond the proximal tubule (e.g., see Carone et al., 1976, Nasjletti et al., 1974). These data imply the existence of kininogen in urine, and Pisano et al. (1978) have reported that incubation of trypsin with urine increases the content of kinins (measured by radioimmunoassay) in urine. Further, Pisano et al. have found that urine contains a protein reactive (in double immunodiffusion) with antibodies to plasma low molecular weight kininogen.

On examination of human urinary proteins separated by chromatography on Sephacryl, we have found further evidence of urokininogen. Fractions were acidified with acetic acid, heated in a boiling H_2O bath, cooled, neutralized, and then incubated with trypsin. Tryptic reactions were terminated by heating. The fractions were assayed for effects on isolated guinea pig ileum. Kinins were formed from protein(s) having an apparent molecular size of 70,000-80,000. However, some kinin-containing protein was eluted with kallikrein itself (~45,000 MW).

Converting Enzymes

The Prados and colleagues (Brandi et al., 1976) have reported that kinin converting enzyme(s) occurs in human urine and is capable of forming bradykinin from Lys-bradykinin. Whether one enzyme can degrade Met-Lys-bradykinin to form bradykinin is less clear. We have found that plasma aminopeptidase enzymes are difficult to separate using molecular sieve and ion exchange chromatography but can be distinguished in terms of responses to specific inhibitors. Curiously, kininase II is also difficult to separate from aminopeptidase enzymes. We have found that guinea pig urine contains an arginine aminopeptidase (measured in terms of hydrolysis of α-L-Arg-β-naphthylamide) that co-chromatographs with an aminopeptidase A-like enzyme (angiotensin aminopeptidase) on Sephacryl. The aminopeptidase A-like enzyme can hydrolyze α-L-Asp-[^{3}H]benzylamide and is inhibited (50%) by α-L-aspartylchloromethylketone, 10^{-6}M(Chung et al., unpublished). The arginine aminopeptidase is not inhibited by the same agent unless >2,000-fold higher concentrations are used.

Kinins

As is well-known, kinins occur in urine (cf. Hial et al., 1976, and their references). Our investigation of urinary kinins was extremely limited: We found that the urinary ultrafiltrate contains basic peptides (adsorbed by Bio Rex 70), capable of contracting rat uterus. The peptides were inactivated by urinary kininase II.

Kininase Enzymes

The urinary proteins concentrated by ultrafiltration contain large amounts of kininase activity, and the net activity can be increased 6- to 30-fold by washing the concentrated proteins with H_2O or 0.9% NaCl (see Ryan, J.W. et al., this volume). In view of the abundant kininase activity, one might well wonder how kinins can be found intact. However, as implied by results of our ultrafiltration studies (activation by washing), the kininase enzymes of crude urine are virtually inactive. The half-life of bradykinin in fresh urine is reported to be >2 h (J. Pisano, personal communication).

When we first began our survey of components of the kallikrein-kinin system in fresh urine, we were mainly concerned with kininase II. As noted above, kininase II is markedly unstable in crude urine. Urinary proteins separated on Sephacryl S-200 yield two distinct fractions of kininase II. The first co-chromatographs with guinea pig lung angiotensin converting enzyme, and the second behaves like a protein having a molecular size of 90,000. Not uncommonly, the activity of the second fraction disappears during storage. Under conditions in which lung kininase II is retained on hydroxylapatite (Das and Soffer, 1975), urine kininase II fraction I is also retained, but fraction II is not. However, there is little doubt that both fractions possess properties of kininase II: Both fractions hydrolyze [3H]Hip-Gly-Gly, [3H]Hip-His-Leu, [3H]benzoyl-Phe-Ala-Pro, [3H]benzoyl-Pro-Phe-Arg, and [3H]benzoyl-Phe-His-Leu to yield the products produced by guinea pig and rabbit lung angiotensin converting enzyme (the latter enzyme provided by Richard Soffer, cf. Das and Soffer, 1975).

Both fractions are inhibited completely by BPP_{9a} at 10^{-7} M (I_{50} 28 nM), and by SQ 14,225 at 10^{-7} M (I_{50} ~20 nM). The two kininase II fractions of guinea pig urine are inhibited, precisely as is guinea pig lung angiotensin converting enzyme, by antibodies to the guinea pig lung enzyme (see Fig.).

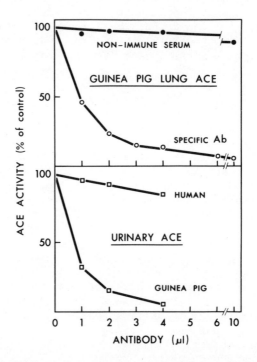

Figure. Inhibition of guinea pig urinary ACE and lung ACE by rabbit anti-guinea lung ACE. Rabbits, rather than goats, were used for immunizations to reduce or minimize cross-reactivity among species (cf. Ryan et al., 1975; Conroy et al., 1976). As shown, dialyzed non-immune rabbit serum had little or no effects on the ability of guinea pig lung ACE to hydrolyze its substrate ([^{3}H]Hip-His-Leu). However, the anti-serum inhibited both guinea pig lung ACE and urinary ACE. There was relatively little inhibition of human urinary ACE.

Although we originally synthesized [^{3}H]benzoyl-Pro-Phe-Arg (the acylated C-terminal tripeptide of bradykinin) as a substrate for kininase II, it has proved to be the least selective of all of our substrates. In fact, several different enzymes of human and guinea pig urine hydrolyze the substrate. The most active of these enzymes (second only to kininase II) behaves like a substance having a molecular size of 63,000, and is inhibited almost completely by

L-arginine at 5×10^{-4} M or bradykinin at 10^{-6} M (cf. Erdös and
Yang, 1970; Erdös et al., 1978). BPP_{9a} and SQ 14,225, each at 10^{-7}
M, do not inhibit the enzyme. Apparently, the enzyme is a carboxy-
peptidase B-like enzyme (cf. Erdös and Yang, 1970; Erdös et al.,
1978). We found that arginine, 5×10^{-4} M, also inhibits kininase
II (~40%).

However, in addition to the major activity, urine contains at
least two other non-kininase II enzymes capable of hydrolyzing [³H]
benzoyl-Pro-Phe-Arg. One is excluded from Sephacryl. The second
is eluted like a substance having a molecular size of ~20,000.

As indicated by the foregoing, [³H]benzoyl-Pro-Phe-Arg proved
to be a poor substrate, in terms of specificity, for kininase II.
However, all other substrates listed above were hydrolyzed by kininase II, and kininase II only, under our assay conditions (cf. Ryan
et al., 1978b).

                          Kallikrein Inhibitors

Beaven et al., (1971) have noted that urine contains a substance or substances capable of inhibiting the hydrolysis of arginine ester substrates by kallikrein. The inhibitor is retained
by Sephadex G-25. We have confirmed that human and guinea pig
urine ultrafiltrates contain a substance or substances capable of
inhibiting the action of highly-purified human urinary kallikrein
on Pro-Phe-Arg-[³H]benzylamide. Urinary kinins do not account for
these results. Even at 10^{-5} M, bradykinin, Lys-bradykinin, or Met-
Lys-bradykinin do not inhibit kallikrein.

The inhibitor is heat stable (100°C, 5 min), and behaves on
Bio-Gel P-2 (5 x 50 cm column developed with H_2O) like a substance
having a molecular size of 300-500. However, we do not know whether
the inhibitor behaves ideally on molecular sieve chromatography.

We also examined for protein inhibitors of kallikrein in guinea
pig urine. In these studies, we assayed each fraction collected from
the Sephacryl column for its ability to inhibit hydrolysis of Pro-
Phe-Arg-[³H]anilide (Chung et al., this volume) by a standard amount
of guinea pig urinary kallikrein (purified from the same urinary proteins). A sharp peak of inhibitory activity was found in fractions
corresponding in molecular size to a substance of 75,000 daltons.
Because of the close correspondence of the inhibitory activity to
urokininogen (see above), it appears distinctly possible that the
apparent enzyme inhibition arose from a competition among substrates:
Pro-Phe-Arg-[³H]anilide vs. urokininogen. However, we cannot, at
this time, rule out that an inhibitor of kallikrein co-chromatographs
with urokininogen.

CONCLUDING REMARKS

Much of our work confirms results obtained by others. Perhaps the most striking of our findings is that voided urine contains kininase enzymes in great abundance, yet one is hard-pressed to conclude that these enzymes are of functional significance. Indeed, the net kininase activity of fresh urine is negligible. In particular, urine contains a great excess of small molecular weight inhibitors of kininase II (Ryan, J.W. et al., this volume), and may contain a proteolytic enzyme that inactivates kininase II. Nonetheless, one cannot make many definitive conclusions about the net activities of components in voided urine.

New substances, like Met-Lys-bradykinin, can be formed after urine is voided (Hial et al., 1976). Furthermore, in addition to materials released by kidneys, urine contains substances released from other sites of the genito-urinary tract. Thus, kininase II may enter urine at the level of renal brush border, and again at the level of the seminal vesicles (cf. Cushman and Cheung, 1971). Kinins within the proximal tubule appear to be inactivated almost instantaneously (cf. Carone et al., 1976), yet are well-protected in the lower nephron.

Nonetheless, it is evident that virtually all of the components of the kallikrein-kinin system occur in voided urine. Thus, the coming challenge is to find out where each component joins the urinary outflow tract, and where conditions exist for one component to react with another.

Our experience in searching for protein inhibitors of kallikrein suggests that a problem exists in terms of measuring urinary kallikrein by functional assay (e.g., that of Beaven et al, 1971, and Chung et al., this volume). The small molecular weight inhibitor(s) can be removed by Sephadex G-25, as performed by Beaven et al., or by dialysis (as we do). However, kininogen and/or a protein inhibitor would not be separated from kallikrein and would be highly competitive with ^{3}H-TAME or Pro-Phe-Arg-[^{3}H]benzylamide. Clearly, varying concentrations of, e.g., urokininogen would influence the rate of hydrolysis of the synthetic substrates by a constant amount of kallikrein.

Inhibition of the action of kallikrein on the synthetic substrates may not be restricted to urokininogen. Sealey et al., (1978) have found that human urinary kallikrein activates inactive renin, and Nakahara (1978) has reported that plasma kallikrein degrades kininase II. Depending on the relative affinities of kallikrein for, e.g., Pro-Phe-Arg-[^{3}H]anilide, and inactive renin or kininase II, other assay artifacts may occur. In fact, there is evidence of discrepancies in terms of the quantities of kinins found in urine in comparison with the varying rates of excretion of kallikrein (cf. Vinci et al., 1978).

ACKNOWLEDGEMENTS

This work was supported in part by grants from the Florida Heart Association, and the U.S. Public Health Service (HL22896 and HL22807). We thank Dr. Richard Soffer, Cornell University Medical College, for providing pure rabbit lung angiotensin converting enzyme.

REFERENCES

Beaven, V.H., J.V. Pierce and J.J. Pisano, 1971. A sensitive isotopic procedure for the assay of esterase activity: Measurement of human urinary kallikrein, Clin. Chim. Acta 32: 67.

Brandi, C.M.W., E.S. Prado, M.J. Prado and J.L. Prado, 1976. Kinin-converting aminopeptidase from human urine partial purification and properties. J. Biochem., 7: 335.

Caldwell, P.R.B., B.C. Seegal, K.C. Hsu, M. Das and R.L. Soffer, 1976. Angiotensin-converting enzyme: Vascular endothelial localization. Science 191: 1050.

Carone, F.A., T.N. Pullman, S. Oparil and S. Nakamura, 1976. Micropuncture evidence of rapid hydrolysis of bradykinin by rat proximal tubule. Am. J. Physiol. 230: 1420.

Chung, A., J.W. Ryan, G.A. Pena and N.B. Oza (this volume). A simple radioassay for human urinary kallikrein.

Conroy, J.M., H. Hoffman, E.S. Kirk, H.O. Hirzel, E.H. Sonnenblick and R.L. Soffer, 1976. Pulmonary angiotensin-converting enzyme, J. Biol. Chem. 251: 4828.

Croxatto, H.R., J. Roblero, R. Albertini, J. Corthorn, M. San Martin and G. Procelli, The kallikrein-kinin system in renal hypertension, 1976. In: Chemistry and Biology of the Kallikrein-Kinin System in Health and Disease, Fogarty Int. Center Proc. No. 27, eds. J.J. Pisano and K.F. Austen (U.S. Government Printing Office, Washington, D.C.) P. 389.

Cushman, D.W. and H.S. Chung, 1971. Concentrations of angiotensin-converting enzyme in tissues of the rat. Biochim. Biophys. Acta 250: 261.

Das, M. and R.L. Soffer, 1975. Pulmonary angiotensin-converting enzyme. Structural and catalytic properties. J. Biol. Chem., 250: 6762.

Elliott, A.H. and F.R. Nuzum, 1934. Urinary excretion of a depressor substance (kallikrein of Frey and Kraut) in arterial hypertension. Endocrinology 18: 462.

Erdos, E.G., D.M. Marinkovic, P.E. Ward and I.H. Mills, 1978. Characterization of urinary kininase. Fed. Proc., 37: 657.

Erdos, E.G. and H.Y.T. Yang, Bradykinin, kallidin and kallikrein,
    1970. In: Handb. Exp. Pharmac., ed. E.G. Erdos (Springer-
    Verlag, New York) p. 289.
Geller, R.G., Urinary kallikrein excretion in normotensive and
    hypertensive rats, 1976. In: Chemistry and Biology of the
    Kallikrein-Kinin System in Health and Disease, Fogarty Int.
    Center Proc. No. 27, eds. J.J. Pisano and K.F. Austen (U.S.
    Government Printing Office, Washington, D.C.) P. 379.
Hial, V., H.R. Keiser and J.J. Pisano, 1976. Origin and content of
    methionyl-lysyl-bradykinin, lysyl-bradykinin and bradykinin
    in human urine. Biochem. Pharmac. 25: 2499.
Keiser, H.R., R.G. Geller, H.S. Margolius and J.J. Pisano, 1976.
    Urinary kallikrein in hypertensive animal models. Fed. Proc.,
    35: 199.
Margolius, H.S., R. Geller, J.J. Pisano and A. Sjoerdsma, 1971.
    Altered urinary kallikrein excretion in human hypertension.
    The Lancet 2: 1063.
Margolius, H.S., D. Horwitz, J.J. Pisano and H.R. Keiser, 1976.
    Relationships among urinary kallikrein, mineralocorticoids
    and human hypertensive disease. Fed. Proc., 35: 203.
McGiff, J.C. and A. Nasjletti, 1976. Kinins, renal function and
    blood pressure regulation. Fed. Proc. 35: 172.
Mills, I.H., N.A.A. MacFarlane, P.E. Ward and L.F.O. Obika, 1976.
    The renal kallikrein-kinin system and the regulation of salt
    and water excretion. Fed. Proc., 35: 181.
Nakahara, M., 1978. Subunits of human plasma kininase II aenerated
    by plasma kallikrein. Biochem. Pharmac., 27: 1651.
Nasjletti, A., J. Colina-Chourio and J.C. McGiff, Effect of
    kininase inhibition on canine renal blood flow and sodium
    excretion. Acta Physiol. latinoam. 24: 587.
Oza, N.B. and J.W. Ryan, 1978. A simple high-yield procedure for
    isolation of human urinary kallikreins. Biochem. J., 171: 285.
Pisano, J.J., K. Yates and J.V. Pierce, 1978. Kininogen in urine.
    Agents & Actions 8: 153.
Ryan, J.W., A. Chung, C. Ammons and M.L. Carlton, 1977. A simple
    radioassay for angiotensin converting enzyme. Biochem. J.
    167: 501.
Ryan, J.W., A. Chung, L.C. Martin and U.S. Ryan, 1978b. New sub-
    strates for the radioassay of angiotensin converting enzyme
    of endothelial cells in culture. Tissue & Cell 10: 555.
Ryan, J.W., L.C. Martin, A. Chung and G.A. Pena (this volume).
    Mammalian inhibitors of angiotensin converting enzyme (kini-
    nase II).
Ryan, J.W., U.S. Ryan, D.R. Schultz, C. Whitaker, A. Chung and F.
    E. Dorer, 1975. Subcellular localization of pulmonary angio-
    tensin converting enzyme (kininase II). Biochem. J. 146: 497.
Sealey, J.E., S.A. Atlas, J.H. Laragh, N.B. Oza and J.W. Ryan,
    1978. Human urinary kallikrein converts inactive to active
    renin and is a possible physiological activator of renin.
    Nature 275: 144.

Ward, P.E., E.G. Erdos, C.D. Gedney, R.M. Dowben and R.C. Reynolds, Isolation of membrane-bound renal enzymes that metabolize kinins and angiotensins. Biochem. J. 157: 643.

Ward, P.E., C.D. Gedney, R.M. Dowben and E.G. Erdos, 1975. Isolation of membrane-bound renal kallikrein and kininase. Biochem. J., 151: 755.

Vinci, J.M., J.R. Gill Jr., R.E. Bowden, J.J. Pisano, J.L. Izzo Jr., N. Radfar, A.A. Taylor, R.M. Zusman, F.C. Bartter and H.R. Keiser, 1978. The kallikrein-kinin system in Bartter's syndrome and its response to prostaglandin synthetase inhibition. J. Clin. Invest. 61: 1671.

PURIFICATION OF HORSE RENAL KALLIKREIN AND CHEMICAL RELATIONS

WITH HORSE URINARY KALLIKREIN

Porcelli, G., Marini-Bettolo, G.B., Croxatto, H.R.,
Di Jorio, M.

Centro Chimica Recettori C.N.R., Instituto di Chimica
Fac. Med. Universita Cattolica, Rome, Laboratorio di
Fisiologia, Universidad Catolica Santiage de Chile,
Chile.

ABSTRACT

Kallikrein was purified from horse kidney by several steps of
chromatographic procedure and by affinity chromatography on Sepharose-
Concanavaline. Horse urinary kallikrein was previously purified by
DE-32 hydroxylapatite and by Sephadex G-100 gel filtration. On the
purified final sample of renal and urinary kallikrein the aminoacid
composition and the gel electrophoretic molecular weight were determined. The ratio in μMoles between each aminoacid residue of both
hydrolyzed renal and urinary kallikrein of horse is about 1,00 ±
0,30. Except for Pro, 1/2Cys and basic aminoacid residues a good
proportion was obtained. It is confirmed that the different molecular weight, respectively 47,500 for renal kallikrein and 28,000
for the urinary enzyme is an artefact of the different procedures
used for the purification of horse kallikrein.

INTRODUCTION

Recently we described the purification of renal rat kallikrein
and the chemical relations (aminoacid composition and molecular
weight) with the most abundant urinary rat kallikrein (Porcelli et
al., 1978). Marked differences were evidenced in the aminoacid
composition and molecular weight between both enzymes. When the
ratio in μMoles of each aminoacid residue of both hydrolyzed protein
amounts was used, a good proportion was obtained, except for Glu,
His and Glucosamine residue (Porcelli et al., same issue).

These results showed that the differences in molecular weight
and in aminoacid composition are probably a consequence of the
different purification procedures used for the enzymes, whose
residues with few exceptions are formed by a similar protein unit.

Considering the importance of urinary kallikrein in hypertension
and the question still pending whether the urinary enzyme is originated in the kidney (for references see Porcelli et al., same issue),
we have purified and characterized horse renal kallikrein and preliminary purified horse urinary kallikrein. The chemical differences
between these enzymes are described in this paper.

MATERIAL AND METHODS

Benzoyl-L-Arginine-ethyl-ester (BAEE) was obtained from Cyclo
Chemicals (USA); DE-32 and CM-32 from Whatman Springfield Mill
(England); Sephadex and Sepharose Concanavaline from Pharmacia
Fine Chemical; trypsin and lysozyme from Sigma Chemical Co. (USA).
Other chemicals used were reagent grade. Protein was measured
either by the method of Lowry et al. (1951) or by the optical
absorption method in a Beckman spectrophotometer, mod. ACTA III C,
at 280 nm.

The molecular weight of horse renal and urinary kallikrein was
estimated by SDS polyacrylamide disc gel electrophoresis, using
bovine albumin, ovoalbumin, trypsin and lysozyme as marker proteins.
Electrophoresis in 10% polyacrylamide gels was done according to
the Weber and Osborn method (1969).

The chemical analysis of the purified enzymes was performed in
Aminoacid Analyzer C. Erba, Mod. 3A27. The sample was previously
hydrolyzed with 6 N HCl at 137°C for 20 hours in an oil bath under
a current of nitrogen. Esterase activity was measured according to
the method of Schwert and Takenaka (1955) using benzoyl-arginine-
ethyl-ester (BAEE) as substrate.

The kinin releasing acitivity of horse renal and urinary kallikrein was determined by incubation of aliquots of the test sample
with horse serum (Prado et al. 1962) and the amount of liberated
kinins was measured on isolated rat uterus. For the purification of
horse renal kallikrein, two separate batches of horse kidney (total
8.9 kg) were used. The procedure to dehydrate the tissue with acetone
and to reduce it to fine powder has been described (Porcelli et al.
1978). The acetone powder obtained from horse kidneys (1.7 kg) was
submitted to 3 successive extractions with 2.1 of 2% NaCl solution
containing 12.7 mg/100 ml of EDTA. After 24 hours of vigorous
stirring in the cold room and centrifugation (12,000 g), the supernatant was dialyzed for 24 hours against running water. The

precipitate obtained in dialysing tubing was separated by centrifugation (12,000 g) and the clear solution containing practically all
kallikrein activity was absorbed on DE-32 column (2 x 20 cm) equilibrated in 0.00 5 M TRIS-PO$_4^-$ at pH 7.3. The column was eluted
with a parabolic chloride gradient (Porcelli and Croxatto, 1971).
The flow was regulated at 40 ml/h (5 fractions/h). After determination on the collected fractions of protein and esterase and kininogenase activities, the most active ones were pooled, dialyzed against
H$_2$O and lyophilized. 1 g of the latter material was suspended in
8 ml of 0.005 M TRIS-phosphate containing 0.9% NaCl, centrifuged
and separated on Sephadex G-100 column (3 x 85 cm) at a flow of
20 ml/h (5 fractions/h). The active product was used for a successive
recycle on Sephadex G-100 column (1.2 x 120 cm).

    Then horse renal kininogenase was separated three times on
concanavaline column (1 x 5 cm) equilibrated in 0.005 M TRIS-Cl
and eluted by 0.01 M TRIS-Cl containing 0.001 M CaCl$_2$ and 0.001 M
MgCl.

    For the purification of horse urinary kallikrein 10 lt. of
horse urine was collected from the bladder of fresh slaughtered
animals. After dialysis for 48 hours against running water this
was centrifuged at 17,000 rpm with superspeed Sorvall centrifuge,
containing a KSB continuous flow system. To the supernatant, dry
Sephadex A 50 (1g/1t of urine) was added and the mixture was stirred
for 2 h in the cold room. The gel, containing the urinary enzyme
was settled on glass wool of a column (5 cm diameter) and eluted by
0.005 M phosphate pH 7.0 buffer, containing 1 M NaCl. On the
collected fractions esterase and kininogenase activities were
measured. The most active ones were pooled and dialyzed against
running water. The precipitate in dialysing tubing was separated
by centrifugation at 12,000 rpm and the clear supernatant fractionated
on DE-32 column (4 x 10 cm) by the usual parabolic chloride gradient.
The fractions containing horse urinary kininogenase, were pooled,
dialyzed and lyophilized. 200 mg of product was dissolved in 5 ml
of 2 M NaCl, absorbed in hydroxylapatite column (2 x 5 cm) equilibrated in 2 M NaCl, and eluted in phosphate gradient (Table 1)
prepared in 2 M NaCl. Successively horse urinary kallikrein was
purified twice on Sephadex G-100 column (0.8x128 cm) at a flow of
0,5 ml/h (5 fractions/h) in 0.005 M TRIS phosphate at pH 7.3
containing 0.9% NaCl.

                          RESULTS

    Starting from acetone powder, a single form of horse renal
kallikrein was purified by procedures combining DE-32 chromatography,
Sephadex G-100 gel filtration and concanavaline affinity chromatography. Results of individual steps in the purification process

TABLE 1

```
I    Cell:    ml 250 2 M NaCl
II   Cell:    ml 250 2 M NaCl in 0.005 M phosfate buffer
                                          pH 7.5
III  Cell:    ml 250 2 M NaCl in 0.01 M phosfate buffer
                                          pH 7.5.
IV   Cell:    ml 250 2 M NaCl in 0.05 M phosfate buffer
                                          pH 7.5.
```

TABLE 2

Fraction	Protein (mg)	Total esterase activity (E.U.)	E.U./mg
Tissue	8,900,000	770	0.00046
DE-32	1,700,000	577	0.048
G-100 (3x85 cm)	12,000	159	0.047
G-100 (1.2x120cm)	600	43	0.071
I Concanavaline	96	22.5	0.23
II Concanavaline	12	15	1.25
III Concanavaline	2	5	2.5

1 E.U. corresponds to the amount of kallikrein esterase activity which, hydrolizing 0.05 µg of BAEE at 25°C and pH 8.0, produces an increment of 0.011 O.D. at 253 nm/min.

are summarized in Table 2.

Figure 1 shows the pattern corresponding to DE-32 cellulose chromatography of kidney extract.

By recycling the active fractions twice on Sephadex G-100 column and three times on concanavaline column, the purified substance obtained from 8.9 kg of horse kidney yielded 5 E.U. of renal kallikrein (2 mg of protein).

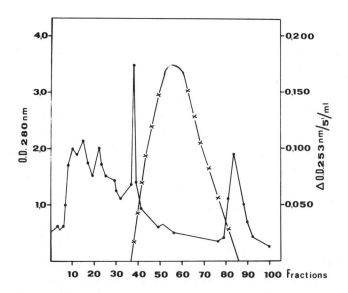

Figure 1.   Protein (—•—•—•—) and BAEE esterase activity (x—x—x—)
on DE-32 chromatography of horse kidney protein (see
RESULTS).   The esterase activity was tested on 0.1 ml
of collected fractions.

Purification procedure of horse urinary kallikrein is summarized
in Table 3. Figure 2 shows the pattern corresponding to DE-32, and
figure 3 shows that of hydroxylapatite chromatography. At this stage
other purification attempts undertaken, using concanavaline chromatography or preparative electrophoresis were unsuccessful.

Recycling the active fraction three times on Sephadex G-100 at
minimum elution column (0.5 ml/h) we obtained from 10 1t of urine
about 0.8 mg of purified kallikrein (73 E.U.).

The molecular weight of renal kallikrein was estimated by gel
electrophoresis as approximately 28,000 and respectively as 47,500
for the horse urinary enzyme. The aminoacid composition of renal
and urinary kallikrein, except for glucosamine, basic aminoacid,
Pro and 1/2 cys residues, is illustrated in Table 4. Considering
the ratio in µmoles of both hydrolyzed amounts of enzymes a good
proportion of about 1,0 ± 0,3 was obtained for almost all acidic
and neutral aminoacid residues.

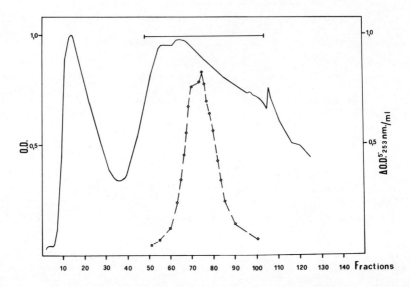

Figure 2.   Protein (————) on DE-32 column of urinary kallikrein.
Esterase activity (—□—□—□—) was determined on 0.1 ml
of collected fractions

TABLE 3

Fraction	Protein (mg)	Total esterase activity (E.U.)	E.U./mg
Urine 10 lt.	-	-	-
A-50-Sephadex	4,500	4900	1.09
DE-32	952	5540	5.82
Hydroxylapatite	68,5	1350	19.75
I G-100 Sephadex (0.8x128cm)	10,7	253	23.62
II G-100 Sephadex	0,8	73	91.20

1 E.U. corresponds to 0.05 µg of hydrolyzed BAEE at
25°C and at pH 8.0 by horse urinary kallikrein activity, producing an increment of 0.011 O.D. at 253 nm/min.

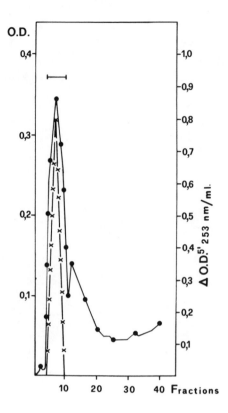

Figure 3.   Separation of horse urinary kallikrein on hydroxy-
            lapatite column. Protein (•—•—•) and Esterase activity
            (—x—x—) determined on 0.1 ml of collected fractions.

DISCUSSION

     Kallikrein extracted from acetone powder of horse renal tissues
proved to bind itself to Sepharose concanavaline, which allowed the
purification of a smaller protein (28,000) than the urinary one
(47,500).

     The inverse results obtained for rat urinary kallikrein (32,000
m.w.), which binds itself to P-200-Trasylol, and for renal rat
kallikrein (40,000 m.w.), suggest that the affinity chromatography
plays a determinant role in the purification procedures of the
protein enzymes.

TABLE 4

Aminoacid residue	Renal Kallikrein (28,000 m.w.)	Urinary Kallikrein (47,500 m.w.)	R.K. in umoles	U.K. in umoles	Ratio R/U in u moles
Asp	22	25	0.071	0.074	0.99
Thr	16	18	0.052	0.051	1.02
Ser	29	26	0.093	0.072	1.22
Glu	31	40	0.100	0.110	0.91
Pro	8	4	0.027	0.010	2.00 +
Gly	27	26	0.087	0.074	1.17
Ala	20	27	0.067	0.075	0.89
½Cys	--	--	--	--	--
Val	6	6	0.026	0.031	0.083
Met	2	3	0.008	0.009	0.089
Ile	10	9	0.033	0.025	1.30
Leu	16	16	0.054	0.041	1.30
Tyr	6	6	0.018	0.015	1.20
Phe	7	6	0.022	0.017	1.30
Glucosamine	3	133	0.010	0.377	--
Galactosamine	2	--	0.007	--	--
Lys	24	--	0.080	--	--
His	9	--	0.031	--	--
Arg	5	--	0.017	--	--

+ Value different than 1,0 $\pm$ 0,3 μmoles

The preliminary purification of horse urinary kallikrein presents some uncommon results in the composition of aminoacid residues (elevated glucosamine and undetectable 1/2Cys, Lys, His, Arg); nevertheless with this purification we defined the electrophoretic molecular weight and the chemical composition of acidic and neutral aminoacid residues.

After the experience achieved during the purification of rat and horse kallikreins some conclusions can be drawn. It is impossible to use an identical procedure for the purification of renal and urinary kallikrein of the same animal species. Each enzyme is influenced by the nature of contaminant components.

The comparison of chemical characteristics (m.w. and aminoacid composition) of two proteins of the same type of enzyme, at different levels of purification, altered the results.

The final amount of each purified kallikrein was not so much to determine at different times the hydrolysis in 6N HCl, which allows a more accurate aminoacid composition of the protein enzyme. In fact, for renal and urinary kallikrein of the same animal species, the identical hydrolysis process was a necessary choice to define in some way the aminoacid residues of hydrolyzed enzymes.

Using the ratio in μmoles of each residue of the hydrolyzed amounts of rat and horse kallikreins, the warps of molecular weight determination and the importance of the exact amount of protein used for the hydrolysis were eliminated. As for the rat renal and urinary kallikrein (Porcelli et al., same issue), except for Pro, 1/2Cys and basic aminoacid residues, the ratio in μmoles of horse kallikreins was equal to 1,0 ± 0,3.

This result could confirm that renal and urinary kallikrein of an animal species may be composed of the same protein unit.

REFERENCES

Lowry, O.H., Rosenbrough, N.J., Farr, A.L., Randall, R.J., 1951. Protein measurement with the folin phenol reagent. J. Biol. Chem., 193: 293.

Prado, E.S., Prado, J.L., Brandi, C.M.W., 1962. Further purification and some properties of horse urinary kallikrein. Arch. Int. Pharmacodyn., 137: 358.

Porcelli, G., Croxatto, H.R., 1971. Purification on kininogenase from rat urine. 20: 66.

Porcelli, G., Marini-Bettolo, G.B., Croxatto, H.R., Di Jorio, M. Chemical relations between renal and urinary kallikrein of rat (same issue).

Porcilli, G., Marini-Bettolo, G.B., Croxatto, H.R., Di Jorio, M., Micotti, G., 1978. Purification of renal rat kallikrein and chemical relations with urinary rat kallikrein. Ital. J. Biochem., 27: 202.

Schwert, G.W., Takenaka, Y., 1955. Spectrophotometric determination of trypsin and chymotrypsin. Biochem. Biophys. Acta. 16: 570.

Weber, K., Osborn M., 1969. The reliability of molecular weight determination by SDS-polyacrylamide gel electrophoresis. J. Biol. Chem., 244: 4406.

SUBSTRATE SPECIFICITIES OF ACID KININOGENASES

Keiko Yamafuji and Makiko Takeishi

Laboratory of Biochemistry, Dept. of Food and Nutrition

Nakamura-gakuen College, Fukuoka, Japan

ABSTRACT

Two kinin forming enzymes were extracted from bovine spleen and separated from cathepsin B1 and B2 by DEAE-Cellulose chromatography. Since these catheptic kininogenases were found to release kinins from kininogens at acidic pH's, these were named acid kininogenase I and II. The presence of SH compounds was not necessary for I to have a kinin forming activity, while it was necessary for II. These have only minor difference for electrophoretic behaviors as can be seen, e.g., from a small difference in pI values, but could be separated by polyacrylamide gel electrophoresis. Their production of kinins from bovine crude bradykininogen was highly reproducible. Kininogenase I was proved to react on bovine HMW kininogen and also to release some kinin from LMW kininogen and leukokininogen. From the study of several substrates, these enzymes were revealed to have very low tryptic and little esterolytic activities and to have affinity to some hydrophobic amino acids.

INTRODUCTION

The enzymes are expected to play important roles for the regulation of kinin levels in tissue injury and also in early stage of inflammation. It has been shown by one of the authors and her coworkers that the acid extract of bovine spleen and the exudate of rabbit polymorphonuclear leucocyte have both the kinin forming and kinin inactivating activities (Greenbaum and Yamafuji 1966, and Greenbaum et al., 1969).

The authors at first separated cathepsin Bl and B2 from the
acid extract of bovine spleen by the use of G-100. In the attempt
to purify each of cathepsin B's using a DEAE-cellulose column, the
authors found two kinin forming enzymes in different protein fractions from those of cathepsin B's. The acid kininogenase which
was separated from the G-100 fraction of cathepsin Bl was called
the kininogenase I. From the G-100 fraction of cathepsin B2, both
the kinin forming and kinin inactivating enzymes were separated.
The former was called the kininogenase II while the latter was the
catheptic carboxypeptidase B, which had been found by one of the
authors and her coworkers (Greenbaum and Yamafuji, 1965; 1966)
and also to which had been attributed a poor kinin detectability
of this acid extract.

The present paper deals with the separation of these acid
kininogenases I and II and a preliminary study on their substrate
specificities. Detailed information on further purification procedure and also on the structure studies will be published elsewhere.

MATERIALS AND METHODS

Sephadex G-100 was purchased from Pharmacia, Uppsala, Sweden.
DEAE-Cellulose (Cellex D) was a product of Bio Rad, Richmond,
Calif., U.S.A. Acrylamide, methylene bis acrylamide and 1=
dimethyl amino-naphthalene-5-sulphonyl chloride (DANS-Cl) were
purchased from Seikagaku Kogyo, Japan. Collagen of bovine achilles
tendon was obtained from Sigma Chemical Co., U.S.A. Oxidized
insulin B chain was obtained from Boehringer-Manheim-Yamanouchi
Co., Trypsin (3.4.4.4), 2X crystallized was a product of Worthington
Biochemical, U.S.A. Phenyl 6-guanidinocaproate p=toluensulfonate
(γ-GCA-Phe) was the generous gift from Dr. Maramatsu of Tokushima
Bunri College. Leukokininogen, human bradykininogen and bradykinin
of Cyclo Chem. were the generous gifts from Dr. Greenbaum of Columbia
Univ., New York. Crude bradykininogen acetone powder was prepared
by the methods of Greenbaum and Hosoda (1963). Bovine HMW and LMW
kininogens were also prepared by the procedures described by
Komiya et al (1974). Benzyloxycarbonyl-glycyl-L-phenylalanine
and glycyl-L-phenylalanine amide were synthesized. Other synthetic
substrates were purchased from Nakarai Chemicals, Ltd.

Extraction of kininogenases

Bovine spleens were obtained at slaughter house and kept
chilling in ice on the way to laboratory. Whole organ was washed
briefly with running water, freed from fat, then cut into pieces
of about 5 cm in size, minced twice, weighed, freezed and kept
frozen until use. The amount of frozen ground tissue treated in
one batch ranged from 800 to 2000g. The following extraction

procedure was repeated to accumulate crude preparation. The frozen
ground tissue (1000g) was defrosted in cold room, then suspended
in cold water (2000 ml) containing 0.001 M EDTA, stirred for 6 hrs.
During the extraction, pH was kept at 3.5 with occasional addition
of 6 N sulfuric acid. The mixture was kept in the cold room overnight. Resulting brown suspension was centrifuged at 6000 rpm
(Tominaga, Model CS-50, Rotor No. 9). Precipitates were discarded.
To the supernatant solution (1850 ml), was added ammonium sulfate
to get 40% saturation. Suspension was stirred for one hour and
stood for one hour. Clear supernatant solution (1920 ml) was
collected by centrifugation as above, then made to 70% saturation
with ammonium sulfate at 4°C. After the centrifugation, the precipitates were taken into solution with water (30 ml) and dialyzed
against 0.001 M EDTA with two changes and then against 0.9% NaCl.
Resulting solution (120 ml, 23.7 mg protein/ml) was designated
as 40~70 SAS.

Gel filtration on Sephadex G-100

One half of above 40~70 SAS fraction was applied on a column
of Sephadex G-100 (5x90 cm) equilibrated with 0.9% NaCl and eluted
by same salt solution. Concentration of protein was monitored by
the absorbancy at 280 nm. Hydrolytic activities of the fractions
were compared on bovine denatured hemoglobin (Hb), benzoyl-L-argin-
ine amide (BAA), benzoyl=DL-arginine-p-nitroanilide (BAPA) and ben-
zoylglycyl-L-arginine (HA). Methods for measuring the hydrolysis
of these substrates will be described later. The cathepsin B1
fraction, which could hydrolyze BAA and BAPA, and the cathepsin B2
fraction, which could hydrolyze BAA and HA but not BAPA, were
collected separately and precipitated with 80% SAS. The 80% SAS
precipitates from two columns were combined, centrifuged and taken
up into solution with 5 ml of water and dialyzed against water
with two changes then against 0.002 M acetate buffer (pH 5.5) in
cold overnight.

Chromatography on DEAE-Cellulose

The solutions thus obtained were 21.3 ml (21.6 mg/ml) for B1
fraction and 20.7 ml (20.8 mg/ml) for B2 fraction and designated
as G-100-B1 and G-100-B2 respectively. Each one was applied onto
a DEAE-Cellulose column (2.5x10 cm) and equilibrated with 0.002 M
acetate buffer (pH 5.5). The column was eluted stepwisely with
the buffers with increasing salt concentrations as shown in figure
2, where the figures demonstrate the results from the pilot runs
starting with 100 mg of protein applied on 0.9 x 50 cm column.
Protein concentration and enzymatic activities were estimated as
above. The fractions in separated peaks were combined and concentrated in collodion bags (Sartorius Membranfilter, SM 13200).

Assay of kinin released

In general, assay was carried out by the following procedure.
2.5 mg of crude kininogen (the amount could be reduced to 0.2~1mg
if the kininogen was only available in diluted solution or was
obtained as pure preparation) was suspended in 0.25 ml acetate
buffer for acidic pH's and Tris buffer for neutral pH, then the
enzyme preparation was added (total amount in the incubation mixture
was 0.1~0.2 mg, though detectable amount of kinin was released even
if the one tenth of this amount was added instead). When the SH
dependent kininogenase was concerned, 0.1 ml of 0.2 M 2-mercapto-
ethanol was added to the mixture. Total volume was made up to
0.5 ml with water. The mixture thus obtained was incubated at
37°C for 120 min., then neutralized with N NaOH, boiled for 5 min.,
and centrifuged to remove insoluble or heat denatured proteins.
Supernatant was used for bioassay on isolated rat uterus. The
muscle was suspended in 5 ml muscle bath filled with the modified
Ringer solution containing dextrose (250 mg/1) and aerated. Contraction was recorded on the kymograph (Harvard Apparatus, Dover,
Mass. Model 600-000) calibrated with the standard solution of
synthetic bradykinin.

Hydrolysis of the synthetic substrates

For BAA, Leucine amide (LeuAm) and glycyl-L-phenylalanine
amide (GlyPheAm), the produced ammonia was titrated by Conway micro
diffusion technique. The hydrolyzed free amino acids from HA,
benzyloxycarbonylglycyl-L-glutamyl-L-tyrosine (ZGluTyr) and benzy-
loxycarbonylglycyl-L-phenyl-alanine (ZGlyPhe) were detected by
Ninhydrin colorimetry. The hydrolysis of BAPA was measured by
reading the increase of absorbancy at 410 nm (Erlanger, 1961).
The hydrolysis of L-leucine-β-naphtylamide (LeuNA) was measured
by the color development of β-naphtylamine in coupling with tetra-
zotized diorthoanisidine (Green et al., 1955). Esterolytic activity
on benzol-L-arginine ethyl ester (BAEE) was estimated by measuring
the increase in absorbancy at 253 nm and by Hestrin method.

Hydrolysis of proteins

The rate of hydrolysis of collagen was measured by Ninhydrin
cclormetry following the instruction appearing in "Enzymes" of
Worthington Biochemical Co. (Mandle et al., 1953). For the
hemoglobin, the increase of absorbancy at 280 nm was read on the
supernatant. Hitachi spectrophotometer Model 100-10 was used
throughout the spectrophotometry.

The analysis of the hydrolysates from oxidized B-chain of
insulin was performed by the method described by Bennet (Bennet,
1967). 5 mg of B-chain was incubated with 0.25 mg of B1-DEAE(1)
(AKI fraction) for 150 min. at 37°C. Then all the solution was

mounted on 3 MM paper (Whatman, 60x60) and subjected to two dimen-
sional paper chromatography. The first dimension was descending
chromatography developed with the upper layer of butanol-acetic
acid-water (4:1:5) and the second dimension was high voltage electrophoresis at pH 3.6 (100 ml of acetic acid and 10 ml of pyridine
were diluted to 3000 ml) for 1 hr. at 3000 V (Fuji Riken, Model
P-A). Dried paper was lightly sprayed with diluted ninhydrin
solution (0.025% in 0.5 N acetic acid in 75% ethanol) and heated
at 80°C. Each spot was cut out and extraced with 3~4 ml of water.
The extract was evaporated and subjected to amino acid analysis
(JOEL, JLC-6AH). N-terminal analysis was also carried out on the
extract obtained with the same procedure, by detecting dansyl
amino acid on the polyamide sheets after ascending chromatography
(Gray, 1972).

Electrophoresis

       Preliminary isoelectric focussing was performed using 110 ml
column and carrier Ampholite (pH 3.5~10)(LKB) according to the
standard procedure (Vesterberg, 1971). Polyacrylamide gel electrophoresis (PAGE) was performed depending on the instruction of
Canal Ind. Co. (1965). Preparative gel electrophoresis was carried
out by the procedure described by Hashimoto and Funatsu (1976).

                              RESULTS

       The elution pattern from Sephadex G-100 is shown in Figure 1.
The first large peak composed of bulk of protein and the next peak
containing cathepsin C were discarded. The enzymes which could
hydrolyze BAA were eluted in the successive two peaks, the first
of which could not hydrolyze BAPA but the second could. This indicates that the first BAA peak contains cathepsin B2 and the second BAA peak contains cathepsin B1. This conclusion is in accordance with the results of Otto (1967), where the notification of
B and B' were used in place of B2 and B1, respectively. From the
collected fraction, the proteins were precipitated, centrifuged,
redissolved and dialyzed, and the resultant solutions were designated
as G-100-B2 and G-100-B1 as mentioned in METHODS.

       The result of DAEA-Cellulose chromatography for G-100-B1 and
G-100-B2 is shown in Figs. 2(a) and 2(b), respectively. The
recovery of protein from 1kg of ground tissue is summarized in
Table 1, and the distribution of enzyme activities is summarized
in Table 2.

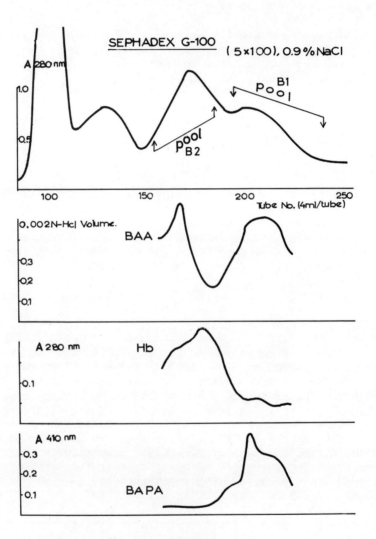

Figure 1.   Gel filtration on Sephadex G-100

        60 ml of dialyzed 40~70 SAS fraction was applied on
the column (5x90 cm) and eluted with 0.9% NaCl, at
the flow rate of 30 ml/hr.   5 ml/tube was collected.

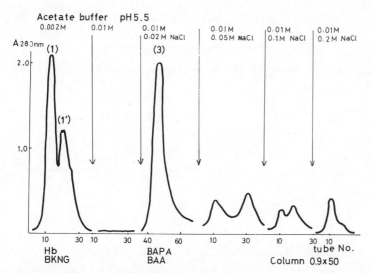

Figure 2(a)   DEAE-Cellulose chromatography of G-100-B1 on D
100 mg of G-100-B1 equilibrated in 0.002 M acetate was applied.
Flow rate was 20 ml/hr. Buffers for stepwise elution were
0.002 M acetate, 0.01 M acetate containing no NaCl, 0.01 M acetate
containing 0.02 M NaCl, and so on, as shown in the figure.

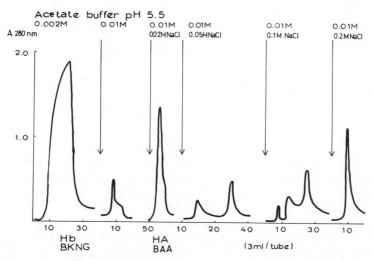

Figure 2(b).   DEAE-Cellulose chromatography of G-100-B2.
100 mg of G-100-B2 equilibrated in 0.002 M acetate was applied.
Flow rate was 20 ml/hr. Buffers for stepwise elution were
0.002 M acetate, 0.01 M acetate containing no NaCl, 0.01 M acetate
containing 0.02 M NaCl, and so on, as shown in the figure.

TABLE 1

RECOVERY OF PROTEIN FROM 1kg OF GROUND TISSUE

40~70 SAS 2,840mg	G-100-B1	460mg	B1-DEAE(1) 75mg B1-DEAE(1') 18mg B1-DEAE(3) 150mg
	G-100-B2	430mg	B2-DEAE(1) 120mg B2-DEAE(3) 40mg

TABLE 2

SPECIFIC ACTIVITY OF THE FRACTION

Fraction	Specific activity				
	(ng BK equiv./mg E) BKNG with SH without SH		$(10^{-2}$ μmoles/mg E) BAA BAPA HA with SH		
	with SH	without SH	BAA	BAPA	HA
40~70 SAS	–	–	4.7	–	–
G-100-B1	30	90	9.4	1.4	0
G-100-B2	0	0	32	0	2.8
B1-DEAE(1)	230	2400	10	0.35	0
B1-DEAE(1')	1350	400	37	1.7	0
B1-DEAE(3)	25	7	64	2.6	0
B2-DEAE(1)	2000	500	0	0	0
B2-DEAE(3)	0	0	25	0	0.4

As can be seen from Fig. 2(a), cathepsin B1 was eluted in the third buffer which consists of 0.01 M acetate containing 0.02 M NaCl, and showed very low kinin forming activity. The major part of the kinin forming activity was found in the first peak (B1-DEAE (1)), which is rich in acid kininogenase I (AKI) and thus may be called the AKI fraction. As was shown in Table 2, the observed kinin forming activity of B1-DEAE(1) was much lower at the exis- tence of SH compound than that at the absence of SH compound. When the inhibitors of kininase were added, SH compound could effect the increase of kinin formation. Furthermore, in the re- action of purified AKI, addition of SH compounds could effect neither increase nor decrease on the formation of kinin. These

findings led to the conclusion that the AKI fraction obtained in
this stage, B1-DEAE(1), is still contaminated with small amounts
of SH dependent kininase and acid kininogenase II (AKII). B1-DEAE-
(3) was composed of almost pure cathepsin B1, which showed one
band in PAGE. As the result of DEAE-Cellulose chromatography
shown in Fig. 2(b), a strong SH dependent kinin forming activity,
AKII, was found in the first peak (B2-DEAE(1)), while cathepsin
B2 and catheptic carboxypeptidase B were eluted in the third peak.
The first peak appeared at a slightly delayed position compared
with that of B1-DEAE(1), and seems to correspond to the sub-peak
B1-DEAE(1') comparing the activity shown in Table 2. Typical
examples of the properties of AKI and II are listed in Table 3.
AKII could be activated by 2-mercaptoethanol (2-ME), dithiothreitol
(DTT), cystein and thioglycolic acid. Among these activators, 2-ME
was chosen to be used in routine assays of AKII, because it is easy
to handle and does not need pH adjustment prior to use. The inhibitory effects of a few reagents were exemplified in this table.
p-chloromercuribenzoate (PCMB and 5,5'-Dithiobis (2-nitro) benzoic
acid (DTNB) showed strong inhibition on both of AKI and II. One
of the cathepsin D inhibitors, Fe, failed to show strong inhibition.
The interactions of AK's with γ-GCA Phe will be discussed later,
and the detailed discussions about the effects of various inhibitors
on AK's will be given elsewhere.

Throughout the present separation procedure of AK's acetone
powder of crude bovine BKNG was used for the screening of the kininogenase activity because it contains both the HMW and LMW kininogens and, furthermore, it is stable and easy to be prepared. The
amount of kinin released by crystalline trypsin from BKNG varied
batch to batch in the range between 0.2 and 1 µg/mg BKNG, while
AKI produced 0.1~0.2 µg BKequiv. of kinin/mg BKNG and AKII produced
0.1~0.4 µg BKequiv. of kinin/mg BKNG. From a purified bovine HMW

TABLE 3

PROPERTIES OF ACID KININOGENASES IN THE REACTION OF BKNG

	Optimum pH	Activator	Inhibitor (Inhibition % at 10^{-3}M)
AKI	5.5	none	PCMB(100), IAA(87), Fe(40), γ-GCA Phe(0)
AKII	4.0	SH compounds 2-ME, DTT	PCMB(100), IAA(60), Fe(0), γ-GCA Phe(0)

kininogen, on the other hand, AKI produced 2 µgBK equiv. of kinin/ mgHMWBKNG. The amount of kinin released from human BKNG or leuko- kininogen is about one tenth of that from bovine BKNG.

The comparison of the activities on various substrates is shown in Table 4 as well as in Table 2. Hb hydrolyzing activity is coexisting with kinin forming activity. Collagen was hydrolyzed by B1-DEAE(1) in the presence of SH compounds, though other enzymes than AKI may also be contributing to this collagenase-like activity.

The activities on several substrates which are typical for known proteases look rather limited. Both of AKI and AKII have no appreciable activity on BAEE even when the enzyme concentration was increased to 25 times of that in the usual condition by the use of a crystalline trypsin. The hydrolyzing activity of B1-DEAE (1) on LeuAm was stronger than that of B1-DEAE(1'), whereas the reaction was SH dependent and preferred neutral pH. Since the results shown in Table 4 are reproducible, the above differences should be reexamined more carefully for purified AKI and II.

TABLE 4

SUBSTRATE SPECIFICITIES OF B1-DEAE(1) and B1-DEAE(1')

| | B1-DEAE(1) | | | | B1-DEAE(1') | | | |
| | pH 4.4 | | pH 7.5 | | pH 4.4 | | pH 7.5 | |
	noSH	SH	noSH	SH	noSH	SH	noSH	SH
BKNG	++++	+	±	+	+	++	±	+
Hb	++	++	±	±	++	++	±	±
Collagen	+	+++	±	+	-	+	-	-
LeuAm	-	+	-	++	-	-	-	-
LeuNA	-	+		++				
Z-GlyPhe	-	+	-	±	-	±	-	±
Z-GluTry	-	±	-	±	-	±	-	±
GlyPheAm	-	-	-	-	-	-	-	-
BAEE	-	-	-	-	-	-	-	-

Phe↑Val AspN GluN His Leu CysO₃H↑Gly Ser His Leu↑Val Glu↑Ala-

-Leu↑Tyr Leu↑Val CysO₃H Gly Glu Arg Gly Phe↑Phe Tyr Thr Pro Lys Ala

Figure 3. Hydrolysis of Insulin B-chain by acid kininogenase I.

The peptide mapping of the hydrolysates of oxidized B-chain of insulin gave fourteen spots. From the amino acid analysis and the N-terminal analysis of peptides, the splitted bonds by the action of AKI are speculated as shown in Figure 3. This preliminary result suggests that the leucyl bond is a preferable target of AKI. Since contaminating enzymes in the AKI fraction is expected to be SH dependent, the reaction occurred in the absence of SH compound can be attributed to AKI alone. By the same reason the reaction occurred in the presence of SH compounds may be the integration of all the SH dependent enzymes, and a more detailed investigation on the reactions of AKI and II had better be postponed until the purification of AKI and II is achieved.

Some other information on the separation of AKI and II is shown in Figures 4 and 5. Figure 4 shows the results from the isoelectric focussing. The protein focussed at pH 6.8 showed a kinin forming activity even in the absence of SH compound, and so assigned to AKI, while the protein focussed at pH 6.1 did not show any kinin forming activity unless 2-mercaptoethanol was added and thus assigned to AKII. Kininase activity could not be detected in any peak.

After the preparative gel electrophoresis was performed on B1-DEAE(1), the purity of each protein was examined by PAGE. The results were shown in Figure 5. The major component, which is the most dense band, was revealed to be AKI itself, while the next mobility to AKI is AKII. The next band, numbered 42, was found to have a strong colleganase activity of 12.2 μmole/mgE on the base of leucine equivalents appeared in the supernatant solution by the action of enzymes, whereas the specific activity of collagenase was 7.0 μmole/mgE for AKI and 2.8 for AKII. Thus, collagenase was concentrated densely in another band than AKI's or AKII's, though AKI still retains a fairly strong activity. The results of further investigation on the purity of PAGE or SDS-PAGE will be published elsewhere.

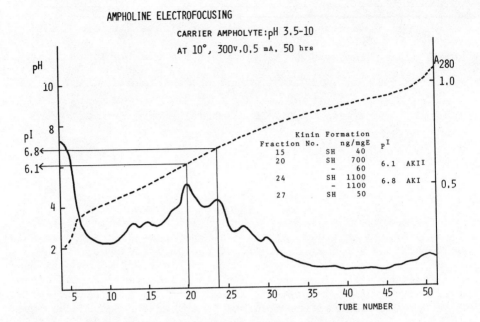

Figure 4. Isoelectric focussing of B1–DEAE(1).

        10 mg of B1–DEAE(1) was applied. Phosphoric acid
and ethylenediamine were used for anode and cathode
solutions, respectively. 2 ml was collected in one
tube by the speed of 2 ml/min.

DISCUSSION

      The present extraction technique is a modified one from that
used in the preparation of cathepsin B (Greenbaum and Fruton,
1957), and the elution condition for gel filtration which we
chose from the beginning of the present work was essentially the
same as Otto's (Otto, 1967).

      The pH value of 5.5 for the elution buffer of DEAE–Cellulose
chromatography was chosen as to separate cathepsin B's, which have
the isoelectric points around 5, from acid kininogenases. This
was also an excellent elution buffer for separating a kinin-
destroying enzyme (catheptic carboxypeptidase B) from kinin-forming
enzymes so as to be able to detect the kinin formed. But this pH
value is obviously not the best one because we now know the isoelectric points of acid kininogenases as 6.8 and 6.1, and hence
should be altered in future works.

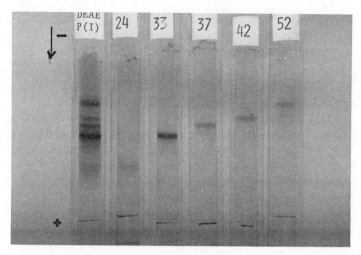

Figure 5.   PAGE of the proteins in B1-DEAE(1) after the separation
            on preparative gel electrophoresis using standard 7%
            gels.

            From the left, PAGE of B1-DEAE(1) before preparative gel
            electrophoresis, the band of largest mobility toward
            anode with no activity, major component: AKI, one of
            the minor components: AKII, the protein having collage-
            nase activity.

        From DEAE-Cellulose, AKI was eluted quickly through the
column while AKII showed a slight delay, which suggests that AKII
is slightly more acidic than AKI. There was no contamination of
SH dependent kininase in AKII fraction, whereas AKI fraction
showed some kininase activity potentiated by SH compounds under
some conditions. The relationship between protein composition
and enzyme activity will be discussed in detail elsewhere.

        Although leucine amide or leucine-β-naphthylamide hydrolyzing
activity had been informed as accompanied by cathepsin B1 (Otto
and Bhakdi, 1969; McDonald et al., 1970), a purified cathepsin B1
(peak 3 of B1-DEAE) did not show such an activity at all. Instead
the AKI fraction was the strongest one to show this activity.

        As for the differentiation of AKI and AKII from cathepsin's,
AKI and AKII were separated from cathepsin C by gel filtration
and from B1 and B2 by DEAE-Cellulose. Furthermore, AKI and AKII
seem to be different from cathepsin A or D, when the behaviours

on activators and inhibitors are concerned. The molecular weights
of AKI and AKII are much smaller than that of cathepsin E.

The pattern of the peptide map of insulin B-chain showed the
difference of AKI and AKII from trypsin or kallikrein. γ-GCA Phe,
which is a potent competitive inhibitor for trypsin, plasmin, plasma
kallikrein and thrombin, did not show any inhibitory effect on
either AKI or AKII. Thus, the actions of AKI and AKII are expected
to be different from that of trypsin or kallikrein.

Provided AKI does produce MetLysBk as we claimed (Yamafuji
and Takeishi, 1974, at the kinin symposium at Reston), it might be
thought as difficult to elucidate the splitting of Arg-Ser bond to
make the C-terminal of BK. One of the possible explanations is
that the action of AKI is initiated with the attachment to the
subsites composed of hydrophobic amino acid. The affinity to
hydrophobic amino acid was also found in a strong inhibition by
leupeptin and TPCK. Another explanation is that the splitting to
form C-terminal arginine is attributed to plasma kallikrein which
contaminates and works on HMW kininogen in the process of purification. Thus, the parts of kininogen molecules had partial
splitting prior to the attack of AKI. The clarification on the
mode of action of AKI in the kinin forming reaction is a future
problem.

ACKNOWLEDGEMENT

The authors wish to express their sincere appreciation to
Prof. L.M. Greenbaum of the Columbia University, U.S.A. for his
valuable suggestions and continuous encouragement throughout this
work.

REFERENCES

Bennet, J.C., 1967. Paper chromatography and electrophoresis;
    Special procedure for peptide maps. Method in Enzymology
    11: 330.
Erlanger, B.F., 1961. The preparation and properties of two
    chromogenic substrates of trypsin. Arch Biophys. 95: 271.
Freer, R., J. Chang and L.M. Greenbaum, 1972. Studies on leuko-
    kinins. III. Pharmacological activities. Biochem. Pharmacol.
    21: 3107.
Gray, W.R., 1972. End-group analysis using dansyl chloride. Methods
    in Enzymology 25: 121.
Green, M.N., K.C. Tsou, R. Bressler and A.M. Seligman, 1955. The
    colorimetric determination of leucine aminopeptidase activity
    with L-leucyl-β-naphthylamine hydrochloride. Arch. Biochem.
    Biophys. 57: 458.

Greenbaum, L.M. and J.S. Fruton, 1957. Purification and properties of beef spleen cathepsin B. J. Biol. Chem. 226: 173.

Greenbaum, L.M. and T. Hosoda, 1963. Studies on the isolation of bradykininogen. Biochem. Pharmacol. 12: 325.

Greenbaum, L.M. and K. Yamafuji. The in vitro inactivation and formation of plasma kinins by spleen cathepsins. Brit. J. Pharmacol. Chemother. 27: 230.

Greenbaum, L.M., R. Freer, J. Chang, G. Semente and K. Yamafuji, 1969. PMN-kinin and kinin metabolizing enzymes in normal and malignant leucocytes. Brit. J. Pharmcol. 36: 623.

Hashimoto, S. and M. Funatsu, 1976. Fractionation of subunits in xylanases from Trichoderma viride with a new simple preparative polyacrylamide gel electrophoresis apparatus. Arg. Biol. Chem. 40: 635.

Komiya, M., H. Kato and T. Suzuki, 1974. Bovine plasma kininogens I. Further purification of high molecular weight kininogen and its physicochemical properties. J. Biochem. 76: 11.

Komiya, M., H. Kato and T. Suzuki, 1974. Bovine plasma kininogens III. Structural composition of high molecular weight and low molecular weight kininogens. J. Biochem. 76: 833.

Mandle, I., J.D. Maclennan and E.L. Howes, 1953. Isolation and characterization of proteinase and collagenase from Cl histolyticum J. Clin. Invest. 32: 1323.

McDonald, K.J., B.B. Zeitmann and S. Ellis, 1970. Leucine naphthyl amide; an appropriate substrate for the histochemical detection of cathepsin B and B'. Nature 225: 1048.

Maramatsu, M. and S. Fujii, 1972. Inhibitory effects of γ-ganidino acid esters on trypsin, plasmin, plasmakallikrein and thrombin. Biochim. Biophys. Acta 268: 221.

Otto, K., 1967. Uber ein neues Kathepsin B. Hoppe-Seyler's Z. Physiol. Chem. 348: 1449.

Otto, K. and S. Bhakdi, 1969. Zur des Kathepsins B'; Spezifitat und Eigenshaften. Hoppe-Seyler's Z. Physiol. Chem. 350: 1577.

Otto, K. and U. Bauer, 1972. Einwirkung von Kathepsin B1 auf Phosphofruktokinase und Hexosediphosphatase. Hoppe-Seyer's Z. Physiol. Chem. 353: 741.

Vesterberg, O., 1971. Isoelectric focussing of proteins. Methods in Enzymology 22: 289.

SOME PROPERTIES OF ACROSIN, A KININOGENASE FROM SPERM ACROSOME

Chiaki Moriwaki and Satoru Kaneko

Faculty of Pharmaceutical Science, Science University
of Tokyo
Ichigaya Funagawara-Machi, Sinjuku-ku, Japan

INTRODUCTION

Acrosin is a protease in the mammalian sperm head, acrosome
(Fritz et al., 1975) and its physiological role in the fertilization processes is thought to participate in the sperm penetration
to ovum. This enzyme is classified as one of the serine proteases,
such as trypsin and kallikreins (Fritz et al., 1975). On the
other hand, it has been reported that administrations of hog pancreatic kallikrein to male infertility patients, especially oligozoospermia and asthenozoospermia caused improvement of sperm counts
and motility (Schill, 1977; Leidl, et al., 1974). Fritz et al.
described that the kinin system enhances sperm motility, O_2-
consumption and fructolysis, in vitro (Schill, 1974).

These findings lead us to a hypothesis that there is a kinin
mimic system in the genital tract and it contributes to the re-
productive function. Acrosin takes part of the kininogenase in
this hypothesis, and we found an enzyme which hydrolyzed bradykinin
in the seminal plasma.

The present investigation deals with the purification of
acrosin from boar sperm by affinity chromatography, and some of
its properties as kininogenase and hemagglutination activity on
sheep erythrocytes.

MATERIALS AND METHODS

The BAEE esterolytic was determined by Schwert and Takenaka's
method (1955) in 0.3 M Tris-HCl containing 0.05 M $CaCl_2$, pH 8.0,

351

at 25°C. The activity is shown in terms of BAEE U which is the
hydrolyzed substrate amount (u moles) in 1 min.

The kinin liberating activity of acrosin was determined by
incubation with the various kininogens, and the amount of kinin
formed was assayed on an isolated rat uterus segment using synthetic
bradykinin as the standard. The crude kininogens were prepared
from heated (60°C, 1 hr) human, boar, bovine and rat plasma
according to Moriwaki et al. (1974), and highly purified bovine HMW-
and LMW-kininogens were donated by Dr. H. Kato, Osaka University.
Human midcycle cervix mucus (CM) was supplied by the Department of
Gynecology and Obstetrics, Keio University.

Hemagglutination was tested by sheep erythrocytes which were
washed 5 times with saline and prepared 5% suspension. The assay
sample (0.1 ml), 0.15 M Tris-HCl, pH 8.0, (0.2 ml) inhibitor or
saline (0.1 ml) and the erythrocyte suspension (0.1 ml) were mixed,
stood for 1 hr at room temperature, and hemagglutination was
observed.

Vasodilator activity was determined by increase of blood flow
at the femoral artery of dog (Moriya et al., 1965). This activity
was expressed in the kallikrein unit (KU).

RESULTS AND DISCUSSION

Frozen boar sperm pellet which was obtained from 140 ml of
freshly ejaculated semen, was thawed and extracted with 2% acetic
acid containing 10% glycerol, pH 2.0, for 1 hr at room temperature.
After centrifugation (105,000 g, 1 hr, 4°C), the supernatant fluid
was concentrated with polyethylene glycol and submitted on the
Sephadex G-100 column (3 x 90 cm) equilibrated with 2% acetic acid,
pH 2.6. The active fractions were adjusted to pH 5.5 by 1 N NaOH,
and further purification was achieved by affinity chromatography
with Phe-Phe-Arg Sepharose, pre-equilibrated with 0.1 M acetate
buffer, pH 5.3. The column was washed with Buffer 1 (0.01 M
ammonium formate, containing 0.3 M NaCl, pH 5.3) until the absorbance at 280 nm of the effluent became 0, and then acrosin was
eluted with Buffer 3 (5 mM HCl, pH 2.6). This acrosin fraction
gave hemagglutination (Fig. 1).

Recently another elution system which could separate agglutinin
from acrosin was developed. Buffer 2 with a composition of 10%
dioxan in Buffer 1, was inserted between Buffer 1 and 3, and the
hemagglutination activity (sperm agglutinin) was eluted with Buffer
2, separately from acrosin which was recovered in 5 mM fraction
(Fig. 1.) Table I tabulated the overall results of the acrosin
purification with the latter elution system. The final acrosin

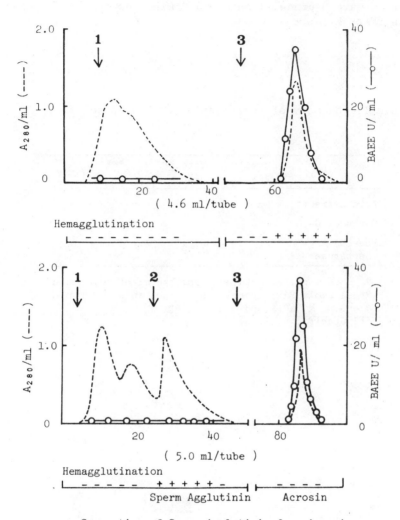

Separation of Sperm Agglutinin from Acrosin

Fig. 1. Affinity Chromatography of Boar Acrosin on Phe-Phe-Arg
         Sepharose.
         Arrows indicate the replacements of elution buffer
         Sample   : Sephadex G-100 active fraction
         Buffer 1: 0.01 M $HCOONH_4$, 0.3 M NaCl, pH 5.5
         Buffer 2: 0.01 M $HCOONH_4$, 0.3 M NaCl, 10% dioxan, pH 5.5
         Buffer 3: 5 mM HCl, pH 2.6

preparation gave a specific activity of 28.9 BAEE U/A$_{280}$, and this
preparation gave 3 bands, 1 main and 2 minor bands on disc electrophoresis (Fig. 2).

Table I. Summary of Purification of Boar Acrosin

	Total A$_{280}$	Total[**] BAEE U	S.A.[***]	Yield %
Acid Extract[*]	435	—	—	—
Sephadex G-100	210	1190	5.67	100
Phe-Phe-Arg-Sepharose	39.8	1149	28.9	96.6

*   Sperm pellet obtained from 140 ml of boar semen
**   1 μmole BAEE hydrolysis / min., in 0.3 M Tris-HCl,
      0.05 M CaCl$_2$, pH 8.3, at 25°C.
*** Specific activity

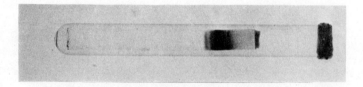

Fig. 2. Disc Electrophoresis of Boar Acrosin
         Purified by Affinity Chromatography

         7.5% polyacrylamide gel, 3 hr.
         Coomasiee brilliant blue stain.

Kininogenase activity of acrosin

    Crude kininogens from various plasma (50 mg) and acrosin (8
BAEE U) were incubated in 2.0 ml of 0.05 M Tris-HCl contained
$CaCl_2$, 0.2 M NaCl and 10 mM 8-hydroxyquinoline, pH 8.0 for 30 min.
at $30°C$. As shown in Table II, acrosin liberated uterus contractile
agent from various crude kininogens, though its ability was rather
low in comparison to those of various kallikreins. Then, as shown
in Fig. 3, acrosin also liberated the uterus contractile agent
from highly purified MHW- and LMW-kininogens. In order to identify
this agent, the incubated mixtures were analyzed on SP-Sephadex
C-25 chromatography (Fig. 3). Synthetic bradykinin (BK) and kallidin (DK) were successively separated by 0-0.5 M NaCl linear gradient
elution, i.e., BK was eluted at 20.2 m mho and KD was recovered in
25.9 m mho fraction (Fig. 3A). The active principle in the incubated mixture of acrosin and highly purified bovine HMW-kininogen
was eluted out in 20.2 m mho fraction, namely BK fraction (Fig. 3B).
Similarly, acrosin liberated BK from highly purified bovine LMW-
kininogen (Fig. 3C). Synthetic kallidin was converted to BK by
incubation with acrosin for 4 hr at $30°C$ (Fig. 3D). The same
conversion was also found by trypsin (Fig. 3E).

Table II. Kinin Forming Activity of Boar Acrosin
           from Various Crude Kininogens

    Kinin amounts were determined on an isolated rat
    uterus segment

Kininogen*	BK ng/A_{280}** /min
Boar	33.5
Bovine	10.9
Human	14.7
Rat	4.5

   * Crude Kininogen : Pseudoglobulin fraction
                        from heated (60°C, 1 hr)
                        plasma
  ** A_{280} : 28.9 BAEE U / A_{280} Acrosin

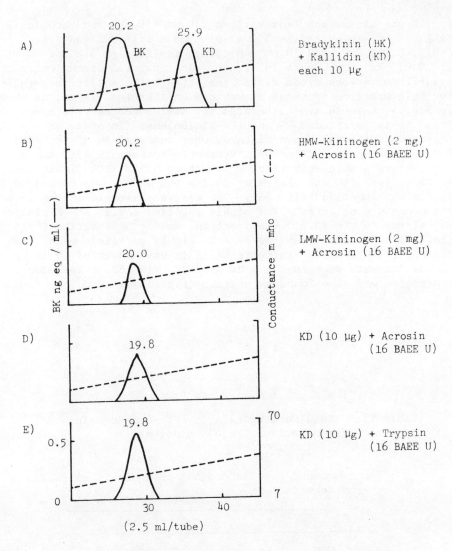

Fig. 3. Identification of Kinin Liberated by Boar Acrosin on
Analytical SP-Sephadex Column Chromatography

All incubations were carried out in 0.05 M Tris-HCl, 0.2M
NaCl, 0.05 M CaCl$_2$, pH 8.0, for 4 hr at 30°C. The reaction
mixtures were applied on SP-Sephadex C-25 column (0.9x10
cm), equilibrated with 0.05 M acetate buffer, pH 5.3, and
eluted by linear gradient (0 - 0.5 M NaCl in equilibrium
buffer).

As mentioned above acrosin yielded BK from both HMW- and LMW-kininogen, and the rates of kinin liberation from these kininogens were similar as shown in Fig. 4, namely 482 ng BK/A_{280} acrosin/min for HMW-kininogen and 340 ng BK/A_{280} acrosin/min for LMW-kininogen.

As shown in Fig. 5, the vasodilator activity of acrosin was 1.7×10^{-2} KU/BAEE U. This activity was much lower than those of various kallikreins, but similar with that of bovine trypsin (1.4×10^{-2} KU/BAEE).

Acrosin (3.2 BAEE U) or trypsin (12 BAEE U) were dissolved in 0.4 ml of 0.3 M Tris-HCl contained 0.05 M $CaCl_2$ and 0.01 M 8-hydro-xyquinoline, pH 8.0, and incubated with human cervical mucus (0.4 ml) for 30 min at 30°C. Both acrosin and trypsin liberated uterus contractile principle from CM, and this principle seemed to be a kinin because it disappeared by treatment with the seminal plasma kininase. However, the liberated kinin from this was only 5 ng BK eq in 30 min respectively, and the kininogen content in CM was considered to be very low in comparison with that of plasma kininogen (Table IV).

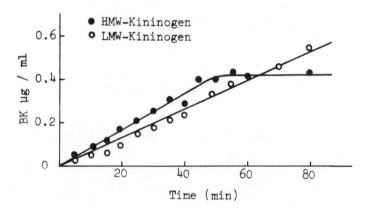

Fig. 4.   Time Courses of Kinin Liberation by Boar Acrosin from Highly Purified Bovine HMW- and LMW-Kininogens

HMW- and LMW-Kininogens (700 µg) were separately incubated with acrosin (16 BAEE U) in 2.5 ml of 0.05 M Tris-HCl, 0.2 M NaCl, 0.05 M $CaCl_2$, pH 8.0, at 30°C.

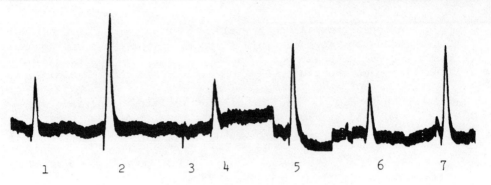

Fig.5   Vasodialator Activity of Boar Acrosin

Hog Pancreatic Kallikrein: 1 and 6: 5×10^{-3} KU,
2: 2×10^{-2} KU,   7: 10^{-2} KU,
Saline: 3: 0.1 ml
Acrosin: 4: 0.31 BAEE U, 5: 0.62 BAEE U,

Table III   Vasodilator Activities of Various Kininogenases

Kininogenase	KU / BAEE U
Acrosin	1.7×10^{-2}
Trypsin	1.4×10^{-2}
Hog Pancreatic Kallikrein	$8 - 9$
Guinea Pig Coagulating Gland Kallikrein	140

Table IV   Kininogen Content in Human Midcycle Cervical Mucus

Kininogenase	BK ng eq / ml CM
Acrosin	$\simeq$ 5
Trypsin	$\simeq$ 5

These results suggest that acrosin is an enzyme quite similar to trypsin but it differs from the kininogenases, such as kallikriens.

Hemagglutination

Acrosin obtained by Sephadex G-100 gel filtration was still
contaminated with sperm agglutinin and both substances were adsorbed
to Phe-Phe-Arg Sepharose. At first we thought that acrosin itself
possessed an agglutination activity, but they were separately eluted
out in 10% dioxan and in 5 mM HCl fractions, respectively.

The minimum concentration for hemagglutination was measured by
the titers system of sperm agglutinin fraction eluted out from Phe-
Phe-Arg Sepharose. In order to investigate the influence of the
surface conditions of erythrocyte for hemagglutination, the erythrocytes were treated by trypsin or neuraminidase. The enzymes
(each 20 mg) were added to 20 ml of 5% erythrocyte suspensions,
pH 7.0, and incubated for 3 hr at 30°C. After the incubation, the
erythrocytes were washed 5 times with saline. The minimum concentration of sperm agglutinin for the intact erythrocyte was 0.06
A_{280}/ml, and that for trypsin- and neuraminidase-treated erythrocyte
were 0.04 and 0.06 A_{280}/ml, respectively. These results indicate
the ineffectiveness of trypsin or neuraminidase treatment of
erythrocyte for the agglutination, while the addition of washed
trypsin-treated erythrocyte to the assay system caused a strong
inhibition of hemagglutination. Hence adding trypsin to the mixture of intact erythrocyte and sperm agglutinin gave the same
inhibition, it was confirmed that trypsin itself inhibited the
sperm agglutinin, but various carbohydrates did not (Table V).

Table V. Effects of Various Carbohydrates, Trypsin,
          and Seminal Plasma Mucin

	Inhibition
Lactose	—
Glucose	—
Galactose	—
Xylose	—
Glucosamine	—
Deoxyglucose	—
Sucrose	—
Maltose	—
Trypsin	+
Boar Seminal Plasma Mucin	+

It is of interest that the inhibition specificity of sperm
agglutinin resembles closely to lysin (Haino, 1971), which is
obtained from the sperm head of Tegula Pfeifferi, a kind of roll
shell. Lysin dissolves vitelline envelope of the sperm non-
enzymatically, and it possesses hemagglutination activity. Such
properties of lysin are thought to relate to the sperm's recognition of the surface in the fertilization process.

SUMMARY

Boar acrosin was purified by acid extract, Sephadex G-100 gel
filtration and affinity chromatography on Phe-Phe-Arg Sepharose.
Sperm agglutinin and acrosin were finally separated by elution
with 10% dioxan and 5 mM HCl from the affinity chromatography.
The final preparation of acrosin gave 28.9 BAEE U/A$_{280}$. Acrosin
liberated kinin from both highly purified bovine HMW- and LMW-
kininogen, and the liberated kinin was identified as bradykinin.
However, the activity was not so potent as kallikreins. Vasodilator
activity of acrosin was lower than those of kallikreins, but almost
the same degree with that of trypsin. These data suggested that
acrosin closely resembled trypsin, but not kallikrein. Hemagglutination activity (sperm agglutinin) and acrosin were separately
eluted out from Phe-Phe-Arg Sepharose, respectively. Sperm agglutinin caused hemagglutination on the intact and trypsin- or
neuraminidase-treated sheep erythrocytes. Trypsin and seminal
plasma mucin inhibited sperm agglutinin but various carbohydrates
reacted negatively.

REFERENCES

Fritz, H., W.D. Schleuning, H. Schiessler, W.B. Schill, V. Wendet
    and G. Winkler, 1975. Boar, bull and human sperm acrosin-
    Isolation, properties and biological aspects: Proteases and
    biological control (Cold Spring Harbor Laboratory, New York)
    p. 715.
Haino, K., 1971. Studies on the egg-membrane lysin of Tegula
    Pfeifferi: Purification and properties of the egg membrane
    lyin. Biochim. Biophys. Acta 229: 459.
Leider, W., R. Prinzen, W.B. Schill and H. Fritz, 1974. The effect
    of kallikrein on motility and metabolism of spermatozoa;
    Kininogenases 2 (F.K. Schattauer Verlag, Stuttgart, New York)
    p. 33.
Moriwaki, C., Y. Hojima and H. Moriya, 1974. A proposal-use of
    combined assays of kallikrein activity measurement. Chem.
    Pharm. Bull. 22: 975.
Moriya,H., K. Yamazaki, H. Fukushima and C. Moriwaki, 1965. Bio-
    chemical studies on kallikreins and their related substances.
    J. Biochem., 58: 208.

Schill, W.B., 1974. Influence of the kallikrein-kinin system on human sperm motility in vitro, Kininogenases 2 (F.K. Schattauer Verlag, Stuttgart, New York) p. 47.

Schill, W.B., 1977. Kallikrein as a therapeutical means in the treatment of male motility, Kininogenases 4 (F.K. Schattauer Verlag, Stuttgart, New York) p. 251.

Schwert, G.W. and Y. Takenaka, 1955. A spectrophotometric determination of trypsin and chymotrypsin. Biochim. Biophys. Acta 16: 570.

STUDIES ON KALLIKREIN-KININ SYSTEM IN BOVINE LUNG

K. Horiuchi, J. Ishikawa, and M. Manabe

Department of Biochemistry, Faculty of Pharmaceutical
Sciences, Tokushima University of Arts and Science,
Yamashiro-cho, Tokushima 770, Japan

Kinins are liberated from their precursor proteins by specific
hydrolysis of kinin-forming enzymes. In blood, there exist two
precursors, the high molecular weight (HMW) kininogen and the low
molecular weight (LMW) kininogen, whose molecular weights are
76,000 and 49,500, respectively (Yano et al., 1967; Komiya et al.,
1974; Nagasawa et al., 1966). Pancreatic kallikrein forms kinins
from both kininogens, while plasma kallikrein acts only on the HMW
kininogen (Nagasawa et al., 1967; Yano et al., 1971). This finding
triggered the idea that in the blood system the genuine substrate
of plasma kallikrein could be HMW kininogen, and the role of LMW
kininogen has been discussed.

It is generally agreed that besides blood system many organs
have their own kallikrein-kinin system based on the existence of
kininogens in many organs. The lung especially contains high concentration of kininogen, its concentration being as high as 80% of
that in blood (Werle and Zach, 1970). It also contains proteinase
inhibitor(s) which inactivates many proteinases related to the
kallikrein-kinin system (Werle, 1964).

We have been studying on the isolation of each components
composing the tissue kallikrein-kinin system from bovine lung.
Some findings on the purification of lung tissue kininogen and the
three proteinase inhibitors found during the purification of the
lung kininogen will be presented here.

Table I. Purification Procedure of Bovine Lung Kininogen

Bovine lung mince
   | homogenized in distilled water (1 : 3, w/v)
   ↓   centrifuged at 4,000 rpm, 20 min.
Homogenate
   | acid treatment (pH 3, 10 min.)
   ↓   centrifuged at 8,000 rpm, 20 min.
Acid supernatant
   | heat treatment (90°C, 10 min.)
   ↓   centrifuged at 8,000 rpm, 20 min.
Heat supernatant
   ↓   fractionated with solid $(NH_4)_2SO_4$
Precipitate between 30 – 60% saturation of $(NH_4)_2SO_4$
   | DEAE-Sephadex A-50 column chromatography
   | 0.01M Tris-HCl buffer, pH 8.5
   ↓   NaCl gradient, 0 – 0.5 M
0.2 – 0.3M NaCl eluate
   | DEAE-Cellulose column chromatography
   | 0.005M phosphate buffer, pH 6.8
   ↓   NaCl gradient, 0 – 0.3 M
0.1 – 0.2M NaCl eluate
   | filtered through Sephadex G-200
   ↓   0.01M Tris-HCl buffer, pH 8.5 containing 0.1M NaCl
Filtrate
   | SE-Sephadex C-50 column chromatography
   | 0.01M acetate buffer, pH 5.0
   ↓   NaCl gradient, 0 – 0.3 M
Unadsorbed effluent

Purification of Bovine Lung Kininogen

Purification procedures of kininogen from bovine lung is out-
lined in Table I. Minced bovine lung was washed thoroughly with
water to remove the blood, and then homogenized with water. The
supernatant was brought to pH 3 with HCl, and after 10 min., the
pH was brought to 7. The supernatant of the acid-treated homogenate
was heated at 90°C for 10 min. and cooled. Through these treatments, significant amount of kininase and proteinase inhibitors
were inactivated despite of minimal loss of kininogen, so that the
recovery of units in these steps surpassed 100% of that in the
homogenate (Table II). The heat treated supernatant was then
fractionated with ammonium sulfate, and the precipitate between
30 - 60% saturation was collected. Crude preparation of kininogen
was thus obtained. Lung kininogen was further purified by the
sequential use of DEAE-Sephadex and DEAE-Cellulose chromatography,
gel filtration on Sephadex G-200, and SE-Sephadex chromatography.
A summary of these purification procedures is shown in Table II.
Nearly 600-fold purification was achieved.

Table II. Summary of Purification of Bovine Lung Kininogen

	Total protein (g)	Total units of kininogen*	Specific activity (units/mg)
Bovine lung (7.5 kg)			
Homogenate	570.0	21,000	0.037
Acid sup.	212.8	30,340	0.142
Heat sup.	104.4	27,000	0.259
$(NH_4)_2SO_4$ 30-60% ppt	24.3	4,500	0.185
DEAE-Sephadex A-50	3.2	3,700	1.155
DEAE-Cellulose	0.87	1,040	1.20
Sephadex G-200	0.43	475	1.11
SE-Sephadex C-50	0.02	438	21.9

* one unit of kininogen will produce active peptides
  equivalent to 1 μg of synthetic bradykinin

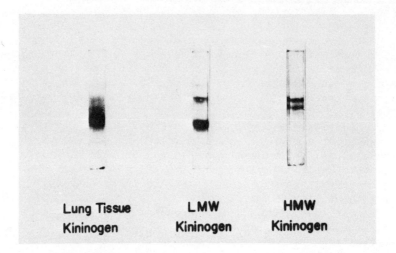

Fig. 1. Polyacrylamide gel electrophoresis of tissue and plasma
         kininogens.

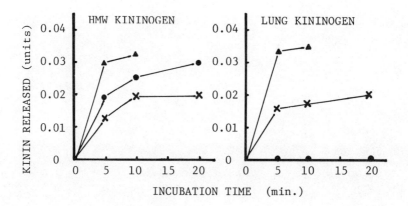

Fig. 2.   The time course of kinin release from kininogens.
          HMW kininogen (0.03 unit) and lung kininogen (0.035
          unit) were incubated with trypsin (———▲———), plasma
          kallikrein (———●———), and pancreatic kallikrein
          (———✕———) at 37°C.

Some Properties of Bovine Lung Kininogen

Purified kininogen preparation from SE-Sephadex C-50 was subjected to disc gel electrophoresis at pH 8.3, and its mobility was
compared with those of HMW and LMW kininogens as obtained by simultaneous run. As shown in Fig. 1, bovine lung kininogen migrated
in a single band, and its position closely coincided with that of
LMW kininogen. Bovine lung kininogen gave single band also on disc
gel electrophoresis in sodium dodecyl sulfate, and its molecular
weight was estimated as 65,000 from its mobility, while those of
HMW and LMW kininogens of the simultaneous run were calculated as
87,000 and 59,000, respectively.

To compare the nature of the lung kininogen with those of the
plasma kininogens, three kinin-forming enzymes were tested for
kinin releasing from lung kininogen and plasma kininogens (Fig. 2).
From HMW kininogen, kinins were released by pancreatic and plasma
kallikreins similar to that of trypsin, while, from bovine lung
kininogen, kinins were formed only by pancreatic kallikrein and by
trypsin, and no kinins were released by plasma enzyme. LMW kininogen, when tested, exhibits quite similar pattern of enzyme susceptibility to that of lung kininogen so that close relationship
was supposed between the lung and the LMW kininogens.

Isolation of Proteinase Inhibitors from Bovine Lung

During the purification of kininogen, we noticed that in the
ammonium sulfate fraction (30-60% sat.) more than one proteinase
inhibitors were contained as they were separable by means of DEAE-
Sephadex chromatography. As acid and heat treatments considerably
inactivate proteinase inhibitors, these procedures were omitted in
the isolation of inhibitors. Crude bovine lung homogenate was
subjected directly to ammonium sulfate fractionation which was
followed by DEAE-Sephadex A-50 chromatography (Fig. 3). When inhibitor activity was assayed by inhibition against hydrolysis of
TAME by trypsin, the activities appeared in three peaks, the first
one was found in unadsorbed fraction, the second eluted with 0.1 -
0.2M NaCl, and the last with 0.2 - 0.3M NaCl. The last active fraction was substantially superimposed with kininogen activity. On
rechromatography, each of these inhibitors were recovered in the
same fractions as in the first chromatography, so that we named
these three proteinase inhibitors as inhibitors I, II, and III in
the order of elution from the DEAE-Sephadex.

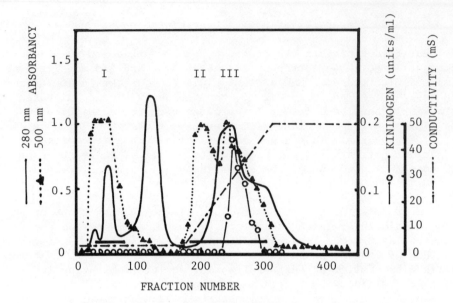

Fig. 3.   Chromatography of ammonium sulfate fraction (30-60% sat.)
of bovine lung homogenate on DEAE-Sephadex A-50 column.
Column:5 x 35 cm; Elution:0.02M phosphate buffer, pH 8,
NaCl gradient 0 - 0.5M; Flow rate: 200 ml/hr.;fractions
of 15 ml/tube were collected.

Characterization of Proteinase Inhibitors

    Three proteinase inhibitors from DEAE-Sephadex were filtered
through Sephadex G-200 (Fig. 4). Inhibitors I and II were eluted
in a single peak, although small contamination was found in I.
Inhibitor III from DEAE-Sephadex gave two nearly equivalent peaks
of inhibitor activity, when, however, these fractions were tested
for kininogen activity it was only found in the first peak, so that
the second peak was considered to be the contamination of inhibitor
II. For comparison, the eluting position of Trasylol (Mol. Wt.
6,500) was indicated by black bars.

    The molecular weights of these inhibitors were estimated from
the eluting position, and they were calculated as 11,000 for I,
13,000 for II, and 80,000 for III.

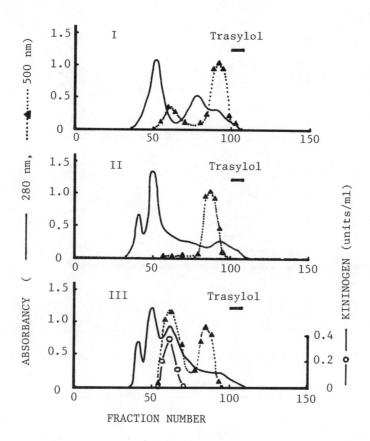

Fig. 4. Gel filtration of DEAE-Sephadex fractions through
Sephadex G-200 column. Column:2.5 x 90 cm;
Elution: 0.02M phosphate buffer, pH 8, containing
0.1M NaCl; Flow rate: 50 ml/hr.; fractions of
5 ml/tube were collected.

In order to clarify the relationship among the three proteinase inhibitors some experiments were carried out taking Trasylol
into special consideration. Using Ampholine three inhibitors from
gel filtration were subjected to isoelectric focusing (pH 3.5-10).
As shown in Fig. 5, isoelectric point of inhibitor I falls on the
alkaline range of pH 9.8 which is, taking into consideration that

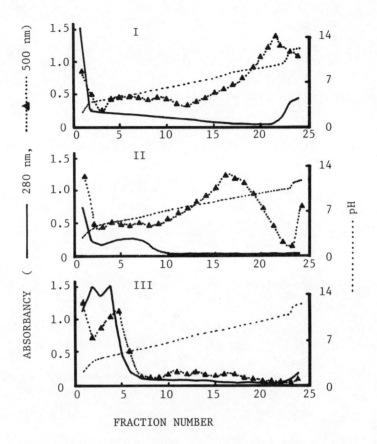

Fig. 5.   Isoelectric focusing of Sephadex G-200 fractions with
          Ampholine (pH 3.5 - 10).
          Electrophoresis was carried out at 500 V for 18 hr.

alkaline extreme of this experiment was pH 10, close to the reported value for Trasylol (pH 10.5).   Isoelectric point of II was
estimated to be pH 8.4.   On the other hand, inhibitor III gave an
isoelectric point at pH 4.8, and in this fraction kininogen activity was also found.   These findings indicate that these inhibitors
were different from the other, and one is not formed by aggregation
or dissociation of the other.

Table III.   Inhibitory Effects of Inhibitors on Several
             Kinin-relating Enzymes

ENZYMES	SUBSTRATES	INHIBITORS			
		I	II	III	TRASYLOL
TRYPSIN	TAME	+	+	+	+
	CASEIN	+	+	+	+
CHYMOTRYPSIN	ATEE	+	−	−	+
	CASEIN	+	−	−	+
PLASMIN	TAME	+	−	−	+
	CASEIN	−	−	−.	+
PLASMA KALLIKREIN*	TAME	−	−	−	−
	KININOGEN**	+	+	+	+
PANCREATIC KALLIKREIN	TAME	+	−	−	+
	KININOGEN**	+	−	−	+
THROMBIN	TAME	−	−	−	+

+ : Inhibition,   − : No inhibition,
* : Glass activated plasma kallikrein, ** : HMW kininogen,
TAME : Tosylarginine methyl ester, ATEE : Acetyltyrosine
ethyl ester.

To confirm the relationship between these inhibitors and
Trasylol, antigen-antibody reaction was carried out between the
three inhibitors and antibody against Trasylol using the
Ouchterlony's method. The precipitation band was recognized only
with inhibitor I, indicating that only I has similar antigenicity
to Trasylol.

We have finally investigated the inhibitory effects of the
three inhibitors on several kinin-relating enzymes. Table III
shows the results together with the known data on Trasylol. Inhibitor I depresses the activities of chymotrypsin as well as trypsin,
while II and III do not inhibit chymotrypsin. The inhibition
pattern of I is very similar to that of Trasylol except the effects
on caseinolysis by plasmin and the hydrolysis of TAME by thrombin.
The similarity of the inhibition patterns of I and Trasylol, that
the molecular weight of I is approximately twice as much as that
of Trasylol, and that, in immunological test, only I reacted with
the Trasylol antibody give the conclusion that inhibitor I is the
dimeric aggregate of Trasylol.

On the other hand, inhibitors II and III gave the identical inhibition pattern which is quite different from that of Trasylol. They do not depress chymotrypsin nor plasmin. It is very interesting that they depress the release of kinins from HMW kininogen by plasma kallikrein but not by pancreatic enzyme. It is quite important whether they or one of them inhibits the release of kinins from bovine lung kininogen, but at present it remains to be investigated. Inhibitors II and III illustrate identical inhibition pattern, but they are distinguishable from each other by the results on isoelectric focusing that II and III have isoelectric points at pH values of 8.4 and 4.8, respectively. The relation between inhibitor III and the overlapping kininogen needs to be investigated as they have similar isoelectric points and behavior on chromatography, but data obtained so far showed that different proteins behave according to their respective activities.

REFERENCES

Komiya, M., H. Kato and T. Suzuki, 1974, Bovine plasma kininogens. I. Further purification of high molecular weight kininogen and its physicochemical properties, J. Biochem. 76, 811.

Nagasawa, S., Y. Mizushima, T. Sato, S. Iwanaga and T. Suzuki, 1966, Studies on the chemical nature of bovine bradykininogen : Determination of amino acid, carbohydrate, amino and carboxyl terminal residues, J. Biochem. 60, 643.

Nagasawa, S., K. Horiuchi, M. Yano and T. Suzuki, 1967, Partial purification of bovine plasma kallikrein activated by contact with glass, J. Biochem. 62, 398.

Werle, E., 1964, Über einen Hemmkörper für Kallikrein und Trypsin in der Rinderlunge, Hoppe-Seyler's Z. physiol. Chem. 338, 228.

Werle, E. and P. Zach, 1970, Verteilung von Kininogen in Serum und Geweben bei Ratten und anderen Säugetieren, Z. klin. Chem. u. klin. Biochem. 8, 186.

Yano, M., S. Nagasawa, K. Horiuchi and T. Suzuki, 1967, Separation of a new substrate, kininogen-I, for plasma kallikrein in bovine plasma, J. Biochem. 62, 504.

Yano, M., S. Nagasawa and T. Suzuki, 1971, Partial purification and some properties of high molecular weight kininogen, bovine kininogen-I, J. Biochem. 69, 471.

Physiological-Pathological
Significance of Kinins

HOW DO KININS AFFECT VASCULAR TONE?

Una S. Ryan, James W. Ryan and Cecil Whitaker

Department of Medicine, University of Miami School
of Medicine, Miami, Florida 33101, U.S.A.

ABSTRACT

Because kinins affect vascular tone, it is assumed that kinins
act directly on smooth muscle. However, a direct interaction is
difficult to conceive. Vessels containing smooth muscle are lined
by a continuous endothelium with tight junctions. In addition,
kinins act on endothelial cells to cause the release of prostaglandin-related substances; possibly through receptors. Furthermore, endothelial cells have a great capacity for hydrolyzing
kinins to inactive products. Hence, even invoking active transport,
less than 1% of kinins might be expected to reach the first layer
of smooth muscle cells. However, kinins may not act directly on
smooth muscle as endothelial cells and smooth muscle cells form
specialized cell contacts. Myoendothelial junctions occur, and we
have shown, in pulmonary arterioles, that smooth muscle cells send
large numbers of projections into the cytoplasm of the endothelial
cells. In addition, smooth muscle cells attach directly to the
abluminal surface of endothelial cells, as do pericytes. Thus,
there is a morphologic basis by which kinins can affect tone of
smooth muscle without acting directly on smooth muscle cells.

INTRODUCTION

Although kinins and angiotensins are classified as hormones
that affect smooth muscle, it is by no means clear how these hormones interact with smooth muscle cells. Furthermore, there are
circumstances in which it is difficult to conceive of means by
which, e.g., bradykinin can reach smooth muscle cells in order to
exert an affect. Thus, bradykinin infused intravenously can dilate

pulmonary blood vessels and can greatly reduce pulmonary vascular
resistance (Rowe et al., 1963), yet little or no bradykinin survives passage from the pulmonary artery to the aortic valves (cf.
Ferreira and Vane, 1967; Ryan et al., 1968, 1970).

As our previous studies have shown, bradykinin is extensively
degraded by enzymes situated on the luminal surface of pulmonary
endothelial cells (Ryan et al., 1968, 1970; Ryan and Smith, 1973;
Smith and Ryan, 1973; Chiu et al., 1975, Ryan et al., 1976b).
Pulmonary endothelial cells in culture provide an excellent model
for defining the means by which intact lungs degrade circulating
bradykinin (cf. Ryan et al., 1976b, 1978a). Indeed, enzymes of
other cell-types need not be invoked. In particular, pulmonary
vascular smooth muscle cells appear to have little ability for
degrading bradykinin, and do not possess kininase II (angiotensin
converting enzyme), (Ryan et al., 1976b and c).

Kininase II is thought to play a major role in the degradation
of bradykinin, but kininase II inhibitors do not preserve bradykinin during passage through the pulmonary circulation, or on
incubation with pulmonary endothelial cells in culture (Ryan et al.,
1968, 1970; see also Ryan, U.S., et al., this volume). In other
words, pulmonary endothelial cells possess a multiplicity of
enzymes capable of inactivating bradykinin.

Thus, one cannot readily conceive of means by which kinins
arriving via the central venous circulation can gain direct access
to receptor sites on or within pulmonary vascular smooth muscle.
Nonetheless, and as indicated above, pulmonary vascular resistance
falls in response to bradykinin. To improve understanding of how
kinins exert their effects on pulmonary vascular resistance, we
have begun to examine for a morphologic basis by which kinins,
acting on endothelial cells, may influence contraction/relaxation
of the adjacent smooth muscle layers.

MATERIALS AND METHODS

Electron Microscopy

Rat lungs were fixed by perfusion with 2.5% glutaraldehyde in
0.05 M cacodylate buffer at pH 7.4 containing 6% sucrose as
described previously (Smith and Ryan, 1970). The lungs were
removed, cut into small blocks and prepared for examination in a
Philips EM 301 electron microscope as described previously (Ryan
et al., 1976b).

Endothelial Cell Isolation and Culture

Endothelial cells were obtained as described previously (Ryan
et al., 1976b and c, 1978a; Habliston et al., in press).

Localization of Prostaglandin Endoperoxide Synthase
by Autoradiography Using [^{3}H]Acetyl-Salicylate

For electron microscope autoradiography, bovine pulmonary
artery endothelial cells were incubated with tritiated aspirin
(New England Nuclear Corp., 50-100 μM, specific radioactivity of
1 Ci/mmole) for 10 min and prepared for electron microscopy either
as monolayers or as pellets. Silver gold sections were cut and
exposed to Ilford L-4 emulsion for periods ranging from 10-150
days as described previously (Ryan et al., 1978c).

RESULTS AND DISCUSSION

As is well known, the pulmonary endothelium is of the continuous type, the cells being linked by tight junctions which are
relatively impermeable (Schneeberger and Karnovsky, 1976). No
evidence has been adduced of a facilitated transport system as
appears to exist for prostaglandins of the E and F series (Ryan and
Smith, 1971; Bito and Baroody, 1975; Eling and Anderson, 1976).
Similarly, there is no evidence of uptake of radiolabelled kinins
by endothelial cells; as occurs with adenosine (Pearson et al.,
1978; see also Ryan, U.S., et al., this volume). Quite to the contrary, the metabolism of bradykinin is accomplished within the
intravascular space (for review, see Ryan and Ryan, 1977). Conceivably, the small fraction of bradykinin which survives
degradation by endothelial cells may gain direct passage to smooth
muscle and yet not be detected by monitoring systems in current use.
However, there are other mechanisms that appear to be far more
likely. Piper and Vane (1971) have shown that lungs perfused with
bradykinin release prostaglandin-related substances, and we have
shown that pulmonary endothelial cells possess cyclo-oxygenase and
synthesize predominantly PGE$_2$ (Ryan et al., 1978a; see also
Gimbrone and Alexander, 1975, in reference to the synthesis of
prostaglandins by human umbilical vein endothelial cells). Our
results are shown in Fig. 1 and Table 1.

Thus, PGE$_2$, for example, could be the final effector for the
action of bradykinin on pulmonary vascular resistance. In terms of
this possibility, it is worth noting that pulmonary artery endothelial cells in culture synthesize surprisingly large amounts of PGE$_2$
and related metabolites of arachidonic acid (Ryan et al., 1978c).
Both McGiff and colleagues (Wong et al., 1977) and Needleman and
colleagues (Blumberg et al., 1977) have adduced evidence to indicate
that effects of bradykinin and angiotensin II may be mediated or
modulated by prostaglandins in other vascular beds.

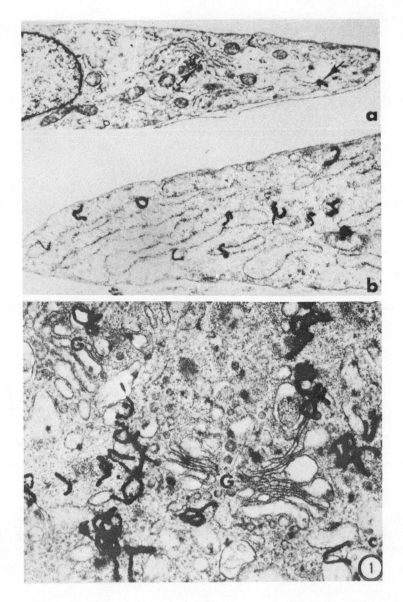

Fig. 1. Autoradiographic localization of prostaglandin endoperoxide
synthase. Bovine pulmonary artery endothelial cells grown in mono-
layer culture were reacted with [^{3}H]acetyl-salicylate and then processed for autoradiography. Silver grains (arrows) developed most
prominently over the endoplasmic reticulum (a). Silver grains over
cisternae of the rough endoplasmic reticulum are shown in b, and in
association with Golgi apparatus (G) in c.
a   x   11,000   b   x   20,000   c   x   48,000
(Reduced 20% for purposes of reproduction.)

Table 1

DISTRIBUTION OF SILVER GRAINS
IN ENDOTHELIAL CELLS PER ORGANELLE

Endoplasmic Reticulum	77%
Nuclei	10
Lipid Droplets	4
Mitochondria	3
Plasma Membrane	0
Background	6

The preponderant labelling occurs in association with endoplasmic
reticulum. None is associated with plasma membrane. This finding
extends previous biochemical work and strongly suggests that prostaglandin endoperoxide synthase is a component of endoplasmic
reticulum.

Myoendothelial Junctions

Possibly one does not have to involve a complex series of reactions in which, e.g., a kinin acts on a cell membrane to activate
a phospholipase which, in turn, makes available arachidonic acid
for the synthesis of prostaglandin-related substances; the latter
substances then being transported to receptor sites on smooth muscle. Conceivably, the kinin could act on the endothelial cell
plasma membrane to elicit an effect transmitted electrically or
ionically directly to smooth muscle. A morphological basis for this
latter possibility may well exist. Several years ago, Rhodin (1967,
1968) described "myoendothelial junctions" between endothelial cells
and smooth muscle cells of microvessels of rabbit skin and fascia of
thigh muscle, and more recently has described similar structures
in cat lungs (Rhodin, 1978).

A small artery, arteriole, precapillary sphincter, venule or
small vein, viewed in cross-section would appear to have its endothelial lining layer clearly separated from the surrounding smooth
muscle by basement membrane. However, at intervals, projections
of one cell-type penetrate the basement membrane to form what
appears to be a junction with the other cell-type. We have found
that the projections may originate from either endothelium or

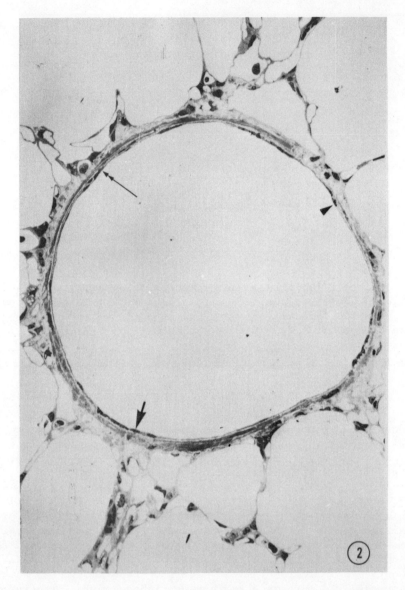

Fig. 2. Low power electron micrograph showing a blood-free small
pulmonary artery (approx. 200 µ in diameter) in tranverse section.
The artery wall is composed of endothelium and from one to three
layers of smooth muscle cells. The artery is surrounded by air-
spaces and smaller vessels. In this section (approx. 600 Å thick),
there are about 150 points of contact between endothelial and smooth
muscle cells. Three areas of cell-cell contact are indicated and
are illustrated at higher magnification as follows: arrow, Fig. 3;
arrowhead, Fig. 4; double arrow, Fig. 7.   x   608
(Reduced 20% for purposes of reproduction.)

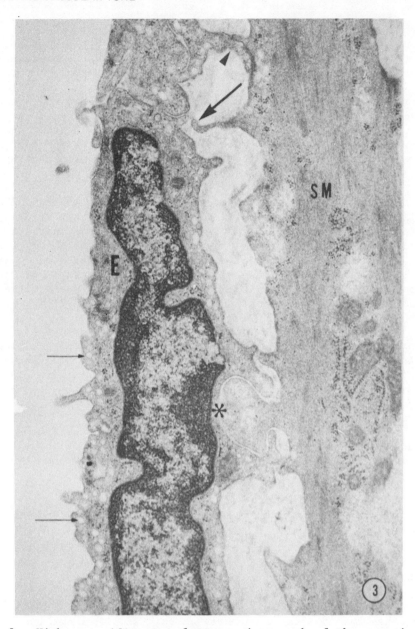

Fig. 3. Higher magnification electron micrograph of the area indicated by an arrow in Fig. 2 showing a myoendothelial junction (*).
A process of the smooth muscle cell (SM) can be seen indenting the
endothelial cells (E), which contains characteristic large numbers
of caveolae (small arrows). The field also shows another smooth
muscle projection approaching the endothelial cell (large arrow) and
an endothelial projection in close apposition with the smooth muscle
cell surface (arrowhead).   x   29,000
(Reduced 20% for purposes of reproduction.)

smooth muscle. Originally, Rhodin (1967) postulated that the appo-
sitions were tight junctions. More recently (1978), he has stated
that these are gap junctions, but no evidence was presented.

We believe that the myoendothelial junctions are likely to be
important to the coordinated activities of endothelial and smooth
muscle cells, and we have begun to investigate their structures in
depth. In addition, there is the distinct possibility that these
junctions provide a path for hormonal, electrical, or ionic transmission of the effects of, e.g., kinins and angiotensins acting at
the endothelial plasma membrane.

We have found that small arteries of the lungs (approx. 200 μ
in diameter) have upwards of 125 points of contact in a single thin
section (approx. 600 Å) (Fig. 2). There are numerous instances of
myoendothelial junctions formed by processes of a smooth muscle
cell indenting an endothelial cell (Fig. 3), but also there are
many instances where an endothelial projection appears embedded in
a smooth muscle cell (Fig. 4). Perhaps the latter would better be
termed "endomyothelial" junctions.

In either case, we have found that the cross-sectional
appearance of the cell-cell interaction may be extremely complex:
The insertions may be of simple peg-like structures, ball-and-
socket configurations or arborizations on a central stalk. In some
planes of section, particularly in venules, the attachment stalk
may not be visible and large numbers of circular profiles of, e.g.,
smooth muscle processes can be found in the endothelial cells
(Fig. 5). However, it should be stressed that the cell membranes
of each cell-type remain distinct. Following Rhodin's lead, we
have termed as "junctions" the associations between endothelial
cells and smooth muscle cells. However, many of the complex insertions are surrounded by an intercellular gap of more than 250 Å,
and are not therefore, junctions in the true sense (Fawcett, 1961;
Farquhar and Palade, 1963).

We have been able to document some instances of close membrane
apposition with associated differentiation of the plasma membrane
of at least one of the cell-types (Figs. 6 and 7).

In some instances (e.g. Fig. 4), the membrane of the smooth
muscle has the appearance normally associated with dense bodies.
Dense bodies are specializations of the smooth muscle cell membrane thought to represent sites of insertion of actin filaments
and are not normally associated with intercellular junctions.

A further association between endothelium and smooth muscle
which appears to be restricted to venules (and collecting vessels)
which lack a complete investment of smooth muscle, consists of a
tendon-like attachment which contains tonofilaments or actin-like

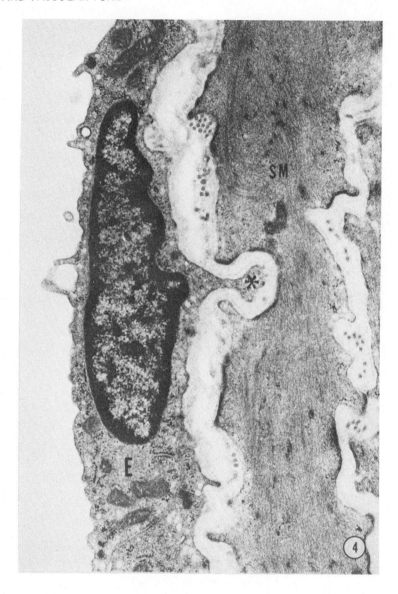

Fig. 4. Higher magnification of the area indicated by an arrowhead
in Fig. 2 showing an endomyothelial junction (asterisk) in contrast
to the myoendothelial junction shown in Fig. 3. An endothelial
cell (E) process can be seen in an indentation of the smooth
muscle cell (SM). In this plane of section, there is no close
membrane contact between the two cells but the indented portion of
the plasma membrane of the smooth muscle cell appears dense (arrows),
similar to the membrane specializations normally referred to as
dense bodies (arrowheads).   x   28,000
(Reduced 20% for purposes of reproduction.)

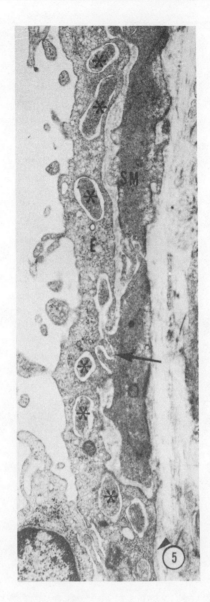

Fig. 5. Electron micrograph illustrating the wall of a pulmonary
venule (approx. 9 μ in diameter). In some regions (arrowhead), the
smooth muscle investment is incomplete. In the region where smooth
muscle cells (SM) are present, the endothelium (E) contains profiles of a large number of smooth muscle processes (*) which do not
show attachment stalks within the plane of section. The complex
interdigitation between finger-like extensions of both cell-types
is apparent (arrow).   x   20,000
(Reduced 20% for purposes of reproduction.)

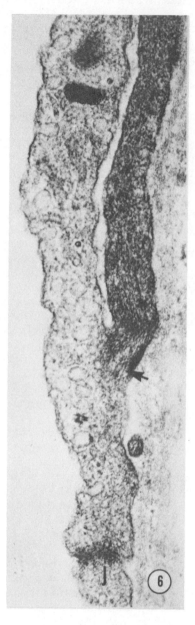

Fig. 6. Another type of myoendothelial junction which appears in
venules consists of a tendon-like attachment. The region of the
junction contains filaments (arrow) similar to those of the smooth
muscle cell. A junction between endothelial cells is shown in the
lower portion of the micrograph (j).   x   78,000
(Reduced 20% for purposes of reproduction.)

filaments (Fig. 6). The diameter of the filaments suggests that
they may be actin, but definitive identification as actin must
await reaction or "decoration" with heavy meromyosin to form the
chevrons or arrowheads characteristic of the actomyosin complex
(Huxley, 1963).

Fig. 7 illustrates a myoendothelial junction where the membranes of both cells appear to be specialized. Superficially, the
junction appears similar to a "nexus" or gap junction linking two
smooth muscle cells (Fig. 8). In both the myoendothelial junction
and the nexus, the density associated with the membrane in the
region of the junction shows a substructural differentiation or
beading.

The exact nature of a junction can only be ascertained by
freeze-fracturing (Friend and Gilula, 1972) and by the use of
tracers, such as colloidal lanthanum (Revel and Karnovsky, 1967).
If the junctions appear by the above techniques to be tight, then
one can begin to postulate that the junction confers impermeability
to water and ions (if the junction is of the desmosomal type and
provides an insertion site for microfilaments, it may bestow
mechanical rigidity). If the junction is a gap junction, the
functional possibilities inferred include low resistance pathways,
transfer of ions and metabolites, and it has recently been postulated that gap junctions may assist in transfer of hormonal
materials (for review see Larsen, 1977) between cells.

It is only when the details of the three-dimensional structure
of myoendothelial interactions are established and the nature of
the membrane or specialization at the junctions become defined that
it will be possible to test hypotheses directly.

As discussed elsewhere in this volume (Ryan, U.S., et al.), it
is not yet clear whether pulmonary endothelial cells possess
receptors for kinins and angiotensins. The ability of bradykinin
to stimulate the release of prostaglandin-related substances may
bespeak receptor sites. However, relevant kinetic studies to explore for high affinity binding sites and hormone-cell interactions
leading to cellular response have yet to be performed. Nonetheless,
the disposition of kinin and angiotensin sites on endothelial cells
would not be without precedent. Gimbrone and Alexander (1977) have
reported that umbilical vein endothelial cells have high affinity
binding sites for insulin, and Buonassisi and Venter (1976) have
found that rabbit aortic endothelial cells in culture also possess
high affinity binding sites for vasoactive hormones. On the other
hand, it should be noted that Jamieson and colleagues (Ives et al.,
1976) have found that fresh isolates of vascular smooth muscle
respond to angiotensin II and norepinephrine by contraction.

Although we have emphasized a mechanical attachment of endo-

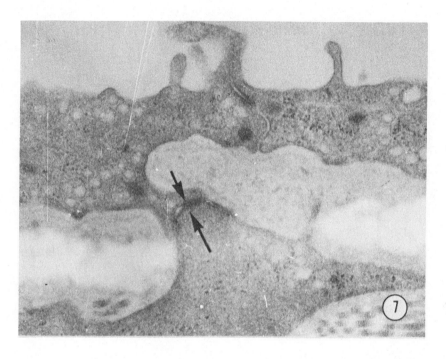

Fig. 7. This micrograph illustrates a myoendothelial junction
(arrow) where the cell membranes of both cell-types appear to show
specialization (arrows). The density associated with the membranes
at the junction is similar to that of a nexus or gap junction between smooth muscle cells such as that illustrated in Fig. 8.

x   49,000

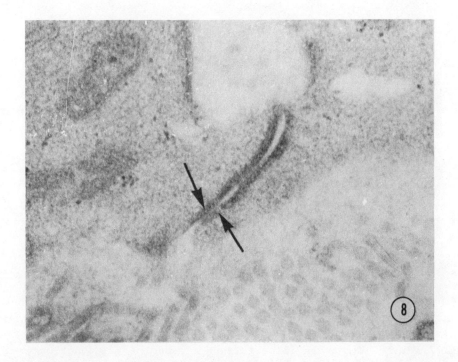

Fig. 8. Nexus or gap junction between two smooth muscle cells
showing a focal increase in density of the junctional membranes.
A beaded or tubular substructure is apparent within the dense
region of the membrane (arrows).   x   88,000

thelium and smooth muscle, we cannot rule out the possibility that myoendothelial junctions carry more than mechanical or electrical messages. Indeed, excitatory agents, such as the prostaglandins, or cyclic nucleotides, may be aided in passing from one cell-type to the other by these junctions.

ACKNOWLEDGEMENTS

This work has been supported in part by grants from the U.S. Public Health Service (HL21568 and HL22087), from the Council for Tobacco Research—U.S.A., Inc. and from the John A. Hartford Foundation, Inc.

REFERENCES

Bito, L.A. and R.A. Baroody, 1975. Inhibition of pulmonary prostaglandin metabolism by inhibitors of prostaglandin biotransport (probenecid and bromcresol green), Prostaglandins, 10: 633.

Blumberg, A.L., S.E. Denny, G.R. Marshall and P. Needleman, 1977. Blood vessel-hormone interactions: Angiotensin, bradykinin, and prostaglandins, Amer. J. Physiol., 323: H305.

Buonassisi, V. and J.C. Venter, 1976. Hormone and neurotransmitter receptors in an established vascular endothelial cell line, Proc. Natl. Acad. Sci., 73: 1612.

Chiu, A.T., J.W. Ryan, U.S. Ryan and F.E. Dorer, 1975. A sensitive radiochemical assay for angiotensin converting enzyme (kininase II), Biochem. J., 149: 297.

Eiling, T.E. and M.W. Anderson, 1976. Studies on the biosynthesis, metabolism, and transport of prostaglandins by the lung, Agents and Actions, 6: 543.

Farquhar, M.G. and G.E. Palade, 1963. Junctional complexes in various epithelia, J. Cell Biol., 17: 375.

Fawcett, D.W., 1961. Intercellular bridges, Exp. Cell Res. Suppl., 8:174.

Ferreira, S.H. and J.R. Vane, 1967. The disappearance of bradykinin and eledoisin in the circulation and vascular beds of the cat, Br. J. Pharmac., 30: 417.

Friend, D.S. and N.B. Gilula, 1972. Variations in tight and gap junctions in mammalian tissues, J. Cell Biol., 53: 758.

Gimbrone, M.A. Jr. and R.W. Alexander, 1975. Angiotensin II stimulation of prostaglandin production in cultured human vascular endothelium, Science, 189: 219.

Gimbrone, M.A. and R.W. Alexander, 1977. Insulin receptors in cultured human vascular endothelial cells, Circulation, 56: 209.

Habliston, D.L., C. Whitaker, M.A. Hart, U.S. Ryan and J.W. Ryan, (in press), Isolation and culture of endothelial cells from the lungs of small animals, Amer. Rev. Resp. Dis.

Huxley, H.E., 1963. Electron microscope studies on the structure of natural and synthetic protein filaments from striated muscle, J. Mol. Biol., 3: 281.

Ives, H.E., R.E. Galardy and J.D. Jamieson, 1976. Isolation of functional aortic smooth muscle cells, J. Cell Biol., 70: 328a.

Larsen W.J., 1977. Structural diversity of gap junctions. A Review, Tissue & Cell, 9: 373.

Pearson, J.D., J.S. Carleton, A. Hutchings and J.L. Gordon, 1978. Uptake and metabolism of adenosine by pig aortic endothelial and smooth-muscle cells in culture, Biochem. J., 170: 265.

Piper, P.J. and J.R. Vane, 1971. The release of prostaglandins from lung and other tissues, Ann. N.Y. Acad. Sci., 180: 363.

Revel, J.P. and M.J. Karnovsky, 1967. Hexagonal array of subunits in intercellular junctions of the mouse heart and liver. J. Cell Biol., 33: C7.

Rhodin, J.A.G., 1967. The ultrastructure of mammalian arterioles and precapillary sphincters. J. Ultrastruct. Res., 18: 181.

Rhodin, J.A.G., 1968. Ultrastructure of mammalian venous capillaries, venules, and small collecting veins. J. Ultrastruct. Res. 25: 452.

Rhodin, J.A.G., 1978. Microscopic anatomy of the pulmonary vascular bed in the cat lung. Microvasc. Res., 15: 169.

Rowe, G.G., S. Afonson, C.A. Castillo, F. Lioy, J.E. Lugo and C.W. Crumpton, 1963. The systemic and coronary hemodynamic effects of synthetic bradykinin. Am. Heart J., 65: 656.

Ryan, James W., A. Chung, L.C. Martin and U.S. Ryan, 1978b. New substrates for the radioassay of angiotensin converting enzyme of endothelial cells in culture, Tissue & Cell, 10: 555.

Ryan, J.W., A.R. Day, U.S. Ryan, A. Chung, D.I. Marlborough and F.E. Dorer, 1976a. Localization of angiotensin converting enzyme (kininase II). I. Preparation of antibody-heme-octa-peptide conjugates. Tissue & Cell, 8: 111.

Ryan, J.W., J. Roblero and J.M. Stewart, 1968. Inactivation of bradykinin in the pulmonary circulation. Biochem. J.,110: 795.

Ryan, J.W., J. Roblero and J.M. Stewart. Inactivation of bradykinin in rat lung., 1970, In: Adv. Exp. Med. Biol. (Bradykinin and related Kinins), Vol. 8, eds. N. Back, F. Sicuteri and M. Rocha e Silva, (Plenum Press, New York) p. 263.

Ryan, J.W. and U.S. Ryan, 1977. Pulmonary endothelial cells. Fed. Proc., 36: 2683.

Ryan, J.W., U.S. Ryan, D.H. Habliston and L.C. Martin, 1978c. (in 1978c. Synthesis of prostaglandins by pulmonary endothelial cells. Trans. Assoc. Amer. Physns., 91, 343.

Ryan, J.W. and U. Smith, 1971. Metabolism of adenosine-5'-mono-phosphate during circulation through the lungs. Trans. Assoc. Physns., 84: 297.

Ryan, J.W. and U. Smith. The metabolism of angiotensin I by endo-
    thelial cells, 1973. In: Protides of the Biological Fluids,
    Vol. 20, ed. H. Peeters, (Pergamon Press, Oxford, England),
    p. 379.
Ryan, U.S., E. Clements, D. Habliston and J.W. Ryan, 1978a. Isola-
    tion and culture of pulmonary artery endothelial cells. Tissue
    & Cell, 10: 535.
Ryan, U.S., J.W. Ryan and A. Chiu, 1976c. Kininase II (angiotensin
    converting enzyme) and endothelial cells in culture. In:
    (Kinins),Vol. 70, eds. F. Sicuteri, N. Back, and G.L. Haberland,
    (Plenum Press, New York), p. 217.
Ryan, U.S., J.W. Ryan, D.L. Habliston and G.A. Pena, (this volume).
    Endothelial cells and components of the kallikrein-kinin
    system, 1979, p. 313.
Ryan, U.S., J.W. Ryan, C. Whitaker and A. Chiu, 1976b. Localization
    of angiotensin converting enzyme (kininase II). II. Immuno-
    cytochemistry and immunofluorescence, Tissue & Cell, 8: 125.
Schneeberger, E.E. and M.J. Karnovsky, 1976. Ultrastructure of
    intercellular junctions in freeze-fractured alveolar capillary
    membranes of mouse lung. Circ. Res., 38: 404.
Smith, U. and J.W. Ryan, 1970. An electron microscopic study
    of the vascular endothelium as a site for bradykinin and ATP
    inactivation in rat lung. In: Adv. Exp. Med. Biol., Vol. 8,
    eds. N. Back, F. Sicuteri and M. Rocha e Silva, (Plenum Press,
    New York), p. 249.
Smith, U. and J.W. Ryan, 1973. Electron microscopy of endothelial
    and epithelial components of the lungs: Correlations of structure
    and function. Fed. Proc., 32: 1957.
Wong, P.Y.-K., D.A. Terragno, N.A. Terragno and J.C. McGiff, 1977.
    Dual effects of bradykinin on prostaglandin metabolism: Relation-
    ship to the dissimilar vascular actions of kinins, Prostaglan-
    dins, 13: 1113.

EFFECT OF BRADYKININ TO CYCLIC AMP LEVELS AND

RESPONSE OF MURINE LYMPHOCYTES

Yoshitami Kimura, Takeo Fujihira, Kazutomi Kato,
Masaichi Furuya, Masahiko Onda* and Akiro Shirota*
Department of Microbiology and Immunology,
*Department of 1st Surgery,
Nippon Medical School
1-1 Sendagi, Bunkyo-ku, Tokyo 113, Japan

ABSTRACT

No information is available on the pharmacological effect of
bradykinin to lymphocytes and immunological responses of them.
In this study it was clarified that bradykinin as well as histamine elevated cyclic adenosine 3',5' monophosphate (cAMP) levels
of murine splenic or lymph node lymphocytes and mature thymocytes
(cortisone-resistant thymus), but did not increase cAMP levels of
immature thymocytes as well as histamine. The increased cAMP
ratios in T cell-enriched splenic lymphocytes by the impulse of
bradykinin were higher than that in splenic and lymph node lymphoid cells by the stimulation of bradykinin. It was also demonstrated that bradykinin as well as histamine suppressed DNA
synthesis by mitogenic (PHA-P, Con-A) stimulation of splenic
lymphocytes, but not a effect to the response of lymphocytes by
mitogenic (LPS) stimulation was observed. These facts suggest
that bradykinin may play an important role in the regulation of
immunologic lymphocyte responses.

INTRODUCTION

It has been considered that bradykinin as well as histamine
is a low molecular weight hormone widely distributed in mammalian
tissues and is released from storage sites or produced by inflammation or allergic reactions. It is also well known that both
bradykinin and histamine, chemical mediators in inflammation or
immediate type hypersensitivity, have similar pharmacological
characteristics.

However, it has also been reported that histamine may exert multiple effects on immune reactions (Lichtenstein et al., 1973; Plaut et al., 1973; Rocklin, 1976).   The most attractive informations reported recently are that histamine may have suppressive effect to proliferative responses of lymphocytes and is associated with the increase of cAMP levels in lymphocytes (Ballet et al., 1976; Wang et al., 1978).

On the other hand, recent numerous studies have suggested that cAMP plays an important role in immune responses (Henney et al., 1971; Abell et al., 1973; Burne et al., 1974; De Ruberts et al., 1974; Bösing-Schneider et al., 1976; Teh et al., 1976). However, no information is available on the effect of bradykinin to cAMP levels of lymphoid cells or to proliferative responses of lymphocytes. The purpose of this study is to clarify the effect of bradykinin to cAMP levels in various lymphoid cells of mice and the suppressive effect to proliferative responses of lymphocytes by mitogenic stimuli.

MATERIALS AND METHODS

Animals

Young adult male C57Bl/6 mice, 8 week of age, purchased from Japan Ohmura Experimental Animal Centre, were mainly used. For some studies, male Balb/c and Balb/c nu/nu mice, 8 week of age, purchased from Japan Clear Laboratory were also employed.

Drugs and Media

Eagle Minimum Essential Medium (Nissui Co., Japan); cAMP assay kit (The radiochemical Center, Amersham, England); bradykinin (Protein Research Institute, Osaka University); histamine (Sigma Co.); ^{3}H-thymidine (The radiochemical Center, Amersham, England); PHA-P (Difco Laboratories, Michigan, U.S.A.); Con-A (Pharmacia Fine Chemicals); LPS (Difco Laboratories, Michigan, U.S.A.); RRMI 1640 medium (Nissui Co., Japan); hyamine hydroxide (New England Nuclear); Bray's solution (New England Nuclear); cortisone acetate (Nippon Merk Co.).

Preparation of Lymphoid Cells

The spleen, thymus and lymph nodes were removed from individual mice after exsanguination. For preparation of cortisone-resistant thymocytes, one group of mice received an intraperitoneal injection of 10 mg of cortisone acetate suspension by

dividing into two. Twenty-four hr later, these mice were exsan-
guinated and thymus were isolated. Single cell suspensions were
prepared from the spleen, thymus and lymph nodes by squeezing the
organs individually through a mesh. Eagle Minimum Essential
Medium (MEM) containing heparin at 5 unit/ml was used for the isolation of all cells. The pellets were washed twice with the
same medium and resuspended in Eagle MEM. However, in the case
of spleen cells, they were previously treated with 0.83 %
ammonium chloride to remove red blood cells. Then, they were
centrifuged and washed twice and the pellets were also resuspended
in Eagle MEM. Thereafter, they were filtered through a glass wool
column to deplete adherent cells and the effluent was adjusted
to 2×10^7 cells/tube lymphocyte suspension. The above all procedures were carried out at 4°C.

Preparation of T Cell-Enriched Splenic Lymphocytes
by the Modified Method of Julius (Julius, 1973)

The splenic lymphocytes isolated as described above were resuspended in 25 ml Eagle MEM containing fetal calf serum (F.C.S.)
at 5 %. Then, they were filtered through a glass wool preincubated at 37°C and then the cell suspension was centrifuged at 160 g
for 10 min. The pellets were resuspended in 6 ml Eagle MEM containing F.C.S. at 5 % and incubated at 37°C for 45 min in nylon
wool column and the effluent, non-adherent cells were obtained.
These cells were designated "T cell-enriched splenic lymphocytes".

Treatment of Lymphocytes with Bradykinin or Histamine

To 1 ml of lymphoid cell suspensions (2×10^7 cells/ml) preincubated at 37°C for 10 min, 1 ml of $2 \times 10^{-11} \sim 10^{-4}$ M bradykinin
(BK) or histamine (H) was added and incubated at 37°C for further
10 min. Then the cell suspensions were centrifuged at 1500 g for
3 min at 4°C and the cell pellets were suspended in 0.5 ml of Tris-
ethylendiaminetetraacetate (EDTA) buffer, pH 7.5. After boiling
for 5 min, it was homogenized and then boiled for further 5 min.
The supernatant after centrifugation at 1500 g for 20 min at 4°C
was used for cAMP assay.

Cyclic AMP Assay

Cyclic AMP contents were measured following protein binding
method, modified method of Gilman (Gilman, 1970) and Brown (Brown
et al., 1971), employing cAMP assay kit. To 50 µl of **super-**
natant separated from cell suspension boiled in Tris-EDTA buffer
50 µl of $8-^3H$ cAMP and 100µl of binding protein (anti cAMP serum)

were added.   After shaking for 5 sec, it was incubated for further
2 hr at 2-4°C.   Then, 100 µl of charcoal suspension was added and
shaken for 10-12 sec.   Within 5 min after shaking it was centrifuged at 1500 g for 20 min and aliquots (200 µl) of the supernatants
were assayed directory for cAMP content.   Cyclic AMP contents of
the samples were evaluated from a linear line prepared with standard cAMP solutions.

Measurement of Incorporation of ^{3}H-thymidine into DNA Synthesis

    Spleens isolated from male Balb/c or same strain of nu/nu
mice, 8 week of age, were minced in Hank's balanced salt solution
and pressed through a 60 mesh screen and suspended in Hank's solution.   It was treated with 0.83 % ammonium chloride to remove red
blood cells.   The pellets after centrifugation were washed twice
and resuspended at the concentration of 1×10^7 cells/ml in RPMI 1640
medium containing F.C.S. at 5 %.   Then each 0.25 ml of mitogen
solutions such as 12.5 µg of Phytohemagglutinin-P (PHA-P), 12.5 µg
of Concanavalin A (Con-A) or 100 µg of Lipopolisaccharide (LPS)
and each 0.25 ml of BK $(6 \times 10^{-11} \sim 10^{-5}M)$ or H $(6 \times 10^{-9} \sim 10^{-4}M)$ were
added to 1 ml of splenic lymphocyte suspension $(1 \times 10^7$ cells/ml)
and incubated at 37°C for 24 hr in a 5 % CO_2 atomosphere.
Then, 0.5 ml of 2 µCi/ml ^{3}H-thymidine (^{3}H-TdR) was added and 24 hr
later the cells were harvested.   After centrifugation at 100 g
for 10 min at 4°C the pellets were washed twice with cold Hank's
solution.   DNA was precipitated by incubating cells in 2 ml of
cold 10 % trichloracetic acid (TCA) for 1 hr in ice-bath.   After
centrifugation 0.6 ml of hyamine hydroxide was added and incubated
at 37°C for a night.   To the precipitate 8 ml of Bray's solution
was added and the radioactivity was measured with a Packard liquid
scientillation counter.

RESULTS

Influence of Bradykinin to the Viability of Lymphocytes

Table 1.   Viability Percents of Lymphocytes After the Treatment
with Bradykinin

min	0	10	30	60
control (non-added)	92.2 %	90.7 %	89.9 %	90.2 %
Bradykinin $10^{-9}M$	92.2 %	90.6 %	91.9 %	90.7 %
Bradykinin $10^{-7}M$	92.2 %	92.3 %	92.0 %	92.6 %
Bradykinin $10^{-5}M$	92.2 %	92.1 %	89.8 %	88.3 %

Bradykinin (BK) at the concentrations of 10^{-9}M, 10^{-7}M and 10^{-5}M were added to splenic lymphocytes in vitro and incubated at 37°C for 10, 30 and 60 min. The cell viability was examined by dye--exclusion test. The percents of the viability were as shown in Table 1. Not a slight decrease in the viability of lymphocytes was observed at the concentrations of less than 10^{-5}M of BK.

The Increase of cAMP Levels in Lymphoid Cells Impulsed with Bradykinin or Histamine

Bradykinin produces a dose-dependent increase in the endogenous cAMP levels of murine splenic lymphocytes. Cyclic AMP levels in splenic lymphocytes began to increase within 5 min and were maximal at 10 min for each dose of BK added. At 30 min, however, seems to return to almost baseline levels (Fig. 1).

The highest increased cAMP levels in lymphocytes (T cell-enriched splenic lymphocytes, splenic lymphoid cells and cortisone-resistant thymocytes) were observed in the cells stimulated with BK at the concentration of 10^{-7}M and the highest cAMP level in lymph node cells stimulated with BK was observed at the concentration of 10^{-5}M. From the points of the increased ratios of cAMP levels in lymphocytes by the impulse of BK, as shown in Table 3, Fig. 2 and 3, T cell-enriched splenic lymphocytes responded the most (3.10-fold), then splenic lymphoid cells (2.75-fold), lymph node lymphocytes (1.89-fold), but not remarkable in immature

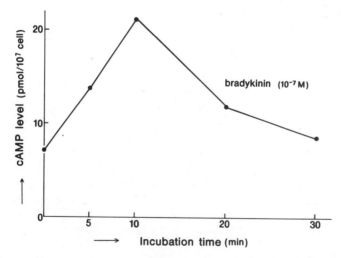

Fig. 1. Cyclic AMP levels in splenic lymphocytes from normal mice after exposure for varying periods of time (5, 10, 20 and 30 min) with 10^{-7}M bradykinin.

thymocytes (1.15-fold). In the case of histamine (H) almost same
patterns of the increased ratios of cAMP in lymphoid cells were
observed. The impulse of H at the concentration of 10^{-4}M produced
an elevation of cAMP levels in T cell-enriched splenic lymphocytes
(3.35-fold), splenic lymphoid cells (2.56-fold) and lymph node
cells (2.09-fold), but not a remarkable increase was observed in
immature thymocytes (1.13-fold).

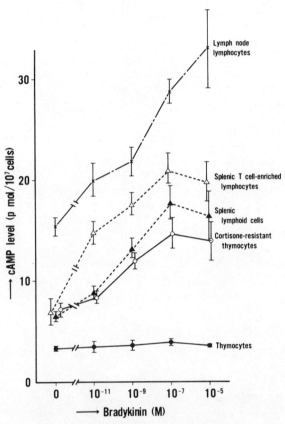

Fig. 2. Effect of bradykinin to cAMP levels of murine lymphocytes
         x-x lymph node lymphocytes; Δ-Δ T cell-enriched splenic
         lymphocytes; ▲-▲ splenic lymphocytes; o-o cortisone-
         resistant thymocytes separated from mice pretreated with
         cortisone acetate suspension; ●-● thymocytes of normal
         mice. Each point represents the mean value ± standard
         deviation of triplicae determinations.

         However, the cortisone-resistant thymocytes isolated from
mice pretreated with cortisone acetate responded to the impulse
with 10^{-7}M BK or 10^{-4}M H and the increased cAMP ratios were 2.06-

fold and 2.22-fold, respectively. These results suggest that immature thymocytes do not respond to BK or H, but mature thymocytes may respond to BK or H.

Table 2. Effect of bradykinin or histamine to cAMP levels in lymphoid cells (thymocytes, splenic lymphocytes, T cell-enriched splenic lymphocytes and lymph node lymphocytes) from normal mice and cortisone-resistant thymocytes separated from cortisone-treated mice.

Lymphoid cells*	cAMP (pmole/10^7cells)**		
	without drug	with Bradykinin (10^{-7}M)	with Histamine (10^{-4}M)
Thymocytes	3.3±0.3	3.8±0.5 (1.15×)***	3.7±0.5 (1.13×)
Cortisone-resistant thymocytes	7.1±1.2	14.6±1.5 (2.06×)	15.7±2.6 (2.22×)
Splenic lymphocytes	6.4±0.6	17.7±3.5 (2.75×)	16.5±1.1 (2.56×)
T cell-enriched splenic lymphocytes	6.8±2.7	21.1±2.7 (3.10×)	22.9±1.7 (3.35×)
Lymph node cells	15.3±1.5	28.8±2.4 (1.89×)	32.1±2.1 (2.09×)

* Lymphoid cells from normal C57Bl/6 mice incubated in vitro for 10 min with or without 10^{-7}M bradykinin or 10^{-4}M histamine.
** Average response levels of cAMP (mean ± standard deviation) in three mice.
*** Number in parenthesis represents increased ratios by stimulation with bradykinin (10^{-7}M) or Histamine (10^{-4}M).

Effect of Bradykinin or Histamine to ^{3}H-thymidine Incorporation in Lymphocyte Mitogenesis

To 1 ml splenic lymphocytes ($1×10^7$cells/ml) 0.5 ml of $3×10^{-5}$M BK or $3×10^{-4}$M H was added without impulse of mitogens and 1 μCi ^{3}H-thymidine was added, respectively. The measurement of ^{3}H-thymidine incorporation in lymphocytes was carried out following the method as described. The results are as shown in Table 3, not a influence by 10^{-5}M BK or 10^{-4}M H on ^{3}H-thymidine incorporation was observed.

Table 3. Effect of bradykinin or histamine to ^{3}H-TdR incorporation in splenic lymphocytes.

cells ($1×10^7$)	BK or H	^{3}H-TdR incorporation (c.p.m.)
splenic lymphocytes	-	825 ± 161
splenic lymphocytes	BK(10^{-5}M)	817 ± 212
splenic lymphocytes	-	1291 ± 101
splenic lymphocytes	H (10^{-4}M)	1225 ± 176

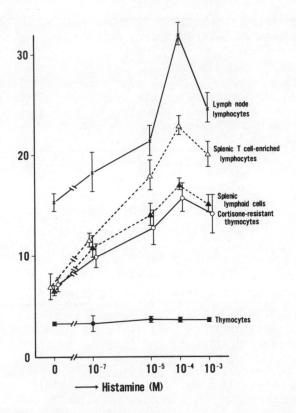

Fig. 3.   Effect of histamine to cAMP levels of murine lymphocytes
          x-x lymph node lymphocytes; Δ-Δ T cell-enriched splenic
          lymphocytes; ▲-▲ splenic lymphocytes; o-o cortisone-
          resistant thymocytes separated from mice pretreated
          with cortisone acetate suspension; ●-● thymocytes of
          normal mice. Each point represents the mean value ±
          standard deviation of triplicae determinations.

Suppressive Effect of Bradykinin or Histamine
to PHA-P or Con-A Induced Lymphocyte Mitogenesis

     Results on the studies of the suppressive effect by the im-
pulse of BK or H to PHA-P or Con-A induced proliferation of splenic lymphocytes are shown in Tables (4,5). Significant suppress-
ions of mitogenic proliferation in lymphocytes by both bradykinin
of 10^{-5}M or less and histamine of 10^{-4}M or less were observed.
However, BK or H at these concentrations were confirmed to exert
no suppressive effect on isotopic incorporation in the above experiment.

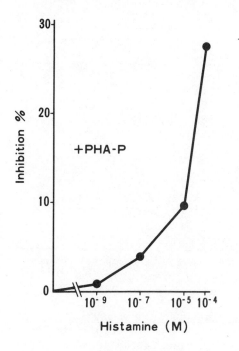

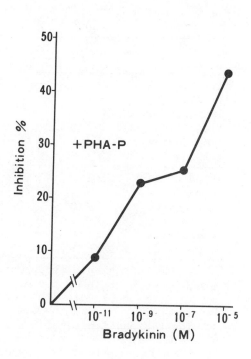

Fig.4 Inhibitory effect of bradykinin of DNA synthesis in
splenic lymphocytes of Balb/c
mice.

Fig.5 Inhibitory effect of histamine of DNA synthesis in splenic lymphocytes of Balb/c mice.

Spleen cells were cultured at a density of 1×10^7 cells/ml and radioactive thymidine incorporation was measured .   Each point represents the inhibition percent of mean value in triplicate experiments.

The increased ratio of ^{3}H-thymidine incorporation in lymphocytes pulsed with PHA-P was 25.2-fold ~ 26.6-fold in two groups
of experiments. However, in the lymphocytes pretreated with BK
(10^{-5} ~ 10^{-11}M) or H (10^{-4} ~ 10^{-7}M) before impulse of PHA-P isotopic
inocorporations were inhibited; the inhibition percents were 44 %
in 10^{-5}M BK, 25.4 % in 10^{-7}M BK, 22.8 % in 10^{-9}M BK, 27.6 % in
10^{-4}M H and 9.6 % in 10^{-5}M H.

Table 5 shows the suppressive effect on Con A-induced proliferation of lymphocytes by BK or H. Almost similar patterns of
suppression by both BK of 10^{-7}M and H of 10^{-4}M were observed.

Table 4. Inhibitory effect of bradykinin or histamine to ^{3}H-TdR
incorporation in PHA-P induced lymphocyte mitogenesis.

cells* (1×10^7)	BK (or H)	PHA-P (12.5μg)	^{3}H-TdR incorpo-** ration (c.p.m.)	inhibition %*** of DNA synthesis
lymphocytes	–	–	825±161	
lymphocytes	–	+	20790±1912 (25.2×)	0
lymphocytes	BK 10^{-11} M	+	18941±1189 (23.0×)	8.7 %
lymphocytes	BK 10^{-9} M	+	16048±2580 (19.5×)	22.8 %
lymphocytes	BK 10^{-7} M	+	15502±764 (18.8×)	25.4 %
lymphocytes	BK 10^{-5} M	+	11635±734 (14.1×)	44.0 %
lymphocytes	–	–	1291±101	
lymphocytes	–	+	34348±763 (26.6×)	0
lymphocytes	H 10^{-9} M	+	34041±2024 (26.3×)	0.9 %
lymphocytes	H 10^{-7} M	+	33023±1744 (25.6×)	3.9 %
lymphocytes	H 10^{-5} M	+	31049±2021 (24.0×)	9.6 %
lymphocytes	H 10^{-4} M	+	24877±571 (19.3×)	27.6 %

* One ml of splenic lymphocytes (1×10^{7}cells/ml) separated from
normal mice were incubated with 0.25 ml of bradykinin ($6×10^{-11}$~
10^{-5}M) or histamine ($6×10^{-9}$~10^{-4}M) and 0.25 ml of PHA-P (50 μg/
ml).
** The radioactive thymidine incorporations were measured.
Each value represents mean ± standard deviation in triplicate
experiments. Number in parenthesis represents the increased
ratios by mitogenic (PHA-P) stimulation and the inhibitory effect
by the presence of bradykinin or histamine.
*** Inhibition percents indicate the inhibitory effect of bradykinin or histamine against PHA-P induced lymphocyte proliferation.

Table 5. Effect of BK (or H) to ^{3}H-TdR incorporation in Con-A
induced lymphocyte mitogenesis.

cells* (1×10^7)	BK (or H)	Con-A (12.5μg)	^{3}H-TdR incorpo-** ration (c.p.m.)	inhibition %*** of DNA synthesis
lymphocytes	–	–	1044±140	
lymphocytes	–	+	39256±2727 (37.6×)	0
lymphocytes	BK 10^{-11} M	+	36870±1518 (35.3×)	6.1 %
lymphocytes	BK 10^{-9} M	+	34614±1083 (33.2×)	11.8 %
lymphocytes	BK 10^{-7} M	+	31313±1088 (30.0×)	20.2 %
lymphocytes	BK 10^{-5} M	+	19382±762 (18.6×)	50.6 %
lymphocytes	H 10^{-9} M	+	36262±906 (34.7×)	7.6 %
lymphocytes	H 10^{-7} M	+	33532±1437 (32.1×)	14.6 %
lymphocytes	H 10^{-5} M	+	31504±1232 (29.2×)	19.7 %
lymphocytes	H 10^{-4} M	+	28102±488 (26.9×)	28.4 %

One ml of splenic lymphocytes (1×10^{7}cells/ml) separated from
normal mice were incubated with 0.25 ml of bradykinin ($6×10^{-11}$~
10^{-5}M) or histamine ($6×10^{-9}$~10^{-4}M) and 0.25 ml of Con-A (50 μg/

ml).

** The radioactive thymidine incorporations were measured. Each value represents mean ± standard deviation in triplicate experiments. Number in parenthesis represents increased ratios by mitogenic (Con-A) stimulation and the inhibitory effect by the presence of bradykinin or histamine.
*** Inhibition percents indicate the inhibitory effect of bradykinin or histamine against Con-A induced lymphocyte proliferation.

Effect of Bradykinin or Histamine to LPS-induced Lymphocyte Mitogenesis

As shown in Table 6, ^{3}H-TdR incorporation in splenic lymphocytes pulsed with LPS increased 15.1-fold $\sim$ 16.6-fold. However, in the cells pretreated with BK ($10^{-5} \sim 10^{-11}$ M) or H ($10^{-4} \sim 10^{-9}$M) not a definite suppression was observed.

Table 6. Effect of bradykinin or histamine to ^{3}H-TdR incorporation in LPS-induced lymphocyte mitogenesis.

cells* (1×10^7)	BK (or H)	LPS (100µg)	^{3}H-TdR incorpo-** ration (c.p.m.)	inhibition %*** of DNA synthesis
lymphocytes	−	−	1011±191	
lymphocytes	−	+	15304±1567 (15.1×)	0
lymphocytes	BK 10^{-11} M	+	13700±1962 (13.6×)	10.5 %
lymphocytes	BK 10^{-9} M	+	15094±1298 (14.9×)	1.4 %
lymphocytes	BK 10^{-7} M	+	15135±1365 (15.0×)	1.1 %
lymphocytes	BK 10^{-5} M	+	13670±1962 (13.5×)	10.7 %
lymphocytes	−	−	1072±226	
lymphocytes	−	+	17796±2526 (16.6×)	0
lymphocytes	H 10^{-9} M	+	18523±2637 (17.3×)	− 4.1 %
lymphocytes	H 10^{-7} M	+	16403±1068 (15.3×)	7.8 %
lymphocytes	H 10^{-5} M	+	19044±5256 (17.8×)	− 7.0 %
lymphocytes	H 10^{-4} M	+	16761±2917 (15.6×)	5.8 %

* One ml of splenic lymphocytes (1×10^7cells/ml) separated from normal mice were incubated with 0.25 ml of bradykinin ($6 \times 10^{-11} \sim 10^{-5}$M) or histamine ($6 \times 10^{-9} \sim 10^{-4}$M) and 0.25 ml of LPS (400 µg/ml).
** The radioactive thymidine incorporations were measured. Each value represents mean ± standard deviation in triplicate experiments. Number in parenthesis represents increased ratios by mitogenic (LPS) stimulation and the effect of bradykinin or histamine.
*** Inhibition percents indicate the effect of the presence of bradykinin or histamine against LPS-induced lymphocyte proliferation.

Effect of BK or H to LPS-induced mitogenesis in splenic lymphocytes isolated from nu/nu mice was also examined. ^{3}H-TdR

incorporation in lymphocytes pulsed with LPS elevated 8.9 ~ 9.1-
fold, but not a change was observed in the lymphocytes pretreated
with BK or H.

Table 7. Effect of bradykinin or histamine to ^{3}H-TdR incorporation
in LPS-induced Balb/c (nu/nu) mice lymphocyte mitogenesis.

cells* (1×10^7)	BK (or H)	LPS (100μg)	^{3}H-TdR incorpo- ration (c.p.m.)**	inhibition %*** of DNA synthesis
lymphocytes	-	-	1745±281	
lymphocytes	-	+	15474±992 (8.9×)	0
lymphocytes	BK 10^{-11} M	+	15884±203 (9.1×)	- 2.6 %
lymphocytes	BK 10^{-9} M	+	14055±1452 (8.1×)	9.2 %
lymphocytes	BK 10^{-7} M	+	13964±1613 (8.0×)	9.8 %
lymphocytes	BK 10^{-5} M	+	14209±1478 (9.1×)	8.2 %
lymphocytes	H 10^{-9} M	+	15891±722 (9.1×)	- 2.7 %
lymphocytes	H 10^{-7} M	+	14792±2206 (8.5×)	4.4 %
lymphocytes	H 10^{-5} M	+	14921±242 (8.6×)	3.6 %
lymphocytes	H 10^{-4} M	+	15935±1032 (9.1×)	- 2.9 %

* One ml of splenic lymphocytes (1×10^{7}cells/ml) separated from
Balb/c (nu/nu) mice were incubated with 0.25 ml of bradykinin (6 ×
10^{-11}~10^{-5}M) or histamine (6 × 10^{-9}~10^{-4}M) and 0.25 ml of LPS (400
μg/ml).
** The radioactive thymidine incorporation were measured. Each
value represents mean ± standard deviation in triplicate experiments. Number in parenthesis represents increased ratios by mitogenic (LPS) stimulation and the effect by the presence of bradykinin or histamine.
*** Inhibitory percents indicate the effect of the presence of bradykinin or histamine against LPS-induced lymphocyte proliferation.

These results showed that not a significant effect by BK or
H on LPS-induced proliferation of splenic lymphocytes was observed.

DISCUSSION

It is now generally accepted that cAMP acts as a second mes-
senger for cells involved in many biological functions, including
immunological reactions (Burne et al., 1974) and the involvement
of cAMP in lymphocyte physiology has been suspected since the
demonstration of the action of cAMP and various drugs or hormones,
known to increase intracellular cAMP levels.
      Now it is also generally accepted that agents which increases
intracellular cAMP have in general an antiproliferative effect on
lymphocytes, whereas an augmentation in intracellular cyclic
guanosine 3',5'-monophosphate (cGMP) stimulates mitogenesis
(Hadden et al., 1972). Various lymphocyte populations have been
studied for their content in cAMP before and after stimulation by

drugs, such isopreterenol or prostaglandin E_1 (Bach, 1975).

As for the influence of histamine to cAMP levels in tissues, it has been reported that histamine increased cAMP levels in mast cells of rats (Sullivan et al., 1975). On the effect of histamine to cAMP levels in lymphoid cells a few reports are available (Roszkowski et al., 1977).

However, it should be emphasized that no information is available on the effect of bradykinin to cAMP levels of lymphoid cells or to the mitogenic proliferation of lymphocytes, though bradykinin and histamine have similar pharmacological characteristics and may have similar receptors in lymphoid cells.

In our studies presented here it was shown that bradykinin as well as histamine elevated cAMP levels in murine lymphoid cells and the highest elevated ratios in cAMP levels in lymphoid cells were observed in T cell-enriched splenic lymphocytes (3.1-fold) and then in splenic cells (2.75-fold), lymph node cells (1.89-fold) and cortisone-resistant thymocytes (2.06-fold), but not a change was observed in normal thymocytes. The patterns of the dose-response curves of splenic lymphocytes, T-cell enriched splenic lymphocytes, and cortisone-resistant thymocytes by bradykinin or histamine were almost similar, with maximal augmentation of cAMP at $10^{-7} \sim 10^{-5}$M of bradykinin and 10^{-4}M of histamine.

The enhanced response to bradykinin or histamine of T cell-enriched lymphocytes suggested that, among the total splenic lymphocyte population, rather T cells may have bradykinin or histamine receptors. Roszkowski et al. suggested from their results that histamine receptor display is associated with the "maturation" of mouse thymus-derived lymphocytes, in that there is a progressive increase in histamine responsiveness from thymocytes to cortisone-resistant thymocytes to T cell-enriched splenic lymphocytes (Roszkowski et al., 1977).

Several recent reports demonstrate that immune activity can be depressed by elevated cAMP levels in lymphoid cells and there is considerable evidence to suggest that cAMP influences lymphocyte mitogenesis in vitro (Cross et al., 1971; MacManus et al., 1970; Makman et al., 1972; Novogrodsky et al., 1970; Smith et al., 1971; Watson, 1976; Vischer, 1976).

Recently, it was reported that in vitro addition of histamine, relatively high (10^{-3}M) concentration suppressed mitogen and antigen-induced lymphocyte proliferation (Ballet et al., 1976; Wang et al., 1978). From our studies on the increase of cAMP levels in lymphoid cells by bradykinin it is conceivable that bradykinin as well as histamine may have some suppressive effect to mitogenic proliferation of lymphocytes. The data presented here demonstrated the suppressive effects of 10^{-5}M bradykinin or 10^{-4}M histamine to PHA-P or Con-A induced mitogenesis of splenic lymphocytes.

However, any significant influence by bradykinin or histamine to LPS-induced mitogenesis of splenic lymphocytes of normal mice

or nu/nu mice was not observed. These results suggest that bradykinin may affect to rather T cells among lymphocyte populations.

REFERENCES

Abell, C. W. and T. M. Monahan, 1973, The role of adenosine 3',
5'-cyclic monophosphate in the regulation of mammalian cell
division, J. of Cell Biol. 59, 549.

Bach, M. A., 1975, Differences in cyclic AMP changes after stimulation by prostaglandins and isopreterenol in lymphocyte sub-
populations, J. Clin. Inv. 35, 1074.

Ballet, J. J. and E. Merler, 1976, The separation and reactivity
in vitro of a separation of a subpopulation of human lymphocytes which bind histamine. Correlation of histamine reactivity
with cellular maturation, Cellular Immunol. 24, 250.

Bösing-Schneider, R. and M. Hang, 1976, Role of cyclic AMP on
differentiation of T- and B-lymphocytes during the immune induction, Cellular Immunol. 27, 121.

Brown, B. L., J. D. M. Albano, R. P. Ekins and A. M. Sgherzi,
1971, A simple and sensitive saturation assay method for the
measurement of adenosine 3:5'-cyclic monophosphate, Biochem.
J. 121, 561.

Burne, H. R., L. M. Lichtenstein, K. L. Melmon, C. S. Henney, Y.
Weinstein and G. M. Shearer, 19 74, Modulation of inflammation and immunity by cyclic AMP, Science 184, 19.

Cross, M. E. and M. G. Ord, 1971, Changes in histone phosphoryla-
tion and associated early metabolic events in pig lymphocyte
cultures transformed by phytohaemagglutinin or 6-N, 2'-0-
dibutyryl-adenosine 3',5'-cyclic monophosphate, Biochem. J.
124, 241.

De Ruberts, F. R., T. V. Zenser, W. H. Adler and T. Hudson, 1974,
Role of cyclic adenosine 3',5'-monophosphate in lymphocyte
mitogenesis, 113, 151.

Gilman, A. G., 1970, A protein binding assay for adenosine 3',5'-
cyclic monophosphate, Proc.Natl. Acad. Sci. 67, 305.

Hadden, J. W., E. M. Hadden, M. K. Haddox and N. D. Goldberg,
1972, Guanosine 3',5'-cyclic monophosphate: a possible intracellular mediator of mitogenic influences in lymphocytes, Proc.
Nat. Acad. Sci. 69, 3024.

Henney, C. S. and L. M. Lichtenstein, 1971, The role of cyclic
AMP in the cytolytic activity of lymphocytes, J. Immunol. 107,
610.

Julius, M. E., E. Simpsone and L. A. Herzberg, 1973, A rapid
method for the isolation of functional thymus-derived murine
lymphocytes, Eur. J. Immunol. 3, 645.

Lichtenstein, L. M. and E. Gilespie, 1973, Inhibition of histamine release by histamine controlled by H_2 receptor, Nature
244, 287.

MacManus, J. P. and J. F. Whitfield, 1970, Stimulation of DNA synthesis and mitotic activity of thymic lymphocytes by cyclic adenosine 3',5'-monophosphate, Exp. Cell Res. 58, 188.

Makman, M. H. and M. I. Klein, 1972, Expression of adenylate cyclase, catecholamine receptor, and cyclic adenosine monophosphate-dependent protein kinase in synchronized culture of Chang's liver cells, Proc. Natl. Acad. Sci. 69, 456.

Novogrodsky, A. and E. Katchalski, 1970, Effect of phytohemagglutinin and prostaglandins on cyclic AMP synthesis in rat lymph node lymphocytes, Biochem. Biophys. Acta. 215, 291.

Plaut, M., L. M. Lichtenstein, E. Gillespie and C. S. Henney, 1973, Studies on the mechanism of lymphocyte-mediated cytolysis, IV. Specificity of the histamine receptor on effector T cells, J. Immunol. 111, 389.

Rocklin, R. E., 1976, Modulation of cellular-immune responses in vivo and in vitro by histamine receptor-bearing lymphocytes, J. Clin. Invest. 57, 1051.

Roszkowski, W., M. Plaut and L. M. Lichtenstein, 1976, Selective display of histamine receptors on lymphocytes, Science 195, 683.

Smith, J. W., A. L. Steiner, W. M. Newberry and C. W. Parker, 1971, Cyclic adenosine 3',5'-monophosphate in human lymphocytes, Alterations after phytohemagglutinin stimulation, J. Clin. Invest. 50, 432.

Smith, J. W., A. L. Steiner and C. W. Parker, 1971, Human lymphocyte metabolism. Effects of cyclic and noncyclic nucleotides on stimulation by phytohemagglutinin, J. Clin. Invest. 50, 442.

Sullivan, T. J., K. L. Parker, W. Stenson and C. W. Parker, 1975, Modulation of cyclic AMP in purified rat mast cells, I. Responses to pharmacologic, metabolic, and physiol stimuli, J. Immunol. 114, 1473.

Teh, H.-S. and V. Paetkau, 1976, Regulation of immune responses, I. Effects of cyclic AMP and cyclic GMP on immune induction, Cellular Immunol. 24, 209.

Vischer, T. L., 1976, The differential effect of cyclic AMP on lymphocyte stimulation by T- or B-cell mitogens, Immunol. 30, 735.

Wang, S. R. and B. Zweiman, 1978, Histamine suppression of human lymphocyte responses to mitogens, Cellular Immunol. 36, 28.

Watson, J., 1976, The involvement of cyclic nucleotide metabolism in the initiation of lymphocyte proliferation induced by mitogens, J. Immunol. 117, 1656.

MECHANISM OF SUBSTANCE P-INDUCED SALIVARY SECRETION IN RATS

Inoki, R., Kudo, T., Kotani, Y., Oka, M., Iwatsubo, K.
and Matsumoto, K.

Department of Pharmacology, Osaka University Dental
School, Osaka 530, Japan

Leeman and Hammerschlag (1,2) found a potent sialogogic substance in the rough extract from bovine or rat hypothalamus.
This sialogogue has been known to be substance P itself. Although
substance P (SP), one of tachykinins, has been recognized as a
neurotransmitter (3,4) or a modulator (5,6) of the primary sensory
neurone, mechanism of sialogogic action of this substance still
remained undissolved.

Leeman and Hammerschlag (2) also demonstrated that SP-induced
salivary secretion was not influenced at all by the pretreatment
with atropine, phenoxybenzamine and propranolol, but by vasopress-
in. They concluded that SP played a role as a neurohormone in
the secretory mechanism of the saliva other than in the autonomic
nervous system. Hökfelt et al. (7) demonstrated that SP-like
immunoreactivity was found in the salivary glands or in the nasal
mucosa of the rat and that these fibers could be observed in relation to secretory elements.

The present study was carried out to investigate mechanism of
SP-induced salivary secretion; that is, changes in salivary flow
and amylase secretion induced by synthetic SP were observed after
some treatments with pharmacological agonists or antagonists in
rats.

METHODS

One hundred and twenty male Wistar strain rats, weighing 200-
300 g, were used. Five to seven animals in a group were usually
employed. The animals were anesthetized with 1.5 g/kg of urethane and the bronchus was cannulated for artificial respiration.

The artificial respiration was controlled against over-ventilation by occasional measurement of blood CO_2. SP and other drugs, unless stated otherwise, were injected via a polyethylene tubing, which was cannulated into the femoral vein. For ventricular administration of SP, animals were fixed on a brain stereotaxic apparatus and scalp was incised to expose a frontoparietal part of skull. A hole, 2 mm in a diameter, was drilled at the cross point of 3 mm line after Bregma and 2 mm line of either side from sagittal line. A small polyethylene tubing was inserted into the hole to 4-5 mm deep from the surface of the skull and was fixed with an instant adhesive. SP was usually administered through this cannula. Animals were placed on the abdominal position.

For the collection of saliva, 3-5 pieces of small cotton globes, which were weighed beforehand, were placed into the oral cavity just before SP administration. These cotton globes were taken out 15 min after the SP administration in order to weigh the wet cotton globes. Weight increase of cotton globes was regarded as secreted salivary volume. Recovery in this method was about 85 % when a relative humidity in the experimental room was 60 %.

For measurement of amylase activity in saliva, the wet cotton globes above mentioned was put in the test tube and the secreted saliva was diluted 1000-2000 fold with distilled water. Amylase activity was measured by blue starch method. Zero point one ml of the diluted saliva was preincubated with 4.0 ml of distilled water for 5 min at 37 °C. One blue starch tablet (Amylase Test Shionogi) was added and then the tablet was broken down by hard shaking of the test tube. After 30 min incubation at 37 °C, reaction was stopped by 0.5M NaOH and the mixture was filtrated by negative pressure. Amylase activity in the filtrate was spectrophotometrically measured at 620 nm wave length.

Approximate ED_{50} of synthetic SP, 5 µg/kg, was administered intravenously at 30 min intervals. The first 2 SP responses were regarded as control. Ten min before the third administration of SP, pharmacological agonists or antagonists were administered intravenously or intraperitoneally and effect of the drugs was obtained from the consecutive 3 SP responses. In the Tables, effects of drugs on SP responses were demonstrated in % of control.

MATERIALS

Drugs used in this study were as follows; synthetic SP (Protein Research Foundation, Mino, Osaka), atropine sulfate (Nakarai Chemicals, Kyoto), alcuronium chloride (Roche, Basel), d-tubocurarine chloride (Yoshitomi, Osaka), hexamethonium bromide (Yamano-

uchi, Tokyo), baclofen (Ciba-Geigy, Basel), phenoxybenzamine hydrochloride (Nakarai Chemicals, Kyoto), phentolamine mesylate (Ciba-
Geigy, Basel), No. 865-123 (4-7-exo-methylene-hexahydroisoindoline
-ethyl-guanidine hemisulfate; Eisai, Tokyo), propranolol hydrochloride (Kowa, Nagoya), isoproterenol hydrochloride (Nikken, Tokyo), prostaglandin E_2 (Ono, Osaka), arachidonic acid (Sigma, St.
Louis) and indomethacin(Sumitomo, Osaka).

All powder drugs, except arachidonic acid were dissolved in
Ringer solution, Arachidonic acid was dissolved in 10 µl/ml of
100 mM Na_2CO_3 solution.

RESULTS AND CONCLUSION

1. Intravenously or Intraventricularly Administered SP-
    Induced Salivary and Amylase Secretions

Intraventricularly administered SP-induced salivary and amylase secretions were much less than intravenously administered SP responses. In comparison of the same dose of SP (5 µg/kg),
the latter responses were 1/10 in salivary secretion and 1/20 in
amylase secretion to the former responses (P<0.05, t test).

2. Effect of Baclofen on SP-Induced Salivary and Amylase
    Secretions

In pretreatment with baclofen (5 mg/kg, i.v.), significant
decrease in SP-induced salivary secretion was observed. The SP-
induced salivary secretion was gradually decreased. Significant
decrease, about 40 % of control was observed at 40-70 min after
the baclofen. On the other hand, SP-induced amylase secretion
was increased rather than decreased (Table 1).

3. Effects of Cholinergic Blocking Agents on SP-Induced
    Salivary and Amylase Secretions

Salivary secretion: Atropine (2 mg/kg, i.v.) inhibited significantly SP-induced salivary secretion 40 min after the administration. The larger dose of atropine was administered, the soon-
er inhibition was observed. d-Tubocurarine (2 mg/kg, i.v.) and
alcuronium (2 mg/kg, i.v.) either inhibited SP-induced salivary
secretion. However, d-tubocurarine showed an early inhibition,
but alcuronium a delayed one. Hexamethonium (3 mg/kg, i.v.) had
no inhibition on SP-induced salivary secretion.

Amylase secretion: Atropine (2-10 mg/kg, i.v.) did not show
any inhibition on SP-induced amylase secretion. d-Tubocurarine
(2 mg/kg, i.v.) and alcuronium (2 mg/kg, i.v.) had no inhibition
on SP-induced amylase secretion (Table 2).

Table 1. Effects of baclofen on SP-induced salivary and amylase secretions

Responses induced by substance P

Time after administration (i.v.) of baclofen

	Before	10	40	70 (min)
Salivary secretion:				
Ringer solution	100	91.3 ± 9.9	95.9 ± 17.2	101.6 ± 29.8
Baclofen (5 mg/kg)		73.3 ± 5.0	54.2 ± 13.3*	58.5 ± 10.9*
Amylase secretion:				
Ringer solution	100	98.4 ± 33.1	105.9 ± 26.9	86.5 ± 19.1
Baclofen (5 mg/kg)		171.4 ± 46.9	137.9 ± 31.6	169.7 ± 72.1

Each value represents the mean ± S.D. of % of control. Salivary and amylase secretions induced by the 2nd injection of SP before drug administration are expressed as 100, respectively. * P <0.05. SP was administered five times intravenously in dose of 5 µg/kg 2 times before and 3 times, 10, 40 and 70 min after drug administration at 30 min intervals.

Table 2. Effects of anticholinergic agents on SP-induced salivary and Amylase secretions

Responses induced by substance P

Time after administration (i.v.) of anticholinergic agents

	Before	10	40	70 (min)
Salivary secretion:				
Ringer solution	100	91.3 ± 9.9	95.9 ± 17.2	101.6 ± 29.8
Atropine (2 mg/kg)		64.4 ± 17.2	55.8 ± 20.0*	61.3 ± 14.1
Atropine (10 mg/kg)		44.4 ± 16.8*	39.5 ± 6.2*	80.3 ± 15.8
Alcuronium (2 mg/kg)		74.5 ± 13.7	45.8 ± 18.1*	34.1 ± 18.4*
d-Tubocurarine (2 mg/kg)		46.6 ± 22.4*	63.7 ± 20.3	61.5 ± 27.6
Hexamethonium (3 mg/kg)		106.4 ± 7.4	114.3 ± 19.9	---
Amylase secretion:				
Ringer solution	100	98.4 ± 33.1	105.9 ± 26.9	86.5 ± 19.1
Atropine (2 mg/kg)		66.8 ± 12.1	72.7 ± 13.1	80.1 ± 23.3
Atropine (10 mg/kg)		69.8 ± 12.1	79.6 ± 23.2	106.0 ± 11.4
Alcuronium (2 mg/kg)		79.5 ± 22.4	83.4 ± 18.1	110.8 ± 43.4
d-Tubocurarine (2 mg/kg)		107.9 ± 29.0	128.9 ± 68.0	111.7 ± 20.7

Each value represents the mean ± S.D. of % of control. Salivary and amylase secretions induced by the 2nd injection of SP before drug administration are expressed as 100, respectively. * P <0.05. SP was administered five times intravenously in dose of 5 μg/kg, 2 times before and 3 times, 10, 40 and 70 min after drug administration at 30 min intervals.

4. Effects of Adrenergic Blocking Agents on SP-Induced
    Salivary and Amylase secretions

Salivary secretion: Phenoxybenzamine (10 mg/kg, i.v.) and
phentolamine (5 mg/kg, i.v.) did not show any significant changes
in SP-induced salivary secretion. Propranolol, single injection
(100 µg/kg, i.v.) and three time injections just before each SP
administration, did not show any inhibition on SP-induced salivary
secretion.

Amylase secretion: Both phenoxybenzamine (10 mg/kg, i.v.)
and phentolamine (5 mg/kg, i.v.) showed a remarkable and durable
increase in SP-induced amylase secretion. On the other hand,
propranolol, single injection (100 µg/kg, i.v.) and three time
injections just before each SP administration either showed no
significant change in SP-induced amylase secretion, but the durable increase by phenoxybenzamine (10 mg/kg, i.v.) in SP-induced
amylase secretion was completely inhibited by 100 µg/kg of propranolol administered just before SP administration(Table 3).

5. Effects of Adrenergic Neuron Blocking Agent on SP-
    Induced Salivary and Amylase Secretions

No. 865-123 (15 mg/kg, i.v.) had no effect on SP-induced
salivary secretion, but it showed significant increase in SP-induced amylase secretion 10, 40 and 70 min after the drug administration (Table 4).

6. Effects of Adrenergic Agents on SP-Induced Salivary
    and Amylase Secretions

Salivary secretion: Phenylephrine (50 µg/kg, i.v.) remarkably inhibited SP-induced salivary secretion. However, isoproterenol (1 µg/kg, i.v.) did not inhibit SP-induced secretion
even when administered immediately before each SP administration.

Amylase secretion: Pheylephrine (50 µg/kg, i.v.) did not
inhibit SP-induced amylase secretion significantly, though the
amylase secretion was inclined to be reduced. On the other hand,
isoproterenol (1 µg/kg, i.v.) remarkably increased the SP-induced
amylase secretion whenever it was administered just before each
SP administration. This increase was very significant from control (Table 5).

7. Effect of Prostaglandin E_2 and Arachidonic Acid on SP-
    Induced Salivary and Amylase Secretions

Salivary secretion: Prostaglandin E_2(10 µg/kg, i.v.) significantly inhibited SP-induced salivary secretion, This effect

Table 3. Effects of adrenergic blocking agents on SP-induced salivary and amylase secretions

Responses induced by substance P
Time after administration (i.v.) of adrenergic blocking agents

	Before	10	40	70 (min)
Salivary secretion:				
Ringer solution	100	91.3 ± 9.9	95.9 ± 17.2	101.6 ± 29.8
Phenoxybenzamine (10 mg/kg)		89.9 ± 41.2	87.9 ± 18.0	98.9 ± 17.2
Phentolamine (5 mg/kg)		79.3 ± 28.0	79.3 ± 38.4	70.4 ± 19.1
Propranolol (100 µg/kg)		89.9 ± 15.0	82.9 ± 9.7	84.3 ± 24.0
Propranolol (3 x 100 µg/kg)		81.1 ± 31.6	90.1 ± 29.1	91.9 ± 30.4
Phenoxybenzamine + Propranolol		69.7 ± 17.8	91.2 ± 29.7	74.8 ± 24.6
Amylase secretion:				
Ringer solution	100	98.4 ± 33.1	105.9 ± 26.9	86.5 ± 19.1
Phenoxybenzamine (10 mg/kg)		138.3 ± 39.4	527.2 ± 54.8**	872.5 ± 57.5**
Phentolamine (5 mg/kg)		167.9 ± 39.4*	231.3 ± 43.5***	210.5 ± 37.8**
Propranolol (100 µg/kg)		104.3 ± 7.5	84.2 ± 28.3	63.9 ± 13.3
Propranolol (3 x 100 µg/kg)		98.4 ± 42.9	88.1 ± 26.7	81.9 ± 42.7
Phenoxybenzamine + Propranolol		56.4 ± 13.1	60.1 ± 15.4	66.7 ± 26.2

Each value represents the mean ± S.D. of % of control. Salivary and amylase secretions induced by the 2nd injection of SP before drug administration are expressed as 100, respectively. * $P < 0.05$, ** $P < 0.01$. SP was administered five times intravenously in dose of 5 µg/kg, 2 times before and 3 times, 10, 40 and 70 min after drug administration at 30 intervals. Propranolol (3 x 100 µg/kg) was administered in dose of 100 µg/kg three times 5 min before the 3rd, 4th and 5th injections of SP.

Table 4. Effects of No. 865–123 on SP-induced salivary and amylase secretions

Responses induced by substance P

Time after administration (i.v.) of No. 876–123

	Before	10	40	70 (min)
Salivary secretion:				
Ringer solution	100	91.3 ± 9.9	95.9 ± 17.2	101.6 ± 29.8
No. 865–123 (15 mg/kg)		101.3 ± 36.8	121.5 ± 50.0	95.1 ± 2.6
Amylase secretion:				
Ringer solution	100	98.4 ± 33.1	105.9 ± 26.9	86.5 ± 19.1
No. 865–123 (15 mg/kg)		190.5 ± 21.3*	736.2 ± 96.2**	1198.7 ± 42.0**

Each value represents the mean ± S.D. of % of control. Salivary and amylase secretions induced by the 2nd injection of SP before drug administration are expressed as 100, respectively. * P <0.05,** P <0.01. SP was administered five times intravenously in dose of 5 μg/kg, 2 times before and 3 times, 10, 40 and 70 min after drug administration at 30 min intervals.

Table 5. Effects of adrenergic agents on SP-induced salivary and amylase secretions

Responses induced by substance P

Time after administration (i.v.) of adrenergic agents

	Before	10	40	70 (min)
Salivary secretion:				
Ringer solution	100	91.3 ± 9.9	95.9 ± 17.2	101.6 ± 29.8
Phenylephrine (50 µg/kg)		30.6 ± 9.9**	63.7 ± 13.3*	60.5 ± 16.1
Isoproterenol (3 x 1 µg/kg)		96.6 ± 40.7	86.0 ± 10.7	70.5 ± 8.7
Amylase secretion:				
Ringer solution	100	98.4 ± 33.1	105.9 ± 26.9	86.5 ± 19.1
Phenylephrine (50 µg/kg)		53.2 ± 19.6	113.7 ± 18.6	112.5 ± 57.9
Isoproterenol (3 x 1 µg/kg)		218.4 ± 31.9**	344.4 ± 56.2**	366.2 ±106.8*

Each value represents the mean ± S.D. of % of control. Salivary and amylase secretions induced by the 2nd injection of SP before drug administration are expressed as 100, respectively. * P <0.05, ** P <0.01. SP was administered five times intravenously in dose of 5 µg/kg, 2 times before and 3 times, 10, 40 and 70 min after drug administration at 30 min intervals. Isoproterenol (3 x 1 µg/kg) was administered in dose of 1 µg/kg three times 5min before the 3rd, 4th and 5th injections of SP.

Table 6. Effects of prostaglandin E_2, arachidonic acid and indomethacin on SP-induced salivary and amylase secretions

| | Responses induced by substance P | | | |
	Before	10	40	70 (min)
Salivary secretion:		Time after administration (i.v.) of PG E_2 and arachidonic acid		
Ringer solution	100	91.3 ± 9.9	95.9 ± 17.2	101.6 ± 29.8
Prostaglandin E_2 (10 µg/kg)		52.8 ± 21.5*	77.1 ± 36.8	115.2 ± 28.9
Arachidonic acid (400 µg/kg)		170.6 ± 35.0*	207.6 ± 58.6*	150.3 ± 15.0*
Indomethacin (5 mg/kg)		131.5 ± 22.8*	133.8 ± 32.8	115.8 ± 29.9
Indomethacin + Arachidonic acid		133.5 ± 32.8	138.3 ± 49.8	120.0 ± 38.9
Amylase secretion:				
Ringer solution	100	98.4 ± 33.1	105.9 ± 26.9	86.5 ± 19.1
Prostaglandin E_2 (10 µg/kg)		110.3 ± 24.4	130.4 ± 24.4	135.2 ± 23.0
Arachidonic acid (400 µg/kg)		128.4 ± 3.6	125.8 ± 34.3	122.2 ± 29.1
Indomethacin (5 mg/kg)		119.5 ± 25.6	105.5 ± 21.8	100.2 ± 48.6
Indomethacin + Arachidonic acid		99.4 ± 27.3	111.9 ± 67.2	97.4 ± 61.9

Each value represents the mean ± S.D. in % of control. Salivary and amylase secretions induced by the 2nd injection of SP before drug administration are expressed as 100,respectively. * P<0.05. SP was administered five times intravenously in dose of 5 µg/kg, 2 times before and 3 times, 10, 40 and 70 min after drug administration at 30 min intervals. In the case of Indomethacin, it was administered intraperitoneally 15 min before the 3rd injection of SP.

was observed 10 min after the drug administration. On the other hand, arachidonic acid (400 µg/kg, i.v.) remarkably increased the SP-induced salivary secretion 10, 40 and 70 min after the drug administration.   Indomethacin (5 mg/kg, i.p.) also showed a remarkable increase in the SP-induced salivary secretion.   Increase in SP-induced salivary secretion by arachidonic acid was shown more predominantly than that by indomethacin.   When arachidonic acid (400 µg/kg, i.v.) was administered after the indomethacin administration, the increasing effect of arachidonic acid on SP-induced salivary secretion could not be observed and the salivary secretion became the similar increase by indomethacin alone.

Amylase secretion: Prostaglandin E_2 (10 µg/kg, i.V.), arachidonic acid (400 µg/kg, i.v.), indomethacin (5 mg/kg, i.p.) and indomethacin plus arachidonic acid did not show any influence on the SP-induced amylase secretion (Table 6).

From these results, the followings were concluded; 1) SP-induced salivary and amylase secretions were involved in the peripheral mechanism not including the central one.   2) SP stimulates not only cholinergic, nicotinic and adrenergic α-receptors, but also another type of receptor, if so-called, as SP-receptor.   3) Enhancement of SP-induced amylase secretion by adrenergic α-blockers may be caused by increasing release of noradrenaline from nerve terminals due to the blockade of the presynaptic adrenergic α-receptor, by which an excitement of postsynaptic adrenergic β-receptor is followed.   In addition, modulation by prostaglandin system of SP-induced salivary secretion was suggested.

REFERENCES

1. Hammerschlag, R. and Leeman, S.E., 1966, Induction of salivation a bovine hypothalamic factor, Fed. Proc. 25, 192.

2. Leeman, S.E. and Hammerschlag, R., 1967, Stimulation of salivary secretion by a factor extracted from hypothalamic tissue, Endocrinol. 81, 803.

3. Lembeck, F.N.S., 1953, Zur Frage der zentralen Übertragung afferenter Impulse.   Das Vorkommen und die Bedeutung der Substanz P in den dorsalen Wurzeln des Rückenmarks, Arch. Pharmacol. 219, 197.

4. Otsuka, M. and Konishi, S., 1976, Substance P and Excitatory transmitter of primary sensory neurons, Cold Spring Harbor Symp. Quant. Biol. XL, 135.

5. Krivoy, W., Lane, M. and Kroeger, D., 1963, The actions of certain polypeptides on synaptic transmission, Ann N. Y. Acad. Sci. 104, 312.

6. Hedqvist, P. and von Euler, U.S., 1977, Effects of substance
    P on some autonomic neuroeffector junctions, in Substance P
    eds. U.S.von Euler and B. Pernow (Raven Press, New York) p. 89.

7. Hökfelt, T., Johansson, O., Kellerth, J.-O., Ljungdahl, Å.,
    Nilsson, G., Nygårds, A. and Pernow, B., 1977, Immunohistochem-
    ical distribution of substance P, in Substance P eds. U.S. von
    Euler and B. Pernow (Raven Press, New York) p. 117.

IMMUNOPHARMACOLOGICAL STUDY OF FORSSMAN SHOCK IN GUINEA PIGS

Hiroichi Nagai and Akihide Koda

Department of Pharmacology, Gifu College of Pharmacy

Mitahora-higashi 5-6-1, Gifu, Gifu, Japan

It has been generally known that similar anaphylactic systemic shock is caused by injection of anti-sheep erythrocyte antibody into guinea pigs. This shock is so-called Forssman shock (FS) because the reaction resulted from the combination of anti-sheep erythrocyte antibody including Forssman antibody and Forssman antigen which exists at the endothelium of capillaries in guinea pigs. The present study was conducted to search for a human disease that is similar to this reaction and the mechanisms of the shock. First of all, the changes of blood components were examined during the shock. Blood cell count, enzyme activity and other components were tested. The results are summarized in Table 1.

Marked drops in CH_{50}, leucocyte count and platelet count and incoagulability of blood are observed. Lactate dehydrogenase activity is slightly increased. Esterase activity and fibrinogen amount are decreased by shock. In addition to the above evidences, smooth muscle contracting substance in serum is diminished after the shock. These observations suggest the similarity of FS in guinea pigs and disseminated intravascular incoagulability (DIC) syndrome in humans. DIC is a bleeding disorder resulting from excessive intravascular clotting with depletion of platelets, fibrinogen and other procoagulants. As a primary event, infectious agents may act, perhaps through immunological mechanisms, to cause this syndrome. Decrease of platelet count, fibrinogen amount and complement level are seen in both reactions. Furthermore, both reactions are caused by immunological injury mechanisms. From the above evidences, the mechanism of FS was investigated by means of the effect of drugs. The effect of drugs on FS is summarized in Table 2.

Table 1   Changes of blood components in
guinea pigs subjected to Forssman shock.

Item		Before	After
Blood cell	White ($\times$ 100)	53.3 $\pm$ 2.80	12.1 $\pm$ 1.26*
	Red ($10^5/mm^3$)	58.2 $\pm$ 3.32	60.0 $\pm$ 3.07
	Platelet ($10^3/mm^3$)	309.2 $\pm$ 44.42	146.3 $\pm$ 27.22*
Enzyme	Complement (CH_{50} U)	205.6 $\pm$ 7.35	157.9 $\pm$ 18.22*
	LDH (U/ℓ)	297.9 $\pm$ 56.34	540.6 $\pm$ 95.48
	Alp ase (mM/ml, B-L)	4.2 $\pm$ 0.31	4.2 $\pm$ 0.21
	Plasmin	0	0
	Esterase activity (TaMe) (μM/ml/h)	7.3 $\pm$ 0.46	6.3 $\pm$ 0.41
Others	Coagulation time (sec)	446.8 $\pm$ 85.40	3572.0 $\pm$ 496.70*
	Fibrinogen (mg/dℓ)	54.1 $\pm$ 6.84	35.9 $\pm$ 7.12
	Smooth muscle contraction	+	—

Each value indicates mean $\pm$ S.E. of 5 animals.
*: Significant from before value at $p < 0.05$.

Table 2   Summary of drug action of Forssman shock

Drug	Action	Forssman shock Symp.	Co-time	C'	WBC	pl.
Control		III	↑	↓	↓	↓
Heparin	Incoagulability	III	↑	↓	↓	↓
Ara C	Decrease of WBC	III	↑	↓	→	→
Colchicine	Inhibition of WBC and platelet	III	→	↓	→	→
Cobra venom factor	Inhibition of C'3 activity	I	→	→	→	→
CCAq	Inhibition of classical pathway	II	↑	→~↓	↓	↓
Cu-chlorphyll	Inhibition of C'2,4 and 5	II	↑	↓	↓	↓
Trasyrol	Inhibition of protease	III	↑	↓	↓	↓
Homochlorcyclizine	Anti-histamine and kinin	III	↑	↓	↓	↓
Chlorpheniramine	Anti-histamine	III	↑	↓	↓	↓
Theophylline	Elevation of c-AMP	III	↑	↓	↓	↓
Isoproterenol	Elevation of c-AMP	III	↑	↓	↓	↓

When 1,000 and 10,000 U/kg heparin was administered by intra-peritoneal injection 1 hr prior to challenge, remarkable prolongation of blood coagulation time is observed. At the same time, other components do not change. Under such conditions, Forssman antibody was challenged. FS and changes of blood components were not pre-vented at all. From the experiments of heparin, incoagulability in FS is the result but not the cause of shock.

Regarding the role of white blood cell and platelet, the effect of citocin arabinoside (Ara C) and colchicine were examined. Daily subcutaneous injections of 37.5 and 70 mg/kg/day Ara C for 5 days resulted in leucopenia in guinea pigs without changes of other blood components. But, FS was not affected by Ara C. The administration of colchicine did not influence the changes of any components in normal guinea pigs. Also, FS was not prevented by administration of 5 and 10 mg/kg colchicine 3 hours before challenge. Under the same conditions, the movement of white blood cell and platelet were interferred in another experiment. These results suggest that a role of white blood cell and platelet in FS is the secondary reaction following the triggering events.

Next, experiments were conducted to search for the role of complement in FS. A potent complement inhibitor, cobra venom factor (CoVF) decrease CH_{50} unit in serum. By intraperitoneal injection of 100 and 200 U/kg CoVF, FS was completely inhibited. Slight shock symptoms and blood component changes were observed. There also appeared clear inhibition when Cu-chlorophyll and aqueous extract of Cinnamomi cassia which inhibit complement activity in vitro were administered intraperitoneally 1 hr prior to challenge. These findings confirm the important role of complement and suggest the triggering mechanism of FS by complement systems.

Concerning the role of kinins in FS, the effect of trasylol, an inhibitor of kallikrein and homochlorcyclizine, kinin antagonist on FS was examined. Their inhibitory effect on FS was not observed. Since esterase activity decreased and kinin-like substance dis-appeared after the shock, contribution of kinin-system to FS was expected. However, the above findings suggest that a role of kinin in FS is uncertain.

In order to compare the mechanisms of anaphylactic shock, the effect of chlorpheniramine, isoproterenol and theophyllin on FS was tested. When each 5 mg/kg drug was administered, IgE mediated anaphylactic shock was prevented. But the same dose of drug was administered, and FS was not inhibited.

A conclusion of the present study, FS was initiated by combi-nation of antigen and antibody at capillary walls with complement activation and following activation of white blood cell and plate-let system. And then as a last event, incoagulability of blood is

induced. There is not, however, included in mediator release
mechanisms or cyclic nucleotides modulation just like IgE mediated
anaphylaxis.

SIGNIFICANCE OF ADRENERGIC α-EFFECT ON SALIVARY KALLIKREIN SECRETION IN THE SUBMANDIBULAR GLAND OF THE DOG

T.Kudo, Y.Kotani, M.Oka, K.Matsumoto and R.Inoki

Department of Pharmacology, Osaka University Dental

School, Osaka, Japan

ABSTRACT

The effects of the sympathetic nerve stimulation and the administrations of sympathomimetics on the secretion of salivary kallikrein induced by the chorda tympani stimulation were examined quantitatively and qualitatively in the submandibular gland of the dog. The secretion of salivary kallikrein may be mediated through both adrenergic α- and β-receptors. The activities of salivary kallikrein secreted by either the chorda tympani stimulation or isoproterenol were not inhibited by soy bean trypsin inhibitor in vitro, but those secreted by the sympathetic nerve stimulation and noradrenaline or adrenaline were markedly inhibited in vitro. These results suggested that secretion of glandular kallikrein was induced by the chorda tympani stimulation and the sympathetic β-stimulation, and secretion of plasma kallikrein was induced by the sympathetic α-stimulation.

INTRODUCTION

It is well known that salivary kallikrein is released not only by parasympathetic nerve stimulation, but also by sympathetic nerve stimulation from salivary gland. In the estimation of kallikrein content in the cat submandibular gland, Beilenson et al(1968) showed that kallikrein content in the gland rapidly reduced when both chorda tympani and sympathetic nerve were stimulated simultaneously, while there was no difference in kallikrein content between the gland which chorda tympani alone was stimulated and the control gland. Gautvik et al(1969, 1972a, 1972b) also showed a similar result to that obtained by Beilenson et al. Further study done by Gautvik et al(1974) showed that the secretion of salivary kallikrein in the cat submandibular gland was mediated only through the sympathetic α-receptor.

The present study was aimed to investigate the effects of sympathetic nerve stimulation and sympathomimetic agents on the activity of salivary kallikrein secreted by the chorda tympani stimulation in the submandibular gland of the dog.

MATERIALS AND METHODS

1. Collection of Saliva

Male and female healthy mongrel dogs, weighing 8 to 12 kg, anesthetized with pentobarbital sodium(35 mg/kg,i.p.) were fixed at dorsal position. Wharton's duct, chorda tympani and cervical sympathetic nerve on the left side were exposed. Wharton's duct was then cannulated with the glass tubing(outside diameter: 1mm) jointed with a polyethylene tubing. Chorda tympani and cervical sympathetic nerve were placed on platinum bipolar electrodes respectively and stimulated using electronic stimulators. Chorda tympani was stimulated with the square wave(frequency 5-100 Hz, duration 1 msec, voltage 1.5-5 V) and cervical sympathetic nerve was stimulated with the square wave(frequency 20 Hz, duration 1 msec, minimum voltage by which mydriasis was able to observe). Administrations of drugs were performed via vein of the foreleg.

Each drop of saliva secreted by the chorda tympani stimulation was recorded on a polygraph, and after the removal of the initial 7 drops(corresponding to a dead space of the tubing), each 8 drops was collected into a siliconized glass test tube as one fraction. Twenty fractions of saliva were successively collected in most experiments. Sympathetic nerve stimulation, increasing voltage for the chorda tympani stimulation and the drug administration were usually performed immediately before the No.8 fraction was collected.

2. Bioassay for Salivary Kallikrein Activity

In measurement of the salivary kallikrein activity, canine citrated plasma which was incubated at 56 °C for 3 hours following centrifugation at 3,000 rpm for 10 min was used as kininogen, and each fraction of saliva diluted 10-fold with saline was used as salivary kallikrein.

Ten µl of the diluted saliva was added to 0.1 ml of the citrated plasma and this mixture was incubated immediately at 36 °C for 1 min. After the incubation, 10 µl of the mixture was applied to a rat uterine muscle strip which was suspended in the bath(bath volume 2 ml). De Jalon's solution at 30 °C, pH 7.4, containing each 10^{-6} g/ml of chlorpheniramine maleate, tryptamine hydrochloride and atropine sulfate was used as bath solution. The kallikrein activities of the fractions were estimated from the contraction of the rat uterine muscle due to kinin which was yielded after the incubation, in reference to the contraction due to the known concentration of synthetic bradykinin.

RESULTS

1. Effects of Chorda tympani Stimulation on Secretion
   of Salivary Kallikrein and Flow Rate of Saliva

A. <u>Change in Frequency of Electric Stimulation.</u>   Among the
stimulus parameters(duration 1 msec, voltage 1.5 V) only frequency
was changed. The secretion of salivary kallikrein and the flow rate
of saliva under different frequencies of 5, 20, 50 and 100 Hz were
examined respectively.
    The salivary kallikrein showed generally a high activity at the
initial stage of the stimulation and then the activity was gradually
reduced to a steady state at No.7 fraction. This tendency was accelerated with higher frequencies of the stimulation and the steady
state came sooner(Fig.1,Upper). Kallikrein activity at the steady
state and the flow rate of saliva showed the highest value at 20 Hz.
Thus, in further experiments, the chorda tympani stimulation was
always performed with 20 Hz frequency and 1 msec duration. Sympathetic nerve stimulation, increasing the voltage of the chorda tympani stimulation and the administrations of drugs were performed at
the time of No.8 fraction after the secretion of salivary kallikrein
arrived at the steady state.

B. <u>Change in Voltage of Chorda tympani Stimulation.</u>   Under
the chorda tympani stimulation(duration 1 msec, frequency 20 Hz),
only the voltage was rapidly increased from 1.5 to 3 V at the time
of No.8 fraction, resulting in an increased salivary kallikrein
activity and an increased flow rate of saliva(Fig.1,Lower).

2. Effects of Sympathetic Nerve Stimulation on Secretion
   of Salivary Kallikrein and Flow Rate of Saliva

    Under the chorda tympani stimulation(frequency 20 Hz, duration
1 msec, voltage 1.5 V), cervical sympathetic nerve was stimulated
electrically for 30 sec at the time of No.8 fraction(frequency 20
Hz, duration 1 msec). After the sympathetic nerve stimulation, the
salivary kallikrein activity showed a remarkable increase. The flow
rate of saliva showed a very slight and transient increase. When
phenoxybenzamine in dose of 8 mg/kg was administered intravenously
15 min before collection of No.8 fraction, the increased activity
of salivary kallikrein induced by the sympathetic nerve stimulation
was markedly inhibited. When the total activity(the integrated
value calculated from an area surrounded between the activity curve
from fraction No.9 to No.13 and 0 line) was compared before and
after phenoxybenzamine, the inhibition of 58.9 ± 6.3 % was demonstrated. When propranolol in dose of 100 μg/kg was administered
intravenously 15 min before collection of No.8 fraction, the increased activity of salivary kallikrein induced by the sympathetic
nerve stimulation was also markedly inhibited. In comparison of the
total activity before and after propranolol, the inhibition of

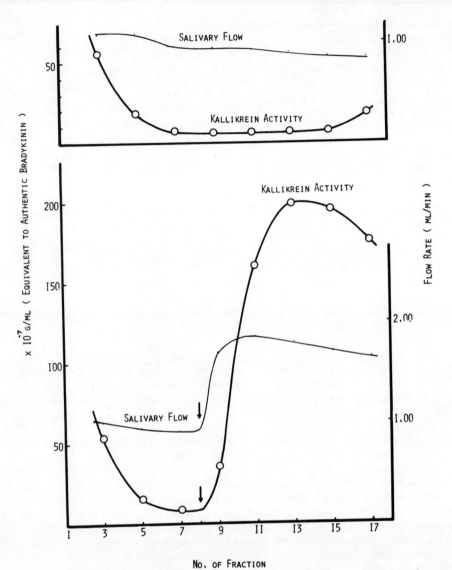

Fig.1. Modes of Salivary Flow and Kallikrein Secretion induced by Chorda tympani Stimulation. Upper: stimulus parameters;frequency 20 Hz, duration 1 msec, voltage 1.5 V. Lower: stimulus parameter; only the voltage was rapidly increased from 1.5 to 3 V at arrows. Abscissa: No. of fraction. Ordinates: left;kallikrein activity expressed as kinin(equivalent to authentic bradykinin) which was produced after the incubation under the experimental conditions in Methods. right;flow rate of saliva. In the further experiments, the total activity of kallikrein means the integrated value calculated from an area surrounded between the activity curve from fraction No.9 to No.13 and 0 line.

67.4 ± 6.8 % was observed(Figs.2 and 3).

With respect to the flow rate of saliva, the flow rate after the pretreatment with phenoxybenzamine was more strongly inclined to decrease than after propranolol. Even after the pretreatment with phenoxybenzamine or propranolol, the flow rate due to the sympathetic nerve stimulation was not so clearly influenced as kallikrein was(Fig.4).

3. Effects of Noradrenaline on Secretion of Salivary Kallikrein and Flow Rate of Saliva

Under the chorda tympani stimulation, noradrenaline in dose of 3 μg/kg was administered intravenously at the time of No.8 fraction. After noradrenaline, the salivary kallikrein activity showed a remarkable increase, but a very slight and transient increase in the flow rate of saliva was observed. After the pretreatment with phenoxybenzamine in dose of 8 mg/kg, the increased activity of salivary kallikrein induced by noradrenaline was markedly inhibited. In comparison of the total activity before and after phenoxybenzamine, the inhibition of 54.5 ± 4.8 % was observed. After the pretreatment with propranolol in dose of 100 μg/kg, the increased activity of salivary kallikrein induced by noradrenaline was also markedly inhibited. The inhibition of 63.3 ± 7.5 % was obtained when the total activity was compared before and after the administration of propranolol(Figs.2 and 3).

With respect to the flow rate of saliva, the slight decreasing effect following the very slight and transient increase due to noradrenaline was not clearly influnced by propranolol, but a little much decrease after phenoxybenzamine(Fig.4).

4. Effects of Adrenaline on Secretion of Salivary Kallikrein and Flow Rate of Saliva

Under the chorda tympani stimulation, adrenaline in dose of 3 μg/kg was also administered intravenously at the time of No.8 fraction. The salivary kallikrein activity showed a remarkable increase and a very slight and transient increase followed by a slight decrease in the flow rate of saliva was observed.

After the pretreatment with phenoxybenzamine in dose of 8 mg/kg, the increased activity of salivary kallikrein induced by adrenaline was markedly inhibited. When the total activity was compared before and after phenoxybenzamine, the inhibition of 71.0 ± 8.7 % was estimated. On the other hand, after the pretreatment with propranolol in dose of 100 μg/kg, the increased activity of salivary kallikrein induced by adrenaline was also markedly inhibited. The inhibition in the total activity was 40.7 ± 5.2 %, when the activity was compared before and after propranolol(Figs.2 and 3).

With respect to the flow rate of saliva, the effect of adrenaline was not clearly influenced after propranolol, but after phenoxybenzamine(Fig.4).

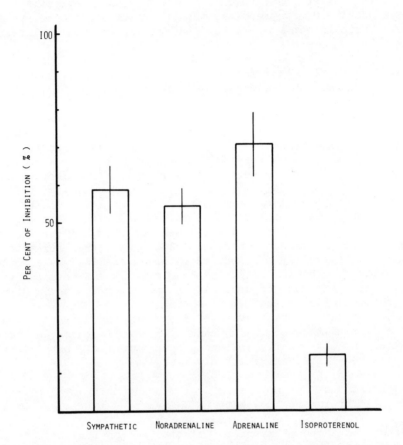

Fig.2. Inhibitions of Various Adrenergic Stimulation-induced Salivary Kallikrein Secretions by Phenoxybenzamine. Abscissa: adrenergic stimulations. Ordinate: per cent of inhibition. Adrenergic stimulus parameters: sympathetic;frequency 20 Hz, duration 1 msec, for 30 sec. Doses of noradrenaline, adrenaline and isoproterenol are 3 μg/kg,i.v., respectively. Dose of phenoxybenzamine is 8 mg/kg, i.v. The total activities of kallikrein secreted by adrenergic stimulations were compared before and after phenoxybenzamine.

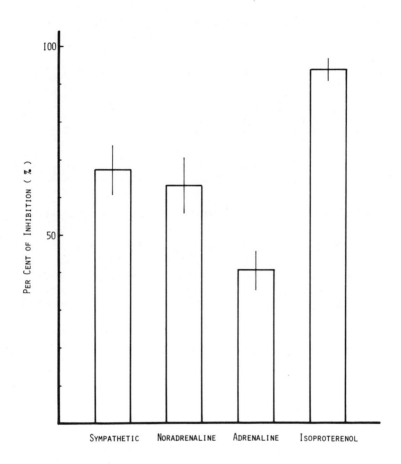

Fig.3. Inhibitions of Various Adrenergic Stimulation-induced Salivary Kallikrein Secretions by Propranolol. Abscissa: adrenergic stimulations. Ordinate: per cent of inhibition. Adrenergic stimulus parameters: as shown in Fig.2. Dose of propranolol is 100 μg/kg,i.v. The total activities of kallikrein secreted by adrenergic stimulations were compared before and after propranolol.

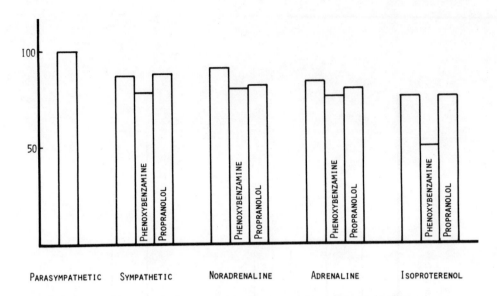

Fig.4. Influences of Various Adrenergic Stimulation-induced
Salivary Flow by Phenoxybenzamine and Propranolol. Abscissa: adrenergic stimulations. Ordinate: per cent of control expressed as
100 for the flow rate of saliva induced only by the chorda tympani
stimulation. Adrenergic stimulus parameters are as shown in Fig.2.
Doses of phenoxybenzamine and propranolol: 8 mg/kg,i.v. and 100 μg
/kg,i.v., respectively. The height of each column indicate B/A x
100 before and after phenoxybenzamine or propranolol. A is average
value from No.3 fraction to No.7 and B is average value from No.9
fraction to No.13.

5. Effects of Isoproterenol on Secretion of Salivary
   Kallikrein and Flow Rate of Saliva

Under the chorda tympani stimulation, isoproterenol in dose of
3 μg/kg was also administered intravenously. The salivary kallikrein activity showed a remarkable increase and the flow rate of
saliva was also clearly changed, as comparing with other cases.
After the pretreatment with phenoxybenzamine in dose of 8 mg/
kg, the increased activity of salivary kallikrein induced by isoproterenol was only slightly inhibited. When the total activity was
compared before and after isoproterenol, the inhibition of 14.8 ±
2.8 % was demonstrated. On the other hand, after the pretreatment
with propranolol in dose of 100 μg/kg, the increased activity of
salivary kallikrein induced by isoproterenol was hardly observed.
The inhibition in the total activity was 97.1 ± 6.5 % when the activities were compared before and after propranolol(Figs.2 and 3).
With respect to the flow rate of saliva, the effects of isoproterenol were clearly influenced after phenoxybenzamine, but

appeared to be not inhibited after propranolol.

6. Effects of Soy Bean Trypsin Inhibitor on Salivary
   Kallikrein secreted by Sympathetic and Parasympathetic
   Stimulations and Various Sympathomimetic Agents

In this experiment, the following fractions were collected for bioassay: (1) No.1, No.7 and No.11 fractions under the chorda tympani stimulation, (2) No.11 fraction after the stimulus voltage for the chorda tympani stimulation was rapidly increased at the time of No.8 fraction and (3) No.11 fraction after the stimulation of the cervical sympathetic nerve and the administrations of **noradrenaline, adrenaline** and isoproterenol at the time of No.8 fraction under the chorda tympani stimulation.

Ten μl of each fraction, which was diluted 10-fold with **saline, was** added to a medium containing 0.1 ml of citrated plasma and 0.1 ml of soy bean trypsin inhibitor (SBTI) in the concentration of 10^{-3} g/ml. This mixture, then, was immediately incubated at 36 °C for 1 min and the activity of the produced kinin was estimated.

In No.1, No.7 and No.11 fractions collected after the chorda tympani stimulation, the inhibition by SBTI of the salivary kallikrein activities was hardly observed. However, in No.11 fractions collected after the sympathetic nerve stimulation and the administration of noradrenaline, the activities of the salivary kallikrein were markedly inhibited by SBTI. Kallikrein activity in No.11 fraction collected after adrenaline was, to a certain extent, inhibited by SBTI. On the other hand, in No.11 fraction collected after the administration of isoproterenol, no inhibition by SBTI of the salivary kallikrein activity was observed(Fig.5).

DISCUSSION

With respect to the release of the salivary kallikrein by adrenergic mechanism, Hilton and Lewis(1956) suggested that the so-called "sympathetic after-vasodilatation" was caused by kinin, which was produced by releasing glandular kallikrein into the interstitial space. However, the fact that the secretion of the salivary kallikrein into the saliva was also probably caused by adrenergic mechanism was first observed by Beilenson et al(1968) who found that under the chorda tympani stimulation, the release of kallikrein into the saliva was considerably increased by the simultaneous stimulation of the cervical sympathetic nerve. Thereafter, Gautvik et al (1969, 1972a, 1972b, 1972c) and Gautvik(1970a, 1970b) suggested in a series of their works that glandular kallikrein was released not only into the saliva, but also into the interstitial space and the marked reduction of kallikrein content in the submandibular gland of the cat was found after the chorda tympani stimulation or the administration of adrenaline.

According to the results obtained in the present study, the increased secretions of salivary kallikrein were found markedly in

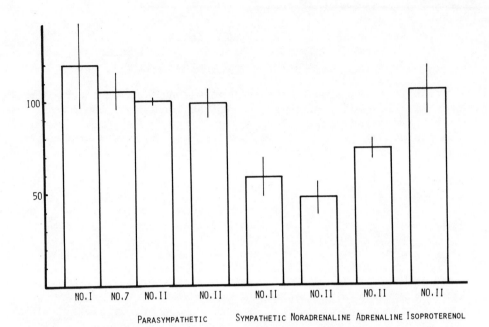

Fig.5. Inhibitions of Various Stimulation-induced Salivary
Kallikrein Activities by Soy Bean Trypsin Inhibitor. Abscissa: Number of fraction collected after the various stimulations. Ordinate:
Per cent of **control** by SBTI. Note that the activities of the
salivary kallikreins induced by the parasympathetic nerve stimulation or isoproterenol are not inhibited by SBTI, but the activities
of the salivary kallikreins induced by the sympathetic nerve stimulation or the administrations of noradrenaline and adrenaline are
markedly inhibited by SBTI in vitro.

every case after the stimulations of the chorda tympani or the cervical sympathetic nerve and the administrations of sympathomimetics.
However, the administration of phenoxybenzamine or propranolol prior
to these adrenergic stimulations did not completely inhibit the
kallikrein secretion into the saliva, except for the pretreatment
with propranolol in the case of isoproterenol. The increased secretion of the salivary kallikrein induced by isoproterenol was not
almost influenced by the pretreatment with phenoxybenzamine, while
it was almost completely inhibited by the pretreatment with propranolol.
    Emmelin et al(1965) suggested that there were both receptors,
α- and β-receptors, for catecholamines in the rat submandibular
gland. The reason was from the following results: (1) the secretion
of saliva induced by adrenaline or sympathetic nerve stimulation was
reduced but not stopped by the pretreatment with dihydroergotamine

or phenoxybenzamine, and (2) the secretion of saliva induced by
methacholine or isoprenaline was not influenced by these pretreatment, and (3) furthermore, the inhibition by adrenergic α-blockers
of the adrenaline-induced secretion of saliva was reinforced or resulted in a stop of the secretion by pronethalol.

In the present study, it is considered, therefore, that the
secretion of kallikrein in the saliva induced by adrenergic action
is also mediated through both α- and β-receptors. On the other hand
, Gautvik et al(1974) suggested that the secretion of salivary kallikrein was accelerated only with adrenergic α-action and that adrenergic β-action was involved in peripheral vasodilatation co-operat-
ing adrenergic α-action. However, since the secretion of salivary
amylase located in zymogen granules is accelerated with adrenergic
β-action(Bdolah and Schramm,1965; Malamud,1972), it can be hardly
explained that salivary kallikrein located in the same zymogen gra-
nules(Bhoola and Ogle,1966; Bhoola,1968; Erdös et al,1968) is secreted only by adrenergic α-action, but not by adrenergic β-action.

It would be possible to assume the other source of the secretion of salivary kallikrein than zymogen granules. Gautvik et al
(1972a, 1972b, 1972c) observed that the content of kininogenase showed about 90 % of reduction rate after the administration of noradrenaline in the cat submandibular gland which was perfused with Krebs-
Ringer's solution, while that of the gland perfused with whole blood
showed only about 50 %(30 - 60 %) of reduction rate. These facts
appear to suggest that kallikrein originated from plasma is included
more or less in the salivary kallikrein secreted by adrenergic mechanism.

In order to make clear these respects, a qualitative analysis
of salivary kallikrein secreted by the stimulations of the chorda
tympani and the cervical sympathetic nerve or after the administrations of sympathomimetics was performed in the present study, using
the properties of SBTI(Vogel and Werle,1970) which inhibits plasma
kallikrein but not glandular kallikrein. In the results obtained,
the activities of the salivary kallikreins collected after the sympathetic nerve stimulation and after the administrations of noradrenaline or adrenaline were found to be markedly inhibited by SBTI,
while the activities of the salivary kallikreins collected under the
chorda tympani stimulation and after the administration of isoproterenol were not influenced by SBTI. These findings suggest that
the former salivary kallikrein contains kallikrein originated from
plasma, secretion of which is mediated through adrenergic α-receptor.
It is also suggested that the salivary kallikrein collected after
the administration of isoproterenol is glandular kallikrein, secretion of which is mediated through adrenergic β-receptor, being similar to that of salivary amylase.

With respect to the flow rate of saliva, although the flow rate
of saliva induced by the chorda tympani stimulation was decreased
after the cervical sympathetic nerve stimulation or the administrations of sympathomimetics, the decreased flow rate of saliva was
more intensively decreased after the pretreatment of **phenoxybenzamine,**

but not after the pretreatment of propranolol. These results
appear to suggest that the adrenergic α-action accelerates the salivary flow, probably via adrenergic α-receptor or prostaglandin synthesis system(Inoki et al,1978).

REFERENCES

Bdolah,A. & Schramm,M.,1965, The function of 3',5'-cyclic AMP in
    enzyme secretion,Biochem.Biophys.Res.Commun.,18,452.
Beilenson,S.C.,Schachter,M. & Smaje,L.H.,1968, Secretion of kalli-
    krein and its role in vasodilatation in the submaxillary gland,
    J.Physiol.,199,303.
Bhoola,K.D. & Ogle,C.W.,1966, The subcellular localization of kalli-
    krein, amylase and acetylcholine in the submaxillary gland of
    the guinea-pig,J.Physiol.,184,663.
Bhoola,K.D.,1968, Intracellular distribution of submaxillary kalli-
    krein,J.Physiol.,196,431.
Emmelin,N.,Holmberg,J. & Ohlin,P.,1965, Receptors for catechol amines
    in the submaxillary glands of rats,Brit.J.Pharmacol.,25,134.
Erdös,E.G.,Tague,L.L. & Miwa,I.,1968, Kallikrein in granules of the
    submaxillary gland,Biochem.Pharmacol.,17,667.
Gautvik,K.M.,Nustad,K. & Vystyd,J.,1969, Kininogenase activity in
    the stimulated submandibular salivary gland in cat,Scand.J.clin.
    Lab.Invest.,24,suppl.107,101.
Gautvik,K.,1970a, The interaction of two different vasodilator me-
    chanisms in the Chorda-tympani activated submandibular salivary
    gland,Acta physiol.scand.,79,188.
Gautvik,K.,1970b, Parasympathetic neuroeffector transmission and
    functional vasodilatation in the submandibular salivary gland of
    cats,Acta physiol.scand.,79,204.
Gautvik,K.M.,Kriz,M. & Lund-Larsen,K.,1972a, Effects of alterations
    in calcium concentrations on secretion and protein synthesis in
    cat submandibular salivary gland,Acta physiol.scand.,85,418.
Gautvik,K.M.,Kriz,M. & Lund-Larsen,K.,1972b, Plasma kinins and adre-
    nergic vasodilatation in the submandibular salivary gland of the
    cat,Acta physiol.scand.,86,419.
Gautvik,K.M.,Nustad,K. & Vystyd,J.,1972c, Kininogenase activity in
    the stimulated submandibular salivary gland in cats,Acta physiol.
    scand.,85,438.
Gautvik,K.M.,Kriz,M.,Lund-Larsen,K. & Waaler,B.A.,1974, Sympathetic
    vasodilatation, kallikrein release and adrenergic receptors in
    the cat submandibular salivary gland,Acta physiol.scand.,90,438.
Hilton,S.M. & Lewis,G.P.,1956, The relationship between glandular
    activity, bradykinin formation and functional vasodilatation in
    the submandibular salivary gland,J.Physiol.,134,471.
Inoki,R.,Kudo,T.,Kotani,Y.,Oka,M.,Iwatsubo,K. & Matsumoto,K.,1978,
    Mechanism of substance P-induced salivary secretion in the rat,
    Proc.Kinin'78 Tokyo.
Malamud,D.,1972, Amylase secretion from mouse parotid and pancreas:
    Role of cyclic AMP and isoproterenol,Biochim.Biophys.Acta,279,373.

Vogel,R. & Werle,E.,1970, Kallikrein inhibitors, in: Handbook of
   Exper.Pharmacol.,Vol.25,edited by Erdös,E.G.,Springer-Verlag,
   Berlin,p.213.

LOCALIZATION OF GLANDULAR KALLIKREINS AND SECRETION OF KALLIKREIN FROM THE MAJOR SALIVARY GLANDS OF THE RAT

Torill B. Ørstavik, K. Nustad, and K.M. Gautvik

Dept. of Physiol. and Biochem., Dent. Fac. (T.B.Ø) and
Inst. Physiol., Med. Fac. (K.M.G.), Univ. of Oslo, Dept.
of Clin. Chem., The Norwegian Radium Hosp. (K.N., K.M.G.)
Oslo, Norway

INTRODUCTION

Glandular kallikreins (E.C.3.4.21.8) are found in major exocrine glands as well as in the kidney. These kinin-forming enzymes
are also present in the glandular secretions and preurine, and, they
are believed to be synthesized in the respective organs (Nustad et
al., 1975). The physiological function of kallikrein in exocrine
glands and the kidney is incompletely understood. However, the
cellular localization and secretory pattern of kallikrein may give
some indication as to the physiological role of kininogenases in
these organs. Moreover, such information is also important for
designing experiments to study the physiological function of glandular kallikreins. The cellular localization of kallikrein was
therefore investigated by means of a direct immunofluorescence
technique in the major salivary glands, the pancreas, the kidney,
and the exorbital lacrimal gland of the rat. The secretion of
kallikrein into saliva from the major salivary glands was investigated after various types of gland activation. Some of these
results have been published previously (Ørstavik et al., 1975;
Ørstavik et al., 1976; Ørstavik and Gautvik, 1977; Ørstavik and
Glenner, 1978).

MATERIALS AND METHODS

Animals: Adult (about 4 months old) Sprague-Dawley and Wistar
rats of both sexes were anesthetized with nembutal (70 mg/kg body
weight by intraperitoneal injections) and tracheotomized.

Immunohistochemistry: The glands were fixed <u>in situ</u> by perfusion
with phosphate buffered saline (PBS: 0.01 M Na-phosphate, pH 7.4,
0.15 M NaCl) followed by 95% ethanol (22°C).   The administration
route for the perfusion fluids was for the submandibular and sublingual glands through the carotid artery; for the parotid gland
retrograde through the posterior facial vein occluded distal to the
posterior auricular vein; for the exorbital lacrimal gland through
the external carotid artery with the cannula pushed close to the
superficial temporal branch; the pancreas was perfused by entering
the superior mesenteric artery and the kidney by a retrograde perfusion through the abdominal aorta which was occluded above the
renal arteries.   After the <u>in situ</u> fixation the organs were dis-
sected out, and the tissues were post-fixed in ethanol and processed
for immunohistochemistry by paraffin-embedding as described previously
(Ørstavik et al., 1975).   Tissue sections (6 μm) were stained to
demonstrate kallikrein by the direct immunofluorescence technique
(Brandtzaeg, 1973) by the use of antisera against rat urinary or
submandibular gland kallikrein conjugated with tetramethylrhodamine
isothiocyanate.   The specificity of the fluorescence reaction was
controlled by either a preincubation with nonimmune serum or by
absorption of the conjugated antibody with purified urinary or
submandibular gland kallikrein.   Morphological orientation was
obtained by histological staining of neighboring sections by methods
described previously (Ørstavik et al., 1975).

Collection of saliva: The main excretory duct of the submandibular,
sublingual, and parotid glands were exposed and cannulated with a
polyethylene tube (Portex, PP 10).   Salivary secretion was stimulated parasympathetically or sympathetically by drugs or by
electrical nerve stimulation as previously described (Ørstavik and
Gautvik, 1977).

Kallikrein quantitation: Kallikrein activity was quantitated by
its Bz-Arg-OEt-esterase activity, and for the submandibular gland
saliva also by its antigenic activity in a single radial immunodiffusion system (Ørstavik et al., 1977).

                                RESULTS

Immunohistochemistry: In the <u>kidney</u> kallikrein was found in the
distal tubular cells of the renal cortex (Fig. 1).   Kallikrein
positive tubules were seen to enter collecting ducts, which were
found to be kallikrein-negative (Fig. 3).   Furthermore, kallikrein-
negative tubules could be observed to change into kallikrein-
positive tubules (Fig. 4) often in the vicinity of the vascular
pole of the glomerulus.   These observations indicate that kallikrein
is located in the convoluted distal tubular cells in the segment
from the macula densa through to the collecting duct.   Kallikrein
could not be detected in the renal marrow, indicating that kalli-

krein was not present in the loop of Henle or in the collecting
duct. In the distal tubular cells kallikrein-specific fluorescence
was found in a granular distribution (Fig. 1 and 3). However, in
some kidneys kallikrein was seen only as a luminal rim and the
granular distribution was not observed. This variation was believed
to be due to differences in the efficiency of the in situ fixation.
In situ fixation was necessary for an immunohistochemical demonstration of kallikrein in the kidney.

In the salivary glands kallikrein was found in the ductal
system, i.e. in the cytoplasm of the intralobular striated ducts
and extralobularly as a luminal rim decreasing in intensity when
the ducts were followed from the lobuli towards the gland hilus.
In the submandibular gland large amounts of kallikrein was also
observed in the secretory granules of the granular tubular cells.
Also, in the submandibular gland (Fig. 5) the amount of kallikrein
seen in the striated duct cytoplasm was less than that seen in the
parotid (Fig. 6) and sublingual (Fig. 7) glands which both are
devoid of granular tubules. Also in the salivary glands the
intensity of the fluorescence reaction was improved by the in situ
fixation compared to in vitro fixation.

In the exorbital lacrimal gland kallikrein-specific fluorescence was not detected. Some granular fluorescence was observed
in the duct system which morphologically resembles the intercalated ducts of the salivary glands. However, this fluorescence
reaction was not prohibited by absorption of the conjugate with
purified kallikrein, and was thus judged as an immunologically non-
specific staining reaction. A similar immunological non-specific
fluorescence was also observed in the intercalated ducts of the
parotid gland.

In the pancreas kallikrein was found in a granular distribution
in the portion of the acinar cells containing the zymogen granules,
thus indicating that kallikrein was located in the zymogen granules
of the acinar cells (Fig. 8). Kallikrein was not seen in the
cytoplasm of the ductal cell but was observed in the lumen and as
a lunimal rim probably representing secreted kallikrein adhering
to the lumen wall (Fig. 9). No kallikrein was observed in the
islets of Langerhans. To demonstrate the intracellular distribution
of kallikrein in the acinar cells, in vivo fixation was found to
be necessary.

Salivary kallikrein secretion: The kallikrein secretory pattern
found in the rat salivary glands resembles that seen in other
species (Gautvik et al., 1974; Barton et al., 1975; Albano et al.,
1976). In the submandibular gland the salivary kallikrein concentration and secretory rate were highest after sympathetic stimulation, particularly following α-adrenergic stimulation.

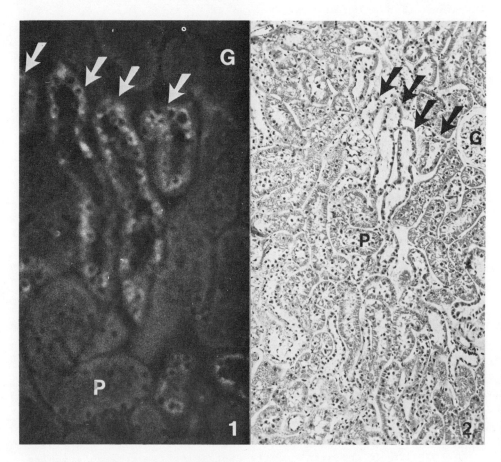

Figure 1.   Tracing of kallikrein in the rat kidney by
            immunofluorescence, demonstrating kallikrein
            in the convoluted distal tubular cells of the
            renal cortex (arrows).

Figure 2.   Neighboring section of that seen in Fig. 1
            stained with haematoxylin-eosin for morphological
            orientation. Arrows point at the same distal
            tubules as in fig. 1.

            Distal tubules: arrows
            Proximal tubules: P
            Glomerulus: G

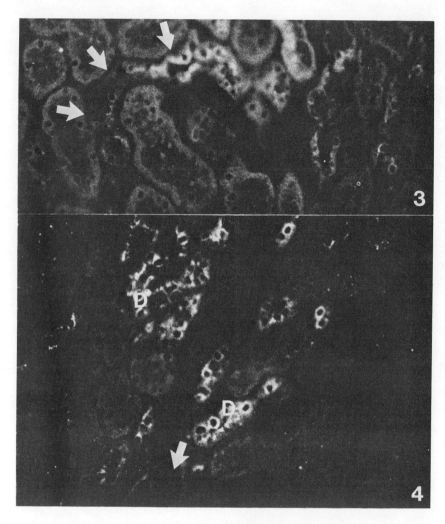

Figure 3. Kallikrein detection in the rat kidney showing
           the transition from kallikrein-negative to kalli-
           krein-positive areas within the same distal tubules
           (arrows).

Figure 4. Kallikrein detection in the rat kidney showing a
           kallikrein-positive distal tubules (D) and a
           kallikrein-negative collecting duct (arrows).

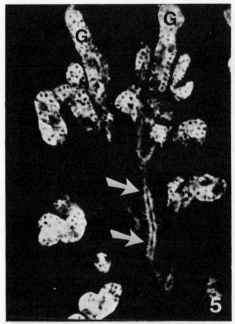

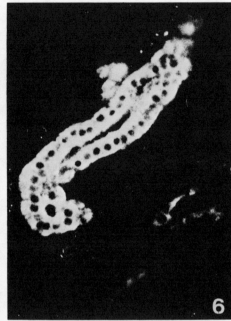

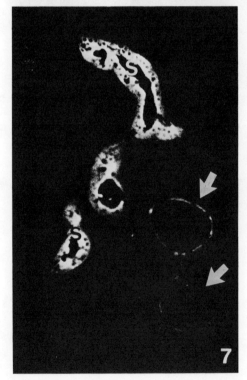

Figure 5. In the submandibular
gland kallikrein is found in
the granular tubular cells
(G) and in the luminal part
of the striated duct cells
(arrows).

Figure 6. A striated duct of
the parotid gland containing
kallikrein.

Figure 7. In the sublingual
gland kallikrein is seen in
the straited duct cell cytoplasm (S) and, like in the
other salivary glands, as a
luminal rim in the extra-
lobular main excretory ducts
(arrows).

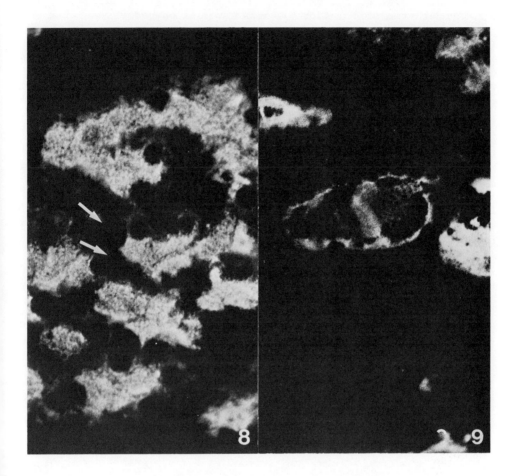

Figure 8. Tracing of kallikrein in the rat pancreas
           by immunofluorescence, showing the presence
           of kallikrein in the zymogen granules of the
           acinar cells. The dark spots (arrows) represent
           the nuclei in the basal part of the acinus cell.

Figure 9. The pancreatic duct. Kallikrein is found in
           the duct lumen and adhering to the lumen wall.
           No kallikrein is seen in the cytoplasm of the
           duct cell.

Also in the parotid and sublingual glands the highest kallikrein concentrations were seen in saliva following sympathetic stimulation. In the parotid gland the secretory rate of kallikrein increased when sympathetic stimulation was superimposed on parasympathetic stimulation. Becuase of the minute amounts of secretion from the sublingual gland, no definite conclusions could be drawn from the observed variations in kallikrein secretory rate in this gland. However, there was a tendency to higher kallikrein secretory rates following sympathetic stimulation compared to parasympathetic stimulation also in this gland.

DISCUSSION

Immunohistochemistry is a sensitive method for the localization of tissue antigens. This technique can be used for a great diversity of substances, and with well characterized reagents and appropriate immunological controls it provides reliable results. The antisera employed in the present studies were produced against highly purified and characterized kallikrein antigens (Nustad and Pierce, 1974; Brandtzaeg et al., 1976). The binding specificity and the immunological specificity of the fluorochrome-conjugated antisera were controlled by preincubation with unlabelled antiserum (blocking test) and by absorption of the conjugate with purified kallikreins and with cross-reacting antigens. Cross-reacting esterases have been isolated from the submandibular gland (Brandtzaeg et al., 1976) but have not been found in urine (Nustad and Pierce,

Table 1.   Concentration and secretory rate of kallikrein in parasympathetic and sympathetic saliva from the submandibular, sublingual, and parotid glands.

	Submandibular gland			Sublingual gland			Parotid gland		
	Kallikrein concentration EU/ml	Kallikrein secretory rate EU/min	n	Kallikrein concentration EU/ml	Kallikrein secretory rate EU/min 10^{-1}	n	Kallikrein concentration EU/ml	Kallikrein secretory rate EU/min	n
Parasympathetic									
Electrical	155.6 ± 130.9	1.76 ± 1.07	6	1.96 · 0.77	19 · 9	5	18.3 · 11.4	0.100 ± 0.047	4
Pilocarpine	42.3 ± 20.3	0.31 ± 0.16	5	0.72 · 0.37	24 · 9	7	8.9 · 3.4	0.073 ± 0.036	15
Sympathetic									
Cervical nerve	113 286 ± 156 720 (7 539–560 367)	1 157 ± 2 706 (38–9 973)	13	22.5 · 17.0	11 · 7	4	85.9 ± 81.9	0.098 ± 0.057	15
Norepinephrine	88 290 ± 111 522 (13 898–274 500)	201 ± 232 (15–494)	5	71.8	14	2	119.6 ± 70.6	0.121 ± 0.048	7
Isoproterenol	1 984 ± 1 669) (725–4 425	1.3 · 1.3 (0.04–3.5)	6	22.1 (8.7–42.3)	16 (2.8–42.3)	3	42.9 ± 19.1	0.052 · 0.017	8

When n = 3, or when the standard deviation is very high due to large individual variations, the range is given below in brackets. n = number of glands investigated. (Modified from Ørstavik, 1978b).

1974). In the rat parotid saliva (Ørstavik, 1978a) and in the rat pancreas (Proud et al., 1977) the detected antigens were immunologically identical and in the pancreas also biologically and enzymatically identical, to the purified submandibular and urinary kallikreins. Moreover, in the submandibular and sublingual glands the demonstration of kallikrein by immunological techniques was supported by alterations in gland morphology and by results of enzyme quantitations following prolonged stimulation with isoproterenol and acute salivary gland stimulations (Ørstavik et al., 1977; Ørstavik and Gautvik, 1977). Also in the submandibular saliva immunological and enzyme quantitations were well correlated (Ørstavik and Gautvik, 1977). A prokallikrein was detected in the pancreas only, and the proenzyme and the active enzyme were immunologically identical (Proud et al., 1977) on the basis of the same antiserum as employed in the present studies. This finding, together with the failure of activation of the submandibular gland to produce alterations in kallikrein localization (Ørstavik and Gautvik, 1977), indicated that the immunofluorescence demonstration of kallikrein was reliable and minimized the possibility that the enzyme might somehow be shielded from intracellular detection. When the immunohistochemical technique produced a negative result, like in the exorbital lacrimal gland, absence of kallikrein was confirmed by the lack of enzyme activity in gland homogenates and secretion (Ørstavik, 1978a and b). It was therefore concluded that the direct immunofluorescence technique was reliable for the study of cellular origin of kallikrein in exocrine organs.

The ductal localization of kallikrein in the submandibular gland has been confirmed by immunohistochemical techniques in the rat (Simson et al., 1978) and in the cat (Hojima et al., 1977). Furthermore, kallikrein was found in homogenates of the ductal cells after ductal and acinar tissue had been isolated by dissection of cultivated pieces of the cat and guinea pig submandibular glands (Uddin and Tyler, 1978). In the cat, physiological studies also indicated a ductal localization of kallikrein (Barton et al., 1975). Similarly, in the mouse submandibular gland trypsin-like esterases have been found in the granular tubular cells (Ekfors and Hopsu-Havu, 1971). However, the latter authors could not demonstrate such enzymes in the striated ducts or in the sublingual gland. This may be explained by species differences, by the in vitro fixation technique, or by a low reactivity of the antiserum used. In the mouse, also, other esterolytic enzymes like the nerve growth factor has been located in the tubular cells (Levi-Montalcini and Angeletti, 1961). In the submandibular gland of the guinea pig, however, an acinar as well as ductal localization of kallikrein has been reported on the basis of immunofluorescent tracing (Bhoola et al., 1977). Thus, it is possible that species variation in the cellular localization of kallikrein may be observed. However, cross-reacting esterases, which are found in the submandibular glands of the rat (Brandtzaeg et al., 1976) and of the mouse (Ekfors and Hopsu-Havu, 1971), represent technical pit-falls. Cross-reacting antigens may well be present in the submandibular acinar cells of the guinea pig, and thus explain the controversial results. Non-specific esterase activity has indeed been detected in the acini of many other species (Chauncey and Quintarelli, 1961). Moreover, an acinar localization of kallikrein in the submandibular gland of the guinea pig does not agree with the above mentioned studies of Uddin and Tyler (1978). In the kidney, the localization of kallikrein in the distal tubular cells has been supported by stop-flow studies on the dog (Scicli et al., 1978).

The rat submandibular gland has long been known to contain extremely high concentrations of kallikrein (Frey et al., 1968). This organ was therefore an obvious choice for initiating studies on glandular kallikreins. However, since the high concentration of kallikrein in this gland was found to be due to the presence of granular tubules, a structure which is not found in other major salivary glands of the rat and which is absent in many species, it was necessary to compare the morphology and behavior of the sub-mandibular gland with other kallikrein containing organs. The submandibular gland granular tubular cells could be compared to the acinar cells of the pancreas; in as much as both types of cells contain esterolytic enzymes (Ørstavik and Glenner, 1978). The secretory granules of these cells may represent a kallikrein store. The enzyme was elsewhere found in relation to cells known to participate in water electrolyte regulations. It seems reason-able to propose that the presence of kallikrein in an organ is connected to the presence of "absorptive" epithelial cells with infoldings of the basal cell membrane associated with a large number of mitochondira. Kallikrein is found in relation to such cells both in the major salivary glands (Ørstavik et al., 1975; Brandtzaeg et al., 1976; Hojima et al., 1977; Ørstavik et al., 1977; Ørstavik, 1978a) and in the kidney (Ørstavik et al., 1976). Similar cells can also be found in sweat glands (Strauss and Matolsky, 1973), and kallikrein has been identified in human sweat (Fräki et al., 1970). Also the toad bladder contains such cells, and recently kallikrein has been isolated from this organ (margolius and Chao, 1978). The mitochondria rich cell is not found in a kallikrein-free organ as the rat exorbital lacrimal gland (electron-microscopy, E.B. Messelt and T.B. Ørstavik, unpublished). They are not found in the pancreas either (Ekholm et al., 1962), but an extraglandular site of function has been suggested for pancreatic kallikrein (Ørstavik and Glenner, 1978). The mitochondria rich cell with numerous infoldings of the basal plasma membrane is involved in transport of water and electrolyties. Thus, the distribution of kallikrein in the body can be related to cells whose function is important for the water-electrolyte balance, functions which have also been assigned to the kallikrein-kinin system.

REFERENCES

Albano, J., K.D. Bhoola, P.F. Heap, and M.J.C. Lemon, 1976. Stimulus-secretion coupling: role of cyclic AMP, cyclic GMP and calcium in mediating enzyme (kallikrein) secretion in the submandibular gland. J. Physiol. 258: 631.

Barton, S., E.J. Sanders, M. Schachter and M. Uddin, 1975. Autonomic nerve stimulation, kallikrein content and acinar cell granules of the cat's submandibular gland. J. Physiol. 251: 363.

Bhoola, K.D., M.J.C. Lemon, and R.W. Matthews, 1977. Immunofluorescent localization of kallikrein in the guinea-pig submandibular gland. J. Physiol. (Lond.) 272: 28P.

Brandtzaeg, P. 1973. Conjugates of immunoglobulin G with different fluorochromes. I. Characterization by anionic-exchange chromatography. Scand. J. Immunol. 2: 273.

Brandtzaeg, P., K.M. Gautvik, K. Nustad, and J.V. Pierce, 1976. Rat submandibular gland kallikreins: purification and cellular localization. Br. J. Pharmacol. 56: 155.

Chao, J. and H.S. Margolius, 1978. Identification of kallikrein in toad urinary bladder and skin and its inhibition by amiloride. Clin. Res. 26: 63A.

Chauncey, H.H. and G. Quintarelli, 1961. Localication of acid phosphatase, nonspecific esterases and β-D-galactosidase in parotid and submaxillary glands of domestic and laboratory animals. Am. J. Anat. 108: 263.

Ekfors, T.O. and V.K. Hopsu-Havu, 1971. Immunofluorescent localization of trypsin-like esteropeptidases in the mouse submandibular gland. Histochem. J. 3: 415.

Ekholm, R., T. Zelander, and Y. Edlund, 1962. The ultrastructural organization of the rat exocrine pancreas. II. Centroacinar cells, intercalary and intralobular ducts. J. Ultrastruct. Res. 7: 73.

Fräki, J.E., C.T. Jansén, and V.K. Hopsu-Havu, 1970. Human sweat kallikrein. Acta Dermat. (Stockholm) 50: 321.

Frey, E.K., H. Kraut, E. Werle, R. Vogel, G. Zickgraf-Fudel and I. Trautschold, 1968. Das Kallikrein-Kinin-System und seine Inhibitoren. Ferdinand Enke Verlag, Stuttgart.

Gautvik, K.M., M. Kriz, K. Lund-Larsen, and K. Nustad, 1974. Control of kallikrein secretion from salivary glands. In: Secretory mechanisms of exocrine glands. Eds. N. A. Thorn and O.H. Petersen. Munksgaard, Copenhagen, pp. 168.

Hojima, Y., B. Maranda, C. Moriwaki, and M. Schachter, 1977. Direct evidence for the localization of kallikrein in the striated ducts of the cat's submandibular gland by the use of specific antibody. J. Physiol. (Lond.) 268: 793.

Levi-Montalcini, R. and P.U. Angeletti, 1961. Growth control of the sympathetic system by a specific protein factor. Quart. Rev. Biol. 36: 99.

Nustad, K. and J.V. Pierce, 1974. Purification of rat urinary
    kallikreins and their specific antibody. Biochem. 13: 2312.
Nustad, K., J.V. Pierce, and K. Vaaje, 1975. Synthesis of kallikrein
    by rat kidney slices. Br. J. Pharmacol. 53: 229.
Ørstavik, T.B., 1978a. An immunohistochemical study of kallikrein
    in the rat parotid and exorbital lacrimal glands. Arch. oral
    Biol. In press.
Ørstavik, T.B., 1978b. The distribution and secretion of kallikrein
    in some exocrine organs of the rat. Acta physiol. Scand.
    Dec. In press.
Ørstavik, T.B., P. Brandtzaeg, K. Nustad, and K.M. Halvorsen, 1975.
    Cellular localization of kallikrein in the rat submandibular
    and sublingual salivary glands. Immunofluorescence tracing
    related to histological characteristics. Acta histochem. 54:
    183.
Ørstavik, T.B. and K.M. Gautvik, 1977. Regulation of salivary
    kallikrein secretion in the rat submandibular gland. Acta
    physiol. Scand. 100: 33.
Ørstavik, T.B. and G.G. Glenner, 1978. Localization of kallikrein
    and its relation to other trypsin-like esterases in the rat
    pancreas. A comparison with the submandibular gland. Acta
    physiol. Scand. 103: 384.
Ørstavik, T.B., K. Nustad, and P. Brandtzaeg, 1977. A biochemical
    and immunohistochemical study of kallikrein in normal and
    isoproterenol-stimulated rat salivary glands during postnatal
    development. Archs. oral. Biol. 22: 495.
Ørstavik, T.B., K. Nustad, P. Brandtzaeg, and J.V. Pierce.
    Cellular origin of urinary kallikreins. J. Histochem. Cytochem.
    24: 1037.
Proud, D., G. Bailey, K. Nustad, and K.M. Gautvik, 1977. The
    immunological similarity of rat glandular kallikreins.
    Biochem. J. 167: 835.
Scicli, A.G., R. Gandolfi, and O.A. Carretero, 1978. Site of
    formation of kinins in the dog nephron. Am. J. Physiol.
    234: F36.
Simson, J.A.V., J. Chao, and H.S. Margolius, 1978. Cytochemical
    localization and secretagogue-induced release of kallikrein
    and nerve growth factor from rodent salivary glands. Anat.
    Rec. 190: 542.
Strauss, J.S. and A.G. Matolsky, 1973. Skin. In: Histology 3. ed.
    Eds. R.O. Greep and L. Weiss. McGraw-Hill Book Company,
    New York, pp. 477.
Uddin, M. and D.W. Tyler, 1978. Localization of kallikrein by a
    direct method. J. Dent. Res. Spec. Issue A, Abstr. nr. 1183.

POSSIBLE RELATIONSHIP BETWEEN SALIVARY KALLIKREIN AND WATER-Na-K

SECRETION STIMULATED BY TITYUSTOXIN (TsTx)

Orlando L. Catanzaro*, Alejandro Martinez Seeber*and
Wilson T. Beraldo
Dept. de Ciencias Biologicas, Orientacion Fisiologia
Humana, Fac. de Farmacia y Bioquimica, U.B.A. and Dept.
de Fisiologia y Biofisica, I.C.B., Univ. Fed. M. Gerais,
Br.

In the salivary glands TsTx can stimulate a number of receptor mechanism(s) including cholinergic, β-adrenergic, α-adrenergic and probably substance P., (Catanzaro, et al., 1976).

The effect of the venom from Brazilian scorpion (Tityus serrulatus) was described as very complex (Magalhaes, 1946).

Intense sialagogue effect was observed after the injection of purified extract of toxin in mice (Diniz and Valery, 1959), and Gomez and Diniz (1966) reported that during assays of toxic activity of the toxin on mice by LD_{50} measurements and by intoxication symptoms, salivation and lacrimation was observed. On the other hand, salivary glands, like most exocrine glands, are known to contain the plasma-kinin forming enzyme kallikrein (E.C. 3.4.4.21) (Frey et al., 1968).

In view of the dramatic effects of tityus toxin on the autonomic nervous systems described by Diniz and Goncalvez (1956) and Freire-Maia et al., (1976), and the preliminary results on salivary glands enzymes, it was decided to study the effect of the toxin (TsTx) on the regulation of kallikrein secretion in parotid and submandibular gland and the relationship with Na-K-water secretion.

MATERIAL AND METHODS

Animals: Female Wistar rats, weighing 180–200 gr. were used. The animals were anesthetized with i.p. injection of urethane (1.4 g/Kg), the trachea was cannulated and a polyethylene cannula was inserted in the jugular vein. The parotid and submaxillary ducts were isolated from different animals, and saliva collected by a micro-pipette from the tip of the duct. Flow rate was measured by determining the interval required to collect a certain volume of saliva. Saliva collected during stimulation period was frozen at -20° for subsequent quantitation of kallikrein. Samples of saliva were simultaneously collected by micropipette, and Na and K were analyzed by flame photometry after appropriate dilution.

Quantitation of kallikrein in saliva: Samples of saliva were measured by its ability to hydrolyze α-N-benzoyl-L-arginine-ethyl ester (Bz-Arg-OEt), as described by Nustad et al., (1975). The kallikrein quantitation by Bz-Arg-OEt-esterase method was also evaluated by comparing the biological assay according to Beraldo et al., (1966) and Nustad and Pierce (1974). All protein measurements were performed by the method of Lowry et al., (1951).

Scorpion toxin and drugs. Tityus toxin (TsTx) was obtained by a combination of extraction and chromatography of the venom of the Brazilian scorpion Tityus serrulatus (Gomez and Diniz, 1966). Atropine sulfate, (Hoffman La Roche), Ouabaina and α-N-benzoyl-L-arginine-ethyl ester (Bz-Arg-OEt)(Sigma), Phenoxybenzamine hydro-chloride (Smith Kline and French Lab.), were used and refer to the weights of the salts.

RESULTS

Effects of TsTx on parotid and submaxillary saliva. Intravenous injection of TsTx in a dose of 0.5 mg/Kg of body weight, produced a profuse salivary secretion within 50 to 60 seconds. Fig. 1 shows the effect of the toxin on Na and K and kallikrein of parotid saliva. Parotid gland secreted a fluid which was usually high in Na concentration per minute and low in K.

After 8 to 10 minutes, Na secretion showed a transient of high level, followed by a decrease of more than 60% of the peak. Potassium in the parotid secretion seemed to behave in a similar manner as Na, but no transient was observed. Samples of saliva were simultaneously taken, and showed that kallikrein activity is corre-lated with the Na output per minute with a maximal activity during the high "rest transient" of Na.

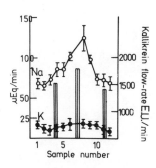

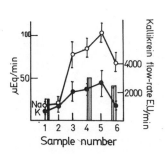

Fig. 1. Effect of tityustoxin
(.5mg/Kg) on parotid
saliva Na-K and kalli-
krein (Bz-Arg-OEt)
esterase activity.

Fig. 2. Effect of tityustoxin
on submaxillar saliva
Na-K and kallikrein (z-
Arg-OEt) esterase
activity.

On the other hand, saliva from submaxillary gland showed an
increase of Na and K during that time, and a close correlation
with salivary kallikrein (Fig. 2.).

However, a marked difference in the composition of electrolites secreted in saliva from parotid and submaxillary glands and
a high kallikrein secretion from submaxillary was always observed.

Effects of ouabain on parotid and submaxillary saliva. Treatment
of rats with ouabain (0.5 mg/Kg i.v.) before the toxin (.5 mg/Kg
i.v.) showed a marked difference with the controls. Fig. 3 shows
that parotid saliva from rats injected with ouabain, have less
output of Na than the controls. Ouabain caused a reduction of 50
to 60% of the Na secreted per minute, and a gradual increase of K
per minute.

It was interesting to observe that kallikrein also started at
high levels and decreased rapidly in the first minutes, to reach a
constant level until the final part of the experiments.

On the other hand, saliva from submaxillary gland showed a
significant reduction of Na secretion, whereas the K secretion
increased progressively on time. The flow-rate of kallikrein showed
a reduction of 50% from the controls, but a consistent activity,
during the experiments (Fig. 4).

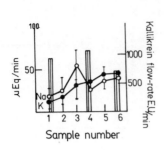

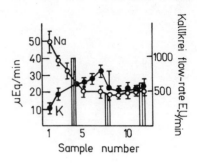

Fig. 3. Effect of ouabain
(.5mg/Kg i.v.) before
TsTx (.5mg/Kg) on
parotid saliva Na-K
and kallikrein (Bz-Arg-
OEt) esterase activity.

Fig. 4. Effect of ouabin (.5mg/Kg)
before TsTx on submaxillar
saliva Na-K and kallikrein
(Bz-Arg-OEt) esterase
activity.

Effects of adrenergic and cholinergic blockers. In order to study
the mechanism of the action of the different blockers on Na and K
secretion and the relationship with the kallikrein output, rats
were injected with 5 mg/Kg of phentolamine or 1 mg/Kg of atropine.
On parotid glands the α-blocker only reduced the concentration of
K, almost 50-60% from the control, with a simultaneous reduction
of kallikrein secretion per minute and concentration per ml of
saliva. On the other hand, atropine, which reduced Na (90%) and
K (40%), also reduced a secretion and concentration of kallikrein.
Estimates of saliva kallikrein activity, measured by Bz-Arg-OEt-
esterase and biological assay, also showed a correlation with
electrolites secretion.

The action of phentolamine and atropine was also observed on
submaxillary glands secretion of Na and K and kallikrein activity.
(Tables 1 and 2).

DISCUSSION

Intravenous injection of TsTx produce a stimulatory effect on
both autonomic branches of the nervous system, but the inorganic
composition of the salivas evoked by the toxin show characteristic
differences. As reported in a previous study (Catanzaro, et al.,
1978 submitted for publication) saliva evoked by TsTx is usually
high in Na and K.

Table 1.

Effects of cholinergic and α–adrenergic
blocker drugs on parotid saliva Na–K and kallikrein

	Kallik.* (ng Bk/min)	Kallik.** Flowrate (E.U./min)	Kallik. E.U./ml	μEq/min Na	K
TsTx	3±0.4	313±75	3475±125	97±0.6	10±.1
+ Phent.	1.4±0.2	121±18	1290±201	93±4	4±.3
+ Atropine	1.7±0.3	183±39	1737±198	15±.89	5±.2

* Biological assay. Phentolamine (Phent.)(5 mg/Kg); Atropine (1 mg/ Kg); TsTx (Tityustoxin).
** Bz–Arg–OEt esterase activity (kallikrein).
Each result is mean of 3-4 samples of saliva from 3-4 rats.
Values are means ± S.D.

Table 2.

Effects of cholinergic and α–adrenergic
blocker drugs on submax. saliva Na–K and kallikrein

	Kallikrein Flowrate (EU/min)	Kallikrein EU/ml	μEq/min Na	K
TsTx	740±90	4200±159	69±3.8	19±2
+ Phent.	190±14	760±79	60±3.1	9±0.2
+ Atropine	512±65	2701±123	30±2.7	8±0.1

* Bz–Arg–OEt–esterase activity–Phentolamine (Phent.) (5 mg/Kg)
Atropine (1 mg/Kg).
Each result is mean of 3-4 samples of saliva from 3-4 rats.
Values are mean ± S.D.

The present results report on a number of characteristic
features of the TsTx induced-Na-K release in parotid and submandibular glands and the possible relationship with the activity of
kallikrein in simultaneous samples of saliva. As far as kallikrein
is concerned in parotid and submaxillary saliva, the in vivo
experiments have shown that the Na and K secretion from the parotid
saliva are correlated with a parallel change in kallikrein esterase
activity. There is no indication in the literature about the
physiological role of kallikrein on salivary glands and the possible
control mechanism(s) involved in active water-electrolyte regulation.
Our data leads to the assumption that the release of Na and K from
parotid and submaxillar saliva is controlled by the activity of
kallikrein, and we can also add that the electrolite's concentration
of saliva and the mechanism of active transport of Na and K to
saliva may be contributed to modulate the activity of kallikrein.

In experiments of Selinger et al., (1973) it was seen that
ouabain did not inhibit the K release by epinephrine. Our results
with rats treated with ouabain and injected with TsTx showed that
this effect is similar to those observed (Selinger et al., 1973) on
parotid gland "in vitro". Elevation of K in saliva of rats with
ouabain and stimulated by pilocarpine was also observed by Schneyer
and Schneyer (1965). The activity of salivary kallikrein on rats
pretreated with ouabin and stimulated by TsTx suggest that the
cardiac glicosides or their aglycones can interfer with accumulation
of K and extrusion of Na, and this effect may produce a regulated
control on kallikrein-kinin-system. On the other hand, it is also
possible that the enzyme acts as a regulatory factor to modulate the
active electrolyte transport in the ductal system. The function
of the active Na-K-ATPase seems to be of great importance in this
process also (Schwartz and Moore, 1968). In considering the effect
of blocker drugs (atropine and phentolamine) the resulting interrelationship between Na-K secretion and kallikrein activity is very
important. A cholinergic blocker, atropine, produced a complete
reduction of Na and partially of K secretion with a significant
difference on kallikrein secretion and concentration on both glands.

Parotid gland seems to be more sensitive to the effect of
cholinergic blocker, since the drug produces an inhibition of 50%
of the enzyme, whereas that of submaxillary gland was only 23%
inhibited. The results above obtained with atropine, show that the
kallikrein activity observed in saliva is partially evoked by a
parasympathetic stimulation of the toxin components; these results
are in accordance with those of Bhoola et al., (1976). The remainder
of activity in the gland, perhaps, helps to equilibrate the secretion
of Na and K in saliva. In contrast, adrenergic blocker, phentolamine,
reduce 50% of K secretion, with any noticeable effect on Na. In
this case, the reduction of activity of kallikrein reached 62%
in parotid saliva and 74% in submaxillary saliva. It shows that
the most effective kallikrein secretion is modulated by α-adrenergic

stimulation.   There is an important point to be solved: since after atropine, kallikrein is reduced and secretion of Na is inhibited almost 90% and K 50%, it is possible to infer that this kallikrein could be involved in the mechanism(s) of water electrolite transport. On the other hand, after phentolamine, kallikrein is also reduced, with a parallel inhibition of K secretion, suggesting that in this way it is possible to have a partial control of water and electrolite secretion.   Another point of interest is to find the role of the kallikrein enzyme and its relation with Na-K ATPase transport enzyme. Secretion of Na and K may occur after primary secretion by the acinar cells (Burgen, 1967).   It is well known that the tubules represent one of the main secretory elements of the gland (Schneyer and Schneyer, 1962), and an active transport apparently occurs in both regions of the gland.   Since the adjustment of ionic concentration to yield a final saliva may occur after primary secretion by acinar cells (Burgen, 1967), it is possible that the higher activity of kallikrein in the ducts modulates the equilibrium with plasma ions and the blood flow (Orstavik et al., 1977).   This point, however, should be taken with some reservations since the primary mechanism of active transport is confined to the acinar cells and probably in those cells, a primary kallikrein is also activated during the secretory process.

The present findings lend the physiological support to the role of salivary kallikrein and their relationship with the active transport system of Na-K and water of saliva.

SUMMARY

Intravenous injection of purified scorpion toxin (TsTx) brings about the appearance of salivary flow with high levels of Na and K and kallikrein in the saliva of the rats.   In experiments performed in vivo a positive correlation between Na and partially with K and kallikrein was observed in parotid and submaxillary saliva.

After ouabaine, saliva K was increasing, whereas Na decreased, and a parallel decrease of kallikrein was observed.   Adrenergic and cholinergic blocking drugs also showed a marked reduction in the output of Na (atropine), and partially of K (atropine or phentolamine), with a correlation in the output of kallikrein per min.   The results of the present investigations support the hypothesis that salivary kallikrein-kinin system is probably involved in salivary control of Na, partially K and water secretion.

ACKNOWLEDGEMENTS

Aided by a grant from the Consejo Nacional de Investigaciones
Cientificas y Tecnicas-Republica Argentina. We are much indebted
to the Butantan Institute and Prof. C.R. Diniz for kindly supplying
the scorpion venom and to Dr. M.V. Gomex for the purified tityustoxin.
* Members of Career Dev. Consejo Nacional de Investigaciones
Cientificas y Tecnicas, Republica Argentina.

REFERENCES

Beraldo, W.T., R.L. Araujo and M. Mares-Guia, 1966. Oxytoxic
    esterase in rat urine. Am. J. Physiol. 211: 975.
Bhoola, K.D., P.F. Heap and M.J.C. Lemon, 1976. The regulation of
    kallikrein secretion from isolated submandibular gland slices
    by neurotransmitters. Cyclic Nucleotides and Calcium. Adv.
    Exper. Med. and Biol. (Eds. Sicuteri, Back and Haberland) 70:
    59.
Burgen, A.S.V., 1967. Secretory mechanism of salivary glands (Ed.
    L. Schneyer and C. Schneyer) N.Y.: Academic. p. 3-10.
Catanzaro, O.L., R.A. Santos, O.M. Parra, L. Freire-Maia and W.T.
    Beraldo, 1978. Effects of Scorpion Toxin (Tityustoxin, TsTx)
    on the salivary gland of the rat, in vivo and in vitro. Agents
    and Action 8: 119.
Diniz, C.R. and J.M. Goncalves, 1956. Some Chemical and Pharmacolo-
    gical properties of Brazilian Scorpion Venom, In: Venoms
    (Ed. E. Buckey and W. Porges). Am. Assoc. Adv. Science. pp.
    131.
Diniz, C.R. and V. Valery, 1959. Effects of a toxin present in a
    purified extract of telson from the scorpion Tityus serrulatus
    on smooth muscle preparation and in mice. Arch. Int. Pharma-
    docyn, Ther., 71: 1.
Freire-Maia, L., J.R. Cunha-Nelo, M.V. Gomex, W.L. Tafuri, T.A.
    Maria, S.L. Calixto and H.A. Futuro-Neto, 1976. Studies on
    the mechanism of action of Tityustoxin In: Animal, Plant and
    Microbiol Toxins, vol. 2 (Ed. A. Ohsaka) pp. 273.
Frey, E.K., H. Krant and E. Werle, 1968. Das Kallikrein-Kinin-
    System und seine Inhibitoren. Ferdinand Enke Verlag, Stuttgart.
Gomez, M.V. and C.R. Diniz, 1966. Separation of toxic components
    from the Brazilian scorpion Tityus serrulatus - venom. Mem.
    Inst. Butantan Simp. Internac. 33: 899.
Lowry, O.H., N.J. Rosebrough, A.L. Farr and R.J. Randall, 1951.
    Protein measurement with the Folin-phenol reagent. J. Biol.
    Chem. 193: 265.
Magalhaes, O., 1946. Escorpionismo Monog. Inst. Oswaldo Crus. 3: 1.

Nustad, K. and J.V. Pierce, 1974. Purification of rat urinary kallikrein and their specific antibody. Biochemistry 13: 2312.

Nustad, K., J.V. Pierce and K. Vaaje, 1975. Synthesis of kallikreins by rat kidney slices. Br. J. Pharmac. 53: 229.

Ørstavik, T.B., K. Nustad and P. Brandtzaeg, 1977. A biochemical and immunohistochemical study of kallikrein in normal and isoproterenol-stimulated rat salivary glands during postnatal development. Arch. oral. Biol. 22: 495.

Selinger, Z., S. Batzri, S. Eimerl and M. Schramm, 1973. Calcium and energy requirements for K+ release mediated by the epinephrine α-receptor in rat parotid slices. J. Biol. Chem. 248: 369.

Schneyer, L.H. and C.A. Schneyer, 1962. Electrolyte and water transport by salivary glands slices. Am. J. Physiol. 203: 567.

Schneyer, L.H. and C.A. Schneyer, 1965. Salivary secretion in the rat after ouabain. Am. J. Physiol. 209: 111.

Schwartz, A. and C.A. Moore, 1968. Highly active Na^+, K^+- ATPase in rat submaxillary gland bearing on salivary secretion. Am. J. Physiol. 214: 1163.

EFFECT OF KALLIKREIN-KININ SYSTEM ON ION TRANSPORT ACROSS RAT SMALL INTESTINE

Chiaki Moriwaki and Hiroyuki Fujimori

Faculty of Pharmaceutical Sciences, Science University of Tokyo
Ichigaya Funakawara-Machi, Shinjuku-ku, Tokyo, Japan

INTRODUCTION

Previously we have reported on the influence of the kallikrein-kinin system on the active transport of amino acids and glucose across the rat small intestines (Moriwaki and Fukimori, 1975; Moriwaki et al., 1977) and the effect of kinin on accumulation of valine into the intestinal segment (Moriwaki et al., 1977). It has been recognized that some amino acids or glucose are co-transported with Na^+ in the small intestines (Crane, 1965; Rosenberg et al., 1965). It is a well-known fact that an active solute transport is associated with an increase in transmural potential difference (PDt) of the small intestines (Barry et al., 1964; Schultz and Zalusky, 1964; Lyon and Crane, 1966; Hoshi and Komatsu, 1968). Meanwhile, Okada et al. (1977b) has demonstrated that the resistance of the intestines was not altered by the addition of glucose and glycine in the mucosal fluid. Therefore, the enhancement of absorption of glucose and amino acids in the intestines seems to be the result of the stimulation of Na^+ flux in the absorptive cells by the kinins.

The present paper deals with the effect of kallidin on PDt and the transepithelial resistance (Rt) between the serosal and the mucosal sides of rat jejunum segment in order to elucidate the mechanism of the enchancement of intestinal transport by the kinins.

MATERIALS AND METHODS

Solutions --- HEPES buffered sulfate solution was used as a control medium throughout the experiment. The control medium

461

contained Na_2SO_4 18.25, NaOH 1.95, $KHCO_3$ 2.5, $CaSO_4$ 2.0, $MgSO_4$ 1.0 and mannitol 243.0 mM. Na^+-free medium was prepared by replacement of Na_2SO_4 with Li_2SO_4. The final pH of both solutions were 7.4 ± 0.05.

Tissue Preparation --- Female Wistar rats, weighing about 200 g, were killed after fasting 12 hr, by a blow on the head and exsanguination from the common carotid artery. About 2 cm length of jejunum was immediately removed and cut open along the mesenteric border. The segment was put into oxygenated HEPES buffered sulfate solution and preincubated for 4 min. A small segment (1x1 cm) was mounted and clamped between two chambers. The mucosal chamber was 1x1x2 cm and the serosal one was 0.75x1x2 cm. The area of the window between both chambers was 0.283 cm^2

Measurement of PDt and Rt --- PDt, by setting the potential of the mucosal side at 0 mV, was measured with a preamplifier connected to the mucosal and serosal fluids by Ag-AgCl electrode via siliconated salt bridge filled with 1.5% agar saturated potassium chloride as shown in Fig. 1. Setting the Ag-AgCl wires close to the segment, the resistance of the intestinal segment was measured by pulses of 1 to 5 μA (around 1 sec.).

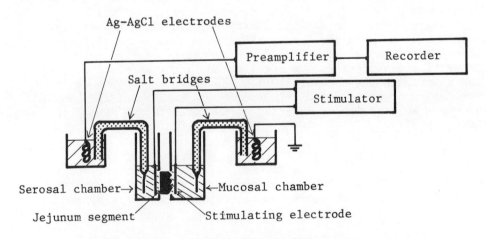

Figure 1.   The Arrangement of the Electrical Circuit Used during the Measurement of Transmural Potential Difference and Transepithelial Resistance.

Experimental Procedures --- The jejunum segment was mounted between two chambers. Both chambers were filled with HEPES buffered sulfate solution, at 37°C, and left standing for 2 min under constant gassing with 95% O_2 - 5% CO_2. This procedure was repeated three times. The mucosal and serosal chambers were filled with 1.0 and 0.75 ml respectively of the above mentioned solution. The salt bridges were poured into them within 1 min. After the DC-level reached a steady state, 0.01 ml of glucose solution was added to the mucosal chamber. During the experimental periods rectangular current was passed through the stimulating electrodes. The effect of kallidin on PDt and Rt was studied as follows: after mounting a jejunum segment between chambers, the serosal surface of it was exposed to various amount of kallidin for 1 min, and then PDt and Rt was measured as described above. A typical recording is shown in Figure 2.

RESULTS

Effect of Kallidin on Glucose-evoked PDt

The mucosal solution was 1.0 ml of HEPES buffered Na_2SO_4 solution and 0.1 to 100 ng of kallidin dissolved in HEPES buffered Na_2SO_4 solution (0.75 ml) was poured into the serosal chamber. Then 0.01 ml of glucose solution was added to the mucosal chamber

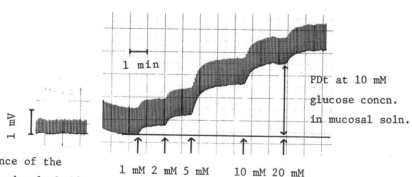

Figure 2. A Representative Recording of Transmural Potential Difference (PDt) and Transepithelial Resistance

Mucosal: HEPES buffered 18.3 mM Na_2SO_4 soln., pH 7.4 + glucose.

Serosal: HEPES buffered 18.3 mM Na_2SO_4 soln., pH 7.4 + 10 ng kallidin.

to prepare a 1 to 20 mM of final glucose concentration. The profile of the glucose-evoked PDt is shown in Fig. 3. The magnitude
of the PDt increased in proportion to the elevation of glucose
concentration. PDt increase was further enhanced by addition of
kallidin to the serosal side of the jejunum. About 2.5 times
greater PDt change than that of the control was observed by 1 ng/
0.75 ml of kallidin at 20 mM glucose concentration. When 20 mM
glucose existed in mucosal chamber, the relationship between
kallidin amount in the serosal chamber and the PDt is shown in
Fig. 4.   The responses became smaller by the larger doses of
kallidin. Lineweaver-Burk plot was applied to the reciprocals of
the PDt against that of glucose concentration in the mucosal chamber
(Fig. 5), and the values of the apparent Km and Vmax were calculated from these plots. The apparent Km at 0, 0.1, 1, 10 and 100
ng/0.75 ml kallidin were 8.04, 28.5, 11.0, 6.02, 11.7 mM and Vmax
were 2.65, 7.63, 7.52, 4.10, 5.03, PDt, respectively. Thus the
apparent Km and Vmax values for the glucose-evoked PDt were
altered by addition of kallidin to the serosal side of the intestinal segment. The Rt were also measured in the same experiments
and the data obtained are summarized in Table 1. The Rt of the
intestine was not significantly changed by addition of glucose
to the mucosal and kallidin to the serodal fluid. PDt and Rt

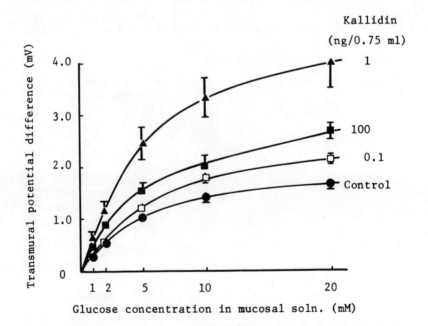

Figure 3.   Effect of Kallidin (serosal) on the mucosal soln. (mM)
            Transmural Potential Difference
            Each bar shows Mean ± S.E. (n = 5 to 7).

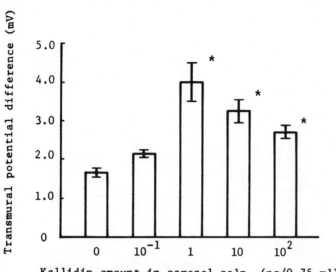

Figure 4.   Effect of Kallidin on Transmural Potential Difference
            Evoked by 20 mM Glucose
            Mean ± S.E. of 4 – 7 experiments
            *Significant difference (P < 0.01)

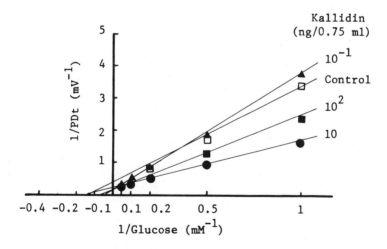

Figure 5.   The Relationship between the Reciprocal of Glucose
            Concentration in Mucosal Solution and the Reciprocals
            of the Glucose–evoked Transmural Potential Difference

Table 1. Effect of Kallidin on Transepithelial Resistance

Glucose concn. (mM)	Transepithelial resistance ($\Omega \cdot cm^2$)				
	Control	KD* 10^{-1} ng	KD 1 ng	KD 10 ng	KD 10^2 ng
0	134.2 ± 8.22 (7)**	133.1 ± 9.74 (5)	127.3 ± 7.37 (6)	132.4 ± 6.07 (5)	144.2 ± 2.90 (5)
1	128.9 ± 8.42 (7)	127.7 ± 9.74 (5)	123.8 ± 6.69 (6)	128.6 ± 7.14 (5)	141.9 ± 2.41 (5)
2	124.9 ± 8.06 (7)	124.9 ± 9.61 (5)	120.2 ± 7.63 (6)	124.8 ± 7.01 (5)	142.0 ± 1.42 (5)
5	126.1 ± 7.91 (7)	124.7 ± 10.1 (5)	120.5 ± 6.93 (6)	122.9 ± 5.84 (5)	139.1 ± 2.73 (5)
10	123.6 ± 7.54 (7)	124.9 ± 10.2 (5)	119.6 ± 7.10 (6)	123.8 ± 5.42 (5)	138.1 ± 3.31 (5)
20	122.1 ± 7.92 (7)	124.9 ± 11.5 (5)	118.8 ± 6.24 (6)	123.6 ± 5.39 (5)	140.7 ± 4.37 (5)

*Kallidin

**Experimental number

were also measured after replacement of Na$_2$SO$_4$ in the serosal
chamber with Li$_2$SO$_4$. In this condition there was Na$^+$-gradient
across the intestinal wall 10 ng/0.75 ml of kallidin in Na$^+$-free
solution was poured to the serosal chamber. The PDt was significantly higher than the control (Fig. 6). Meanwhile, there was
no shift in Rt under these experimental conditions. Differed
from the above mentioned two experiments, 10 and 100 ng of kallidin
was added to the mucosal side of the intestines (Fig. 7). In
these experiments HEPES buffered Na$_2$SO$_4$ solution was used in both
mucosal and serosal solutions and the final glucose concentration
was made up to 1 and 2 mM in the mucosal side. There was no
significant difference between PDt of kallidin treated and nontreated jejunum segment.

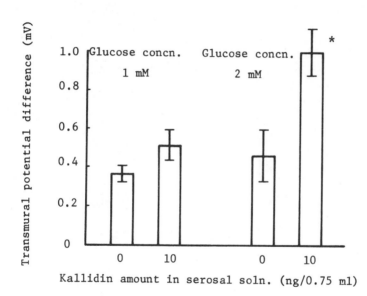

Figure 6. Effect of Kallidin on the Glucose-evoked Transmural
           Potential Difference
           Mean ± S.E. of 4 intestinal segments
           * Significant difference (P < 0.05)

Effect of Kallidin on the Valine-evoked PDt

    Valine is one of the amino acids which are actively trans-
ported and which could evoke the PDt between the mucosal and
serosal sides of the intestines. Whether the magnitude of the
valine (5 mM)-evoked PDt elevation was influenced by the addition
of 10 ng kallidin to the serosal surface of the jejunum segment
was also investigated. As shown in Fig. 8, higher PDt values were
found in kallidin treated segment than in the control.

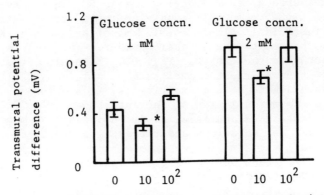

Figure 7.   Effect of Kallidin (mucosal) on the Glucose-evoked
            Transmural Potential Difference
            Mean ± S.E. of 4 intestinal segments
            * Significant difference (P < 0.01)

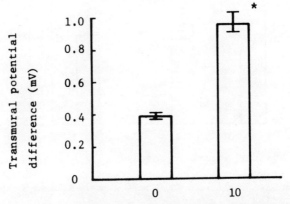

Figure 8.   Effect of Kallidin (serosal) on Transmural
            Potential Difference Evoked by 5 mM Valine
            Mean ± of 4 intestinal segments
            *Significant difference (P < 0.01)

DISCUSSION

There are quite a few papers that deal with the relationship between active solute transport and active solute-evoked PDt or Rt of the small intestine (Barry et al., 1964; Schultz and Zalusky, 1964; Lyon and Crane, 1966; Hoshi and Komatsu, 1968; Okada et al., 1977). Okada (1977a,b) has demonstrated that the presence of actively transported glucose or glycine which can evoke significant PDt changes scarcely affected tissue resistance. It has become clear that extracellular shunt pathway in the small intestine is highly conductive (Rose and Schultz, 1971; White and Armstrong, 1971), and it plays an important role in the transport of ions, water and solutes (Schultz et al., 1974). In the present investigation PDt and Rt were measured under low Na^+ concentration, replacement Cl^- with SO_4^{--} and high resistance of the fluid in order to repress the conductance of the extracellular shunt pathway and of the ions, especially anions which were transported into the epithelial cells. Intra-luminal administration of kallikrein, a kinin-forming enzyme, enhanced the intestinal absorption of valine, methionine, and glucose (Moriwaki and Fujimori, 1975). The same enchancement was observed by the infusion of bradykinin into the mesenteric blood vessels (Moriwaki et al., 1978). Na^+ flux in the intestinal epithelia is closely related to the active transport of some amino acids and sugars, and it also causes PDt of the intestine. Dennhardt and Haberich (1973) reported that the net transport rates of Na^+ and water from the intestinal lumen to the blood vessels were increased by the perfusion of the intestines with kallikrein. Hence the kallikrein-kinin system seems to stimulate Na^+ metabolism and active solute transport.

As shown in Fig. 3, 4 and 6, addition of kallidin to the serosal side of jejunum elevated the PDt values under presence of glucose but kallidin was not affected from the mucosal side (Fig. 7). Valine-evoked PDt change was also elevated by kallidin. The Km and Vmax values calculated from the PDt and glucose concentration were also changed by addition of kallidin (Fig. 5). Meanwhile, Rt was not altered by addition of kallidin (Table 1), and this suggested that the ion permeability through the extracellular shunt pathway was not influenced. Therefore, these data imply that at least the co-coupled ion and glucose or valine transport from mucosal to serosal sides are stimulated by kallidin.

According to an equivalent circuit model for intestinal epithelium, the origin of PDt change consisted of the difference of the electromotive force which is present in the brush border and basolateral membrane, and the potential difference derived from diffusion or leak potential. The diffusion and the leak potentials could be negligible because the mucosal and serosal solution were of the same ionic composition. The PDt should be derived from the difference of the electromotive forces between the serosal and mucosal sides.

The bell-shaped dose-response curve as shown in Fig. 4 is similar to that obtained by bradykinin infusion into mesenteric blood vessels (Moriwaki et al., 1978). The data obtained from the electrophysiological procedure suggested that a suitable amount of kinin elevates the electromotive force located along the serosal basement of the epithelial layer and stimulates the mucosa-serosal net cation flux. However, the effect was lowered by higher doses of kinin. As far as our experimental observations are concerned it seems most likely that the kallikrein-kinin system gives a stimulating effect on ion transport and therefore the solutes transport across the various biological membrane are enhanced.

ABSTRACT

The flow of glucose and valine from the mucosal to the serosal side of rat intestine was stimulated significantly by kallikrein-kinin system. To elucidate the mechanism of this function the effects of kallidin on the transmural potential difference (PDt) between the serosal and the mucosal sides and the transepithelial resistance (Rt) of rat jejunum segment were investigated by electrophysiological procedures.

The glucose-evoked PDt was not significantly altered by addition of kallidin to the mucosal fluid. Meanwhile, PDt which evoked by glucose was significantly shifted under the presence of 10^{-1}-10^2 ng kallidin in the serosal fluid. The valine-evoked PDt was also changed by addition of 10 ng kallidin into the serosal fluid. However, the addition of glucose to the mucosal and kallidin to the serosal fluid did not affect on the Rt of the jejunum segment. These results suggest that kinin stimulated Na^+ transport at the baso-lateral membrane of the intestinal absorptive cells, and the transports of other substances were enhanced consequently.

ACKNOWLEDGEMENTS

A part of this investigation was carried out in the Dept. of Physiology, Teikyo University School of Medicine. The authors express their deep gratitude to Prof. S. Obara for his courtesy and helpful suggestions.

REFERENCES

Barry, R.J.C., S. Dickstein, J. Matthews, D.H. Smyth and E.M. Wright 1964. Electrical potentials associated with intestinal sugar transport, J. Physiol. (London). 171: 316.

Crane, R.K., 1965, Na$^+$-dependent transport in the intestine and other animal tissue, Fed. Proc. 24, 1000.

Dennhardt, R. and F.J. Haberich, 1973, Effect of kallikrein on the absorption of water, electrolytes, and hexoses in the intestine of rats, in: Kininogenases, eds. G.L. Haberland and J.W. Rohen (F.K. Schattauer Verlag·Stuttgart,New York) p. 81.

Hoshi, T. and Y. Komatsu, 1968, Sugar-evoked potential in isolated toad intestine, Jpn. J. Physiol. 18, 508.

Lyon, I. and R.K. Crane, 1966, Studies on transmural potentials in vitro in relation to intestinal absorption. I. Apparent Michaelis constants for Na$^+$-dependent sugar transport, Biochim. Biophys. Acta 112, 278.

Moriwaki, C. and H. Fujimori, 1975, Further observations on the influence of the kallikrein-kinin system on the intestinal absorption, in: Kininogenases 3, eds. G.L. Haberland, J.W. Rohen, G. Blümel and P. Huber (F.K. Schattauer Verlag Stuttgart, New York) p. 57.

Moriwaki, C., H. Fujimori, H. Moriya and K. Kizuki, 1977, Studies on kallikrein. IV. Enhancement of valine transport across the rat small intestine, Chem. Pharm. Bull. 25, 1174.

Moriwaki, C., H. Fujimori and Y. Toyono, 1977, Intestinal kallikrein and the influence of kinin on the intestinal transport, in: Kininogenases 4, eds. G.L. Haberland, J.W. Rohen and T. Suzuki (F.K. Schattauer Verlag.Stuttgart, New York) p.283.

Okada, Y., W.Tsuchiya, A. Irimajiri and A. Inouye, 1977a, Electrical properties and active solute transport in rat small intestine I. Potential profile changes associated with sugar and amino acid transports, J. Membrane Biol. 31, 205.

Okada, Y., A. Irimajiri and A. Inouye, 1977b, Electrical properties and active solute transport in rat small intestine II. Conductive properties of transepithelial routes, J. Membrane Biol. 31, 221.

Rosenberg, I.H., A.L. Coleman and L.E. Rosenberg, 1965, The role of sodium ion in the transport of amino acids by the intestine, Biochim. Biophys. Acta 102, 161.

Rose, R.C. and S.G. Schultz, 1971, Studies on the electrical potential profile across rabbit ileum. Effects of sugars and amino acids on transmural and transmucosal electrical potential differences, J. Gen. Physiol. 57, 639.

Schultz, S.G., R.A. Frizzell and H.N. Nellans, 1974, Ion transport by mammalian small intestine, Annu. Rev. Physiol. 36, 51.

Schultz, S.G. and R. Zalusky, 1964, Ion transport in isolated rabbit ileum II. The interaction between active sodium and sugar transport, J. Gen. Physiol. 47, 1043.

White, J.F. and W. McD. Armstrong, 1971, Effect of transported solutes on membrane potentials in bullfrog small intestine, Am. J. Physiol. 221, 194.

PULMONARY ANAPHYLAXIS AND THE KALLIKREIN-KININ SYSTEM

Narendra B. Oza, James W. Ryan, Una S. Ryan, Pierre
Berryer and Guillermo Pena
Department of Medicine, University of Miami School of
Medicine, Miami, Florida 33101, U.S.A.

ABSTRACT

The kallikrein-kinin system has been thought to participate in
the pathogenesis of anaphylaxis. Kallikrein, released from lungs,
has been postulated to contribute to cardiovascular collapse.
Further to test the hypothesis, we examined for the occurrence of a
kallikrein-like enzyme in guinea pig lungs and examined for release
of such an enzyme by isolated, perfused lungs of guinea pig sensitized to and challenged with egg albumin. In addition, we treated
guinea pigs with the bradykinin potentiating agents, BPP_{9a} and
SQ 14,225. In parallel experiments, we examined for effects of
non-steroidal anti-inflammatory agents on the supposition that
prostaglandin-related substances may mediate or modulate actions of
kinins during anaphylaxis. A plasma kallikrein-like enzyme was
found in lung homogenates and occurred in concentrations greater
than that of plasma itself. Similarly, a store of kininogen occurs
in lungs. However, using a sensitive radioassay for kallikrein-
like enzymes, we were unable to confirm that antigenic challenge of
sensitized lungs causes the release of enzyme into pulmonary venous
effluent. Further, we were unable to modify the acute course of
anaphylaxis by pretreatment of guinea pigs with bradykinin
potentiating agents. However, indomethacin and aspirin at 20-40
mg/kg were found to greatly increase the severity of pulmonary
anaphylaxis in terms of increased resistance to ventilation and
increased numbers of lung hemorrhages. Paradoxically, aspirin or
sodium salicylate at 80-100 mg/kg prevents the characteristic rise
of insufflation pressure and the formation of lung hemorrhages.

INTRODUCTION

From the time of its discovery, bradykinin has been thought to play a role in acute inflammation (Rocha e Silva et al., 1949). Beraldo et al. (1950) considered the possibility that bradykinin contributes to the vascular collapse sometimes seen in anaphylaxis. Subsequently, Brocklehurst and Lahiri (1962, 1963) adduced evidence to indicate that lungs of sensitized guinea pig respond to antigenic challenge by releasing a kininogenase enzyme. Jonasson and Becker (1966) extended the studies of Brocklehurst and Lahiri to show that the kininogenase released by isolated lung resembles plasma kallikrein. The enzyme was inhibited by SBTI and DFP and by C'1 esterase inhibitor. The lung and plasma enzymes behaved similarly on electrophoresis and on molecular sieve chromatography.

However, a precise role for bradykinin or one of its higher homologs in the pathogenesis of anaphylaxis in general and pulmonary anaphylaxis in particular has not been defined. Further, the effects of bradykinin on mast cells have led to the hypothesis that kinins modulate mast cell release (Austen, 1974). In addition, Levi and colleagues (1976) have adduced evidence to indicate that sudden cardiovascular collapse, at least in guinea pigs, is likely to be owing to cardiac anaphylaxis and not to pulmonary anaphylaxis. The latter investigators have reported an association of the fatal ventricular arrhythmias of anaphylaxis with the dysrrhythmic effects of histamine; a substance that occurs abundantly in mast cells of the sinus node.

On the other hand, Newball and colleagues (1975, 1978) have reported that basophils respond to antigenic challenge by releasing a kinin-generating enzyme; an enzyme that may then activate the plasma kallikrein-kinin system.

Our studies were begun with three goals in mind: 1) to examine for a kallikrein-like enzyme in blood-free lung tissue, 2) to develop simple means of monitoring the release of kallikrein-like enzymes by antigenic challenge of sensitized lungs, and 3) to determine whether pretreatment of sensitized guinea pigs with an inhibitor of kininase II (angiotensin converting enzyme) makes anaphylaxis better or worse. By using kininase II inhibitors, it should be possible to potentiate the effects, if any, of bradykinin. Thus, if bradykinin is a primary mediator of anaphylaxis, inhibitors such as BPP9a or SQ 14,225 should increase the severity of the anaphylactic reaction. However, if bradykinin is an important modulator, the reaction should be lessened.

MATERIALS AND METHODS

Guinea pigs (450–700 g body weight) of the Hartley–Ft. Dietrich strain were used in all of the studies to be described. The animals were immunized with egg albumin according to the protocol of Vargaftig and Dao (1971). Guinea pigs were immunized in groups of 12, and 2 of each group were used to test the adequacy of sensitization. The remainder of each group received drug treatment (e.g. BPP_{9a} of aspirin) before antigenic challenge.

Except where noted for studies using isolated lungs, the animal preparations were as follows: Guinea pigs were anesthetized with sodium pentobarbital, 30 mg/kg i.p. Tracheostomy was performed, and the animal was ventilated with a Harvard small animal respirator. A femoral vein was exposed and heparin, 1,000 units, was injected i.v. The femoral vein was cannulated. The femoral artery of the opposite leg was cannulated. Insufflation pressure (resistance to inflation) and arterial blood pressure were measured via pressure transducers. Lead II of the electrocardiogram was monitored throughout each experiment. Each animal was observed until death or for 30 min following antigenic challenge. Approximately 35% of the animals died within 15 min of antigenic challenge (egg albumin, 2 mg in 0.2 ml of saline administered intravenously). Death was always associated with ventricular fibrillation. Cardiovascular collapse ("shock") was never observed in the absence of severe atrio-ventricular block or ventricular fibrillation.

Aspirin and sodium salicylate were obtained from Sigma Chemical Co. BPP_{9a} was synthesized in this laboratory. SQ 14,225 was the kind gift of Dr. Zola Horowitz, Squibb Institute of Medical Research.

RESULTS AND DISCUSSION

Kallikrein–Like Enzymes of Lungs

Guinea pig lungs were either soaked in saline or perfused with saline until free of blood. The lungs were homogenized in 0.1 M sodium phosphate buffer, pH 8.5 (5 ml/g) and the homogenate was centrifuged at 9,000 r.p.m. for 45 min at 4°C. The supernatant was saved and was incubated with acetone (20% by vol.) at 37°C for 4 h. The reaction mixture was dialyzed against 20 mM sodium phosphate buffer, pH 8.0. After centrifugation at 10,000 r.p.m. for 30 min to remove a precipitate, the solution was applied to a column (5.2 x 40 cm) of DEAE–cellulose equilibrated with 20 mM sodium phosphate buffer, pH 8.0. The column was washed with 2 liters of starting buffer. A linear gradient was developed, 0 to 1.0 M NaCl. The active fractions (assayed for arginine esterase activity) were pooled, dialyzed against 0.1 M $NaHCO_3$ plus 0.5 M NaCl, pH 9.5 and

Table I

PURIFICATION OF KALLIKREIN-LIKE ENZYME OF LUNG

Steps	Procedure	EU/mg/h*	Purification	Per Cent Recovery
1	Lung Homogenate	17.4	1	100
2	DEAE-Cellulose	83.6	4.8	51
3	SBTI-Sepharose followed by Sephadex G-25	1164	67	1.8

*EU: μmoles of TAME hydrolyzed

then applied to a SBTI-Sepharose affinity gel (5 ml/g of settled gel; 16 ml of solution; 5 mg of SBTI/ml of settled gel). The gel was washed with the bicarbonate buffer until the $A_{280 \, nm}$ of the eluate was less than 0.07. The gel was then developed with bicarbonate buffer containing 1 M benzamidine. The resulting eluate was dialyzed against the original bicarbonate buffer to remove benzamidine. The nondiffusible material was chromatographed on Sephadex G-25 to remove final traces of benzamidine. Results are shown in Table I.

Jonasson and Becker (1966) have reported that the lung kallikrein-like enzyme resembles plasma kallikrein. Therefore, plasma was treated in parallel.

In addition to the ability of the lung enzyme(s) to hydrolyze arginine esters, the enzyme was also found to hydrolyze Pro-Phe-Arg-[3H]benzylamide to release [3H]benzylamine (e.g. see Chung et al., this volume). The arginine esterase activity of lung homogenate was only partially inhibited by Trasylol (52%) or SBTI (58%). However, the activity obtained by chromatography on DEAE-cellulose (eluted between 0.3-0.5 M NaCl was inhibited by >90% when SBTI (500 μg/ml) or Trasylol (500 μg/ml) was added to enzyme 1 h before addition of substrate.

Tables II and III show relative activities of lung homogenate and plasma (guinea pig and rat). Rat lung contains >100 times more arginine esterase activity than does rat plasma. Guinea pig lung contains approximately twice as much as guinea pig plasma. Further, the apparent specific activities (EU/mg of prot.) are 10- to 20-times greater for lung than for plasma. Thus lungs of both guinea pig and rat contain kallikrein-like enzymes in quantities much greater than could be accounted for by trapped blood.

Lung Kininogen

If the intrapulmonary formation of kinins contributes to the course of anaphylaxis, conditions must exist under which lung kallikrein may act on kininogen. The kininogen could be supplied by blood, but it is also possible that lungs have a store of kininogen independent of blood. To test the latter possibility, we tested guinea pig and rat lung supernatants (prepared as described above) for their abilities to react with trypsin to yield kinins.

Kinins were assayed using isolated guinea pig ileum. For comparison, we also measured kininogen of rat and guinea pig sera. Both rat and guinea pig lungs contain kininogen (expressed as kinin equivalents/mg of protein) at approximately twice the specific activities of their respective sera (see Table IV). Total quantities of lung kininogen (kinin equivalents/g wet weight) exceeded those of sera by almost 9-fold (Table V).

Table II

KALLIKREIN-LIKE ACTIVITY OF LUNG VERSUS PLASMA

(Specific Activities)

Source	EU*	EU after 20% Acetone	Per Cent Activation	Free Lung/Plasma	Total Lung/Plasma
Guinea pig lung	9.1	11.7	22		
				18.4	11.5
Guinea pig plasma	0.5	1.02	52		
- -					
Rat lung	4.0	12.4	67		
				71.2	21.8
Rat plasma	0.06	0.6	90		

*EU: μmoles of TAME/mg protein/h
      Incubation in 0.75 M Tris·HCl, pH 8.5, 37°C

Table III

COMPARISON OF KALLIKREIN-LIKE ACTIVITY IN LUNGS VERSUS PLASMA

(Activities/g of Tissue)

Source	Units of Activity/g Wet Weight	Lung/Plasma
Guinea pig lung	129	
		1.8
Guinea pig plasma	71.2	
Rat lung	620	
		111
Rat plasma	5.6	

Release of Kallikrein-Like Enzymes during Anaphylaxis

Having found evidence of a kallikrein-like enzyme in lungs, we then examined for release of the enzyme by isolated, blood-free lungs of sensitized guinea pigs perfused with saline or saline containing antigen (egg albumin). For comparison, we also examined lungs of non-immunized guinea pigs perfused with antigen in saline. Kallikrein-like activity was assayed using Pro-Phe-Arg-[3H]benzylamide (Chung et al., this volume). Plasma kallikrein-like activity was measured by conducting incubations at pH 8.0. Glandular kallikrein activity was measured by conducting reactions at pH 9.5. Plasmin has little effect on the substrate. Chymotrypsin, urokinase and thrombin do not hydrolyze the substrate (Chung et al., this volume).

Lungs were isolated from guinea pigs anesthetized with pentobarbital (30 mg/kg i.p.). Tracheotomy was performed, and lungs were ventilated mechanically. Heparin, 1,000 units, was injected via a femoral vein. Thoracotomy was performed and a cannula was inserted into the pulmonary artery. A large bore cannula was inserted via the left ventricle into the left atrium. The lungs and heart were removed en bloc. The lungs were pumped with Krebs-Henseleit solution (maintained at 38°C and aerated with 95% CO_2; 5% O_2) until the venous effluent was free of blood.

Perfusion was continued for 3 min and the entire venous effluent was collected in 1 min fraction (10 ml/fraction). At time zero, egg albumin in saline (1 mg/10 ml) or saline alone was added to the pump line. The venous effluent was collected in 1 min fractions for 15 min. All fractions were assayed for kallikrein-like activity.

In all cases (n=7), sensitized lungs perfused with antigen developed marked hyperinflation and gross pulmonary edema within 3 min of beginning antigenic challenge. In addition, insufflation pressure rose more than 5-fold. None of the sensitized lungs (n=6) perfused with saline alone developed discernible edema, hyperinflation or increased insufflation pressure. However, neither group showed any changes in terms of the release of kallikrein-like activity. In general, specific activities (% hydrolysis of Pro-Phe-Arg-[^{3}H]benzylamide/mg of prot.) remained constant or fell while total activities declined progressively through the experiment. Lungs of non-sensitized guinea pigs perfused with egg albumin (n=6) did not differ from the test groups in terms of release of kallikrein. Thus, we were unable to confirm that kallikrein-like enzyme is released by induction of anaphylaxis in isolated guinea pig lung (cf. Jonasson and Becker, 1966).

Release of Kininase II during Anaphylaxis

Pulmonary venous effluents of the isolated lung preparations were assayed for their contents of kininase II (angiotensin converting enzyme) using [^{3}H]hippuryl-His-Leu as substrate (Ryan et al., 1978). Induction of anaphylaxis did not cause changes in the

Table IV

KININOGEN CONCENTRATION OF LUNG VERSUS PLASMA

Source	ng Kininogen/mg Protein	Lung/Plasma
Guinea pig lung	31.0	
Guinea pig plasma	17.7	1.8
Rat lung	45.7	
Rat plasma	26.7	1.7

Table V

COMPARISON OF KININOGEN CONCENTRATION IN LUNG VERSUS PLASMA

Source	ng Kininogen/g Wet Weight	Lung/Plasma
Guinea pig lung	775	8.8
Guinea pig plasma	87.7	
Rat lung	1142.5	8.7
Rat plasma	131.9	

rate of release of kininase II. As was the case for kallikrein-like activity, the quantities of kininase II released into the lung effluent decreased slowly throughout the experiment. Lungs of non-immunized animals could not be distinguished from those of sensitized animals, and neither of these control groups could be distinguished from anaphylactic lungs in terms of kininase II release. At every time interval, the specific activity of kininase II in lung effluent was but a small fraction (less than 1/100th) of that of guinea pig serum.

We considered the possibility that isolated perfused lungs might yield misleading results. Although isolated lungs developed marked hyperinflation and edema, they did not develop the diffuse patchy hemorrhages seen following induction of anaphylaxis in anesthetized guinea pigs. Therefore, under the assumption that capillary damage is more severe in lungs of intact animals, we measured kininase II activity in arterial blood of sensitized guinea pigs infused with saline or with egg albumin in saline. In neither case was there a rise or fall of kininase II activity detectable within 30 min of the beginning of infusion.

Effects of Bradykinin Potentiating Agents on the Course of Anaphylaxis

As discussed above, if bradykinin is a primary mediator of anaphylaxis, preservation of bradykinin should worsen the disease process. If bradykinin is a modulator, its preservation might decrease the severity of anaphylaxis.

Therefore, we examined BPP$_{9a}$ (n=6) and SQ 14,225 (2-D-methyl-3-mercaptopropanoyl-L-proline) for their effects on the course of anaphylaxis. BPP$_{9a}$ at 4 mg/kg (i.v.) invariably lowered serum kininase II activity to unmeasurably low values (cf. Ryan et al., 1977). However, guinea pigs appeared to be markedly resistant to SQ 14,225 and required the drug at 30 mg/kg i.v. to inhibit kininase II by >90%. However, even at these dose levels, neither drug affected the course of anaphylaxis in terms of blood pressure rise, insufflation pressure, changes in the electrocardiogram or onset of sudden cardiovascular collapse. On the latter point, our observations did not differ from those of Levi and colleagues (Levi et al., 1976): Sudden cardiovascular collapse always followed the onset of ventricular fibrillation or severe A-V block.

Within the limits of these studies, we were unable to obtain evidence that indicated a role for kinins in anaphylaxis. However, it must be added that enzymes other than kininase II can inactivate bradykinin (e.g. see Ryan et al., 1968, 1970). Hence, inhibition of kininase II may not suffice to preserve or allow the accumulation of kinins. In addition, it is not known at present whether BPP$_{9a}$ or SQ 14,225 are efficiently delivered to sites at a distance from the vascular space (e.g. to the immediate environment of mast cells in lungs).

Effects of Cyclo-oxygenase Inhibitors

There are no fewer than eleven different excitatory agents thought to act as humoral mediators of anaphylaxis (cf. Collier, 1976). Further, it is thought that one mediator may act to stimulate the release of other mediators and modulators. The complexity of mediators is such that inhibition or augmentation of the effects of a single mediator may not change the overall course of the anaphylactic reaction. However, if one could inhibit the release or formation of several different classes of mediators, then the influence of a single class, e.g. kinins, might be more readily defined.

Thus, we examined for the effects of nonsteroidal anti-inflammatory agents on the course of anaphylaxis in anesthetized guinea pigs. In adequate dosages, aspirin and indomethacin should prevent the formation of prostaglandin endoperoxides, prostaglandins, thromboxanes and prostacyclins--but probably at the expense of increased production of hydroperoxy-fatty acids (cf. Adcock et al., 1978). In addition, indomethacin has been shown to be capable of augmenting the release of mediators such as SRS-A from isolated perfused lung tissue (e.g. see Engineer et al., 1978). Adcock et al., (1978) have suggested that the augmentation may be owing to increased

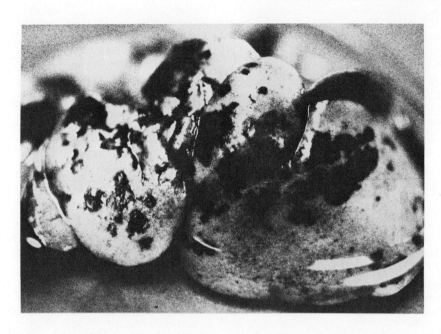

Fig. 1. Effects of indomethacin on pulmonary anaphylaxis. A
sensitized guinea pig, prepared as described in Materials and
Methods, was injected (i.v.) with indomethacin, 40 mg/kg. Three
minutes later, 2 mg of egg albumin was injected intravenously to
induce anaphylaxis. Fifteen minutes later, the animal was killed
with an overdose of pentobarbital and the lungs were removed. Note
the occurrence of hemorrhages in all lobes of the lungs.   X   2

formation of the fatty acid hydroperoxide, HPETE.

    In our first studies, we pretreated sensitized guinea pigs
with both indomethacin (25 mg/kg) and a kininase II inhibitor,
SQ 14,225 at 30-60 mg/kg or BPP$_{9a}$ at 4 mg/kg, before antigenic
challenge. Both drugs were administered intravenously. In all experiments (n=7), anaphylaxis was made worse as compared to that seen
in guinea pigs not pretreated (n=5). Insufflation pressure was
increased in terms of the absolute rise in pressure and in terms of
duration. Characteristically, all sensitized guinea pigs reacted to
antigenic challenge to produce patchy lung hemorrhages of the lower
and, sometimes, middle lobes. However, those animals pretreated
with indomethacin and a kininase II inhibitor developed extensive
hemorrhages throughout all lobes of the lungs (cf. Figs. 1 and 2).

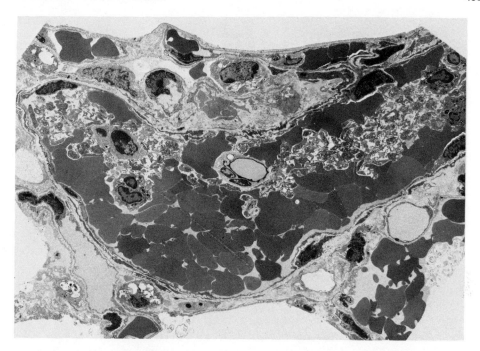

Fig. 2.   Low power electron micrograph of lungs shown in Fig. 1.
Note stasis of blood in small vessel and abundance of platelet
aggregates.   X   2,700

The marked increases in severity of anaphylaxis were not
dependent on pretreatment with BPP_{9a} or SQ 14,225. Indomethacin
given alone, 3 min before antigenic challenge, sufficed to produce
the same effects (Figs. 1 and 2).

For comparison, we used aspirin at 20-40 mg/kg. Of 6 sensitized guinea pigs thus treated, 3 did not respond to antigenic
challenge with a discernible rise of insufflation pressure. In
addition, lung hemorrhages did not develop. However, the remaining
3 developed severe anaphylaxis and consequent diffuse lung hemorrhage.

We considered the possibility that we had reached a critical
dose level and proceeded to examine for effects of aspirin at
80-100 mg/kg. At the higher dosage, none of the guinea pigs (n=6)
developed objective signs of pulmonary anaphylaxis. Inadequacy of
sensitization was not a factor: All of the guinea pigs not treated
with aspirin (n=7), immunized at the same time by the same protocol,
developed the typical 4- to 7-fold increase in insufflation pressure
and patchy lung hemorrhages.

However, we were unable to invoke inhibition of cyclo-oxygenase as a major factor: Sodium salicylate at 80 mg/kg conferred the same protection (n=5; no change in insufflation pressure, no lung hemorrhages).

Clearly, enormous doses of aspirin or salicylate were required to protect against major changes in lung function following induction of anaphylaxis. We have not yet ruled out changes in blood pH that may be induced by acetyl salicylate and salicylate itself. Nonetheless, it should be emphasized that the pH change inducible by hyperventilation was not a factor: All animals were ventilated with a mechanical respirator throughout the experiments.

CONCLUDING REMARKS

We set out to define the role of the kallikrein-kinin system in the acute phase of pulmonary anaphylaxis in guinea pigs. By examining lung homogenates, we found evidence of one or more kallikrein-like enzymes and a store of kininogen. However, we were unable to find evidence of release of kallikrein-like activity into the venous effluent of anaphylactic lungs perfused with Krebs-Henseleit solution. In addition, there was no release of kininase II, an enzyme of endothelial cells (e.g. see Ryan and Ryan, 1977). When we began our studies, it seemed possible that the release of kininase II might be useful as an index of lung capillary injury. Since the capillary injury of anaphylaxis is much more severe in lungs of intact animals than in isolated lungs perfused with a salt solution, we also examined for changes in kininase II of arterial blood following induction of anaphylaxis. No changes were found.

Our results do not support the concept that kallikrein, released from lungs, participates in the cardiovascular collapse of anaphylaxis. Whether the kallikrein-kinin system plays a role within the lungs is less clear. Neither BPP$_{9a}$ nor SQ 14,225, drugs which can potentiate the actions of kinins, made anaphylaxis better or worse. On the other hand, it is not yet known whether BPP9$_a$ or SQ 14,225 can be delivered efficiently to sites within the lungs where mast cells occur in greatest abundance.

Quite incidentally we found that aspirin and sodium salicylate in high dosage can protect completely against major pulmonary changes of anaphylaxis; namely, increased insufflation pressure and development of lung hemorrhages. Our results cannot be taken as a recommendation that anaphylaxis be treated with the salicylates or other nonsteroidal anti-inflammatory agents. Aspirin, at lower dosage, and indomethacin, at all dosage levels used, greatly enhanced the effects of anaphylaxis on lung structure and function. The present challenge is to define how aspirin at high dosage confers it protective effects.

ACKNOWLEDGEMENTS

This work was supported in part by grants from the U.S.P.H.S (HL22087 and HL21568), the John A. Hartford Foundation, Inc., The Council for Tobacco Research-U.S.A., Inc. and the American Heart Association (Palm Beach County Chapter, Inc.).

REFERENCES

Adcock, J.J., L.G. Garland, S. Moncada and J.A. Salmon, 1978. Enhancement of anaphylactic mediator release from guinea-pig perfused lungs by fatty acid hydroperoxides, Prostaglandins 16: 163.

Adcock, J.J., L.G. Garland, S. Moncada and J.A. Salmon, 1978. The mechanisms of enchancement by fatty acid hydroperoxides of anaphylactic mediator release. Prostaglandins 16: 179.

Amundsen, E., L. Svendsen, A.M. Vennerød and K. Laake, Determination of plasma kallikrein with a new chromogenic tripeptide derivative, 1976 In: Chemistry and Biology of the Kallikrein-Kinin System in Health and Disease. Fogarty Int. Center Proc. No. 27, eds. J.J. Pisano and K.F. Austen (U.S. Government Printing Office, Washington) p. 215.

Austen, K.F., 1974. Reaction mechanisms in the release of mediators of immediate hypersensitivity from human lung tissue. Fed. Proc. 33: 2256.

Beraldo, W.T., 1950. Formation of bradykinin in anaphylactic and peptone shock. Am. J. Physiol., 163: 283.

Brocklehurst, W.E. and S.C. Lahiri, 1962. The production of bradykinin in anaphylaxis, J. Physiol., 160: 15.

Brocklehurst, W.E. and S.C. Lahiri, 1963. Formation and destruction of bradykinin during anaphylaxis. J. Physiol., 165: 39.

Chung, A.C., J.W. Ryan, G. Pena and N.B. Oza (this volume). A simple radioassay for human urinary kallikrein.

Collier, H.O.J. Role of the kallikrein-kinin system in lung diseases, 1976 In: Chemistry and Biology of the Kallikrein-Kinin System in Health and Disease. Fogarty Int. Center Proc. No. 27, eds. J.J. Pisano and K.F. Austen (U.S. Government Printing Office, Washington) p. 495.

Engineer, D.M., U. Niederhauser, P.J. Piper and P. Sirois, 1978. Release of mediators of anaphylaxis: Inhibition of prostaglandin synthesis and the modification of release of slow reacting substances on anaphylaxis and histamine. Br. J. Pharmac. 62: 61.

Jonasson, O. and E.L. Becker, 1966. Release of kallikrein from guinea pig lung during anaphylaxis. J. Exp. Med., 123: 509.

Levi, R., G. Allan and J.H. Zavecz, 1976. Cardiac histamine receptors. Fed. Proc., 35: 1942.

Newball, H.H., S.D. Revak, C.G. Cochrane, J.H. Griffin and L.M. Lichtenstein, 1978. Cleavage of hageman factor (HF) by a basophil kallikrein of anaphylaxis (BK-A). Clin. Res., 26:519A.

Newball, H.H., R.C. Talamo and L.M. Lichtenstein, 1975. Release of leukocyte kallikrein mediated by IgE, Nature 254: 635.

Rocha e Silva, M., W.T. Beraldo and G. Rosenfeld, 1949. Bradykinin, a hypotensive and smooth muscle stimulating factor released from plasma by snake venoms and by trypsin. Am. J. Physiol., 156: 261.

Ryan, J.W., A Chung, C. Ammons and M.L. Carlton, 1977. A simple radioassay for angiotensin converting enzyme. Biochem. J., 167: 501.

Ryan, J.W., A. Chung, L.C. Martin and U.S. Ryan, 1978. New substrates for the radioassay of angiotensin converting enzyme of endothelial cells in culture. Tissue & Cell. 10: 555.

Ryan, J.W., J. Roblero and J.M. Stewart, 1968. Inactivation of bradykinin in the pulmonary circulation. Biochem. J., 110: 795.

Ryan, J.W., J. Roblero and J.M. Stewart, 1970. Inactivation of bradykinin in rat lung. Adv. Exp. Med. Biol., 8: 263.

Ryan, J.W. and U.S. Ryan, 1977. Pulmonary endothelial cells. Fed. Proc., 36: 2683.

Vargaftig, B.B. and N. Dao, 1971. Release of vasoactive substances from guinea pig lungs by slow-reacting substance C and arachidonic acid. Pharmacology 6: 99.

STUDIES ON THE EFFECTS OF BRADYKININ AND ITS FRAGMENTS ON THE CENTRAL NERVOUS SYSTEM

K. Kariya, H. Okamoto, H. Iwaki, A. Hashimoto, M. Yagyu*,
Y. Tsuchiya* and Y. Okada*
Department of Pharmacology and Department of Chemistry*
Faculty of Pharmaceutical Sciences, Kobe-Gakuin Univ.
Igawadani-cho, Tarumi-ku, Kobe 673, Japan

Kininases were separated by DEAE-cellulose column chromatography with stepwise gradient of sodium chloride from rat whole brain. F-A which developed with 70 mM NaCl cleaved Phe-Ser bond, F-B with 100 mM NaCl hydrolyzed post-proline site and F-C with 150 mM NaCl broke down bradykinin to amino acids. F-A activity was inhibited by Arg-Pro-Pro-Gly-Phe, Ser-Pro-Phe-Arg and Gly-Phe-Ser-Pro, and the two formers blocked F-B activity.

INTRODUCTION

It is well known that bradykinin (Arg^1-Pro^2-Pro^3-Gly^4-Phe^5-Ser^6-Pro^7-Phe^8-Arg^9) injected intracerebrally produces a short-lasting excitation followed by sedation in experimental animals (Graeff et al. 1969; Iwata et al. 1970; De Silva et al. 1971). To study the relationship between these phenomena and the peptide fragments of bradykinin, we synthesized a number of fragments and observed that a fragment Ser-Pro of bradykinin prolonged pentobarbital induced sleeping time in the mouse (Okada et al. 1977). Also, some effects of bradykinin and its fragments on spontaneous electroencephalogram activity were observed in the rat with chronically implanted electrodes and cannula on the skull (unpublished data).

On the other hand, enzymatic degradation of bradykinin in the brain has been studied in many species (Shikimi et al. 1970; Shikimi and Iwata 1970; Marks and Pirotta 1971; Camargo et al. 1973). Oliveira et al (1976) separated two endopeptidases including thiol group from the rabbit cerebral cortex. These enzymes were temed kininase A which cleaved a Phe-Ser bond and kininase B which hydrolyzed Pro-Phe in bradykinin. Furthermore, they concluded

that the properties of kininase B differed from those of other
peptidyl peptidases, such as plasma kininase II or angiotensin
converting enzyme.

However, the physiological and pharmacological significances
of bradykinin in the central nervous system is not clarified as yet.
Therefore we have studied the relationship between the behavioural
changes and the degradation system of bradykinin in the rat brain.

MATERIALS AND METHODS

Peptides: Bradykinin was purchased from Protein Research
Foundation, Osaka, Japan. The peptide fragments derived from
bradykinin were synthesized by liquid phase synthesis as described
previously (Okada et al. 1977).

Enzyme preparation: Male S.D. strain rats weighing 200 to 300
g were anesthetized with pentobarbital Na (30 mg/kg, i.p.) and
were infused with cold saline through a cannula inserted in both
carotid arteries. After blood was flowed from jugular veins, the
whole brain was removed and homogenized with four volumes of 0.25
M sucrose. The homogenate was centrifuged at 25,000 g for 60 min.
The supernatant was adjusted to pH 5.0 with 0.5 M acetic acid,
held for 2 hr at 4°C and recentrifuged at 900 g for 15 min. This
supernatant was applied to a DEAE-cellulose column as shown by
Oliveira et al. (1976). Each fraction obtained from the chromatography was concentrated in a collodion bag under reduced pressure
for enzyme preparation.

Measurement of kininase activity: The reaction mixture, consisting of enzyme preparation (0.8-1.0 μg), 1 nmole bradykinin,
50 mM sodium phosphate buffer (pH 7.5) and 100 mM NaCl in a total
volume of 0.5 ml, was incubated for 20 min at 37°C. The reaction
was stopped by an addition of 10 μl 0.5 N HCl. Kininase activity
was measured by a contraction of the guinea-pig ileum with residual
bradykinin. The isolated ileum was bathed in Tyrode's solution
consisting 1.7 μM atropine sulfate at 28°C using the Mangus method.

Determination of fragments derived from bradykinin: Thin-
layer chromatography was used for this experiment. The mixture,
containing 10-20 μg protein as enzyme preparation, 40 nmoles bradykinin and 4 nmoles dithiothreitol in 100 μl Tris-HCl buffer (50 mM,
pH 7.4), was incubated for 60 min at 37°C. After the incubation,
10 μl of 0.5N HCl was added and dansylation was carried out by
the method of Gray (1972). Dansylated peptides and amino acids
were applied to silica gel G layer and the gel plate was developed
with the solvent (n-butanol:acetic acid:water = 4:1:5). After
the chromatography, dansylated compounds were visually detected as
fluorescent spots by the irradiation of UV light (360 nm) and the

spots were recorded by sketch.

Determination of protein concentrations: Protein concentrations
in the above experiments were assayed spectrophotometrically by
the method of Lowry et al. (1951) using bovine serum albumin as
a standard.

RESULTS

DEAE-Cellulose column chromatography and kininase activities:
Fig. 1 shows protein concentrations and kininase activities in the
elution diagram. Kininase activities appeared with stepwise gradient in various sodium chloride concentrations. The activities of

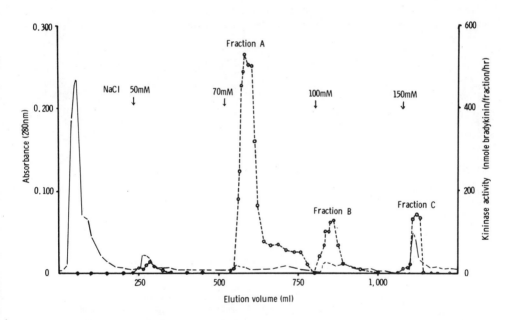

Fig. 1. Chromatography on DEAE-cellulose of pH 5.0 supernatant
fraction from rat brain. The pH 5.0 supernatant fraction was dialyzed against 50 mM Tris-HCl buffer (pH. 7.5), 30 mM NaCl and applied
to the column (0.9 x 40 cm) previously equilibrated with the same
buffer. After the sample application, the column was developed by
stepwise gradient of NaCl as shown in the figure. The sample was
eluted at the rate of 13 ml/hr and fractions of 5.0 ml were collected. Kininase activity was determined with the isolated guinea-pig
ileum. (————) Absorbance at 280 nm; (o---o) kininase activity.
Each fraction of kininase activity was termed A, B and C as a matter
of convenience.

fraction A kininase (F-A) was detected in eluate with 70 mM NaCl gradient, fraction B (F-B) with 100 mM and fraction C (F-C) with 150 mM. Little kininase activity was observed in eluate with 50 mM NaCl at the first step. Purification of kininases from the rat whole brain homogenate are summarized in Table 1. The specific activity of F-A was increased about 126 times as that of the homogenate and about 60 times as that of the 25,000 g supernatant fraction. The activity of F-B was about 30% of F-A. And the activity of F-C was less than those of F-A and F-B.

Then we attempted to determine the site of hydrolysis of bradykinin by each kininase on thin-layer chromatography. Fluorescent spots of dansylated sample are shown in Fig. 2. F-A produced Arg-Pro-Pro-Gly-Phe and Ser-Pro-Phe-Arg from bradykinin. F-B cleaved Pro-Gly and Pro-Phe bonds in the peptide. Furthermore, it was observed that Phe and Arg were dansylated. However, F-C broke down bradykinin to amino acids composed of the one and the spot of bradykinin as substrate was not detected visually during this incubation period.

Effects of pH on F-A and F-B activities. The effects of pH on kininases activities were assayed in different buffers according to pH ranges, such as Na-phosphate (pH 6.0-8.0), Tris-HCl (pH 7.5-10.0) and carbonate-bicarbonate (pH 9.0-10.5) buffers in the concentration of 50 mM. As shown in Fig. 3, the optimal pH for F-A was 7.5 and also showed a weak peak at pH 9.5. A suitable pH value of F-B was similar to that of F-A but F-B was less active than F-A.

Table 1. Purification of kininase from rat brain

Fraction	Protein (mg)	Specific activity (µg/mg protein/hr)	Degree of purification	Yield (%)
Homogenate	460	75	1	100
25,000 g Supernatant	120	146	1.9	50
pH 5.0 Supernatant	20.6	846	11.2	50
DEAE-Cellulose column				
A	0.73	9,520	126	20
B	0.32	3,063	41	2.8
C	0.99	889	12	2.5

Effect of various compounds on kininases activities of the
rat whole brain. After the incubation with each enzyme preparation,
bradykinin and a compound, a portion of the mixture was tested for
the contracting response of the isolated guinea-pig ileum. Effects
of some SH blockers and metal chelating agents on kininases activities were given in Table 2. F-A was inhibited by 8-hydroxyquinol-
ine, o-phenanthroline and N-ethylmaleimide in the concentration of
10^{-3}M, but in the concentration of less than 10^{-4}M, 8-hydroxyqui-
noline activated the enzyme. The kininase activity of F-B was
inhibited markedly by o-phenanthroline and N-ethylmaleimide in the
concentration of more than 10^{-4}M. Ethylenediaminetetraacetic acid
at the concentration of more than 10^{-4}M increased the activity of
both enzymes, but p-chloromercuribenzoate strongly inhibited these
enzymes. However, diethyldithiocarbamate did not influence the
activity.

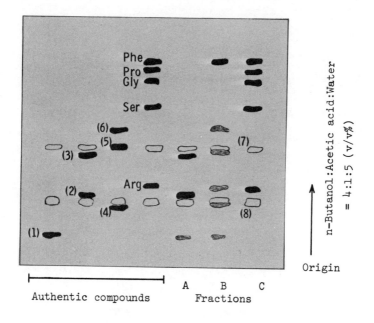

Fig. 2. Thin-layer chromatogram of dansylated peptides derived from
bradykinin. DEAE fraction A (17.4 μg protein), B (7.8 μg protein)
and C (23.8 μg protein) were incubated in 50 mM Tris-HCl buffer
(pH 7.4)containing 4 nmoles dithiothreitol and 40 nmoles bradykinin
at 37°C for 60 min. The 20 μl of reaction mixture was dansylated
according to the method of Gray. Numbers in chromatogram show (1)
Arg-Pro-Pro-Gly-Phe-Ser-Pro-Phe-Arg(bradykinin); (2) Arg-Pro-Pro-
Gly-Phe; (3) Ser-Pro-Phe-Arg; (4) Arg-Pro-Pro; (5) Phe-Arg;
(6) Gly-Phe-Ser-Pro; (7) DNS-NH_2 and (8) DNS-OH.

The effects of SH protectors on kininases are shown in Table
3. In the concentration of less than 10^{-4}M, dithiothreitol increased the activity of F-A but glutathione in the concentration
of 10^{-3}M inhibited the activity strongly. In the case of F-B, cysteine, glutathione and 2-mercaptoethanol increased the activity.
Dithiothreitol inhibited the F-B activity in the concentration of
10^{-3}M but did not affect the activity in the concentration less
than 10^{-4}M.

Observed effects of peptide fragments derived from bradykinin
on these enzymes were shown in Table 4. Both of the kininases activities were inhibited by Arg-Pro-Pro-Gly-Phe and Ser-Pro-Phe-Arg
in the concentration of more than 10^{-4}M. Gly-Phe-Ser-Pro did not
block F-B but inhibited F-A in the concentration of 10^{-3}M. However, Phe-Arg did not influence the bradykinin inactivation by both
kininases. Higher concentrations of Ser-Pro-Phe-Arg could not be
tested in this experiments, because the fragment potentiated the
contraction of the ileum by bradykinin.

Table 2. Effects of SH blockers and metal chelating agents on kininases activities. Results are expressed as percentage changes from
the activity without added compound. Each compound was added at the
same time with bradykinin in the incubation medium.
EDTA : ethylenediaminetetraacetic acid.
    + : activation   - : inhibition

Reagents	Concentration (M)	Fraction A (%)	Fraction B (%)
EDTA	10^{-5}	+27	+2
	10^{-4}	+40	+37
	10^{-3}	+38	+41
o-Phenanthroline	10^{-5}	+7	-3
	10^{-4}	-26	-41
	10^{-3}	-47	-65
8-Hydroxyquinoline	10^{-5}	+70	+57
	10^{-4}	+55	-4
	10^{-3}	-66	-65
Diethyldithio-carbamate	10^{-5}	0	+22
	10^{-4}	0	0
	10^{-3}	-27	-10
N-Ethylmaleimide	10^{-5}	+2	+14
	10^{-4}	-11	-37
	10^{-3}	-41	-74
p-Chloromercuri-benzoate	10^{-6}	-58	-94
	10^{-5}	-100	-100
	10^{-4}	-100	-100

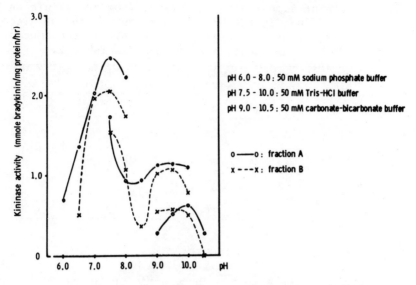

pH 6.0 - 8.0 : 50 mM sodium phosphate buffer
pH 7.5 - 10.0 : 50 mM Tris-HCl buffer
pH 9.0 - 10.5 : 50 mM carbonate-bicarbonate buffer

o——o : fraction A
x---x : fraction B

Fig. 3. Effects of pH on kininases activities.

Table 3. Effect of SH reagents on the activities of kininases in rat brain. The conditions are same as Table 2.

Reagent	Concent-ration (M)	Fraction A (%)	Fraction B (%)
Dithiothreitol	10^{-5}	+71	+16
	10^{-4}	+67	+18
	10^{-3}	-8	-42
Cysteine	10^{-5}	+30	+29
	10^{-4}	+32	+100
	10^{-3}	-13	+100
Glutathione	10^{-5}	+6	+36
	10^{-4}	+12	+85
	10^{-3}	-64	+52
2-Mercaptoethanol	10^{-5}	-4	+12
	10^{-4}	-27	+55
	10^{-3}	-31	+107

Table 4.   Effects of some fragments derived from bradykinin on the
activities of kininases in rat brain. (*); Contraction of ileum
by bradykinin was potentiated by Ser-Pro-Phe-Arg in the concentration
of more than 10^{-4}M.   The conditions are same as Table 2.

Peptides (M)	Fraction A (%)			Fraction B (%)		
	10^{-5}	10^{-4}	10^{-3}	10^{-5}	10^{-4}	10^{-3}
Arg-Pro-Pro-Gly-Phe	-9	-43	-100	0	-32	-100
Ser-Pro-Phe-Arg	-22	-84	* -	-17	-78	* -
Gly-Phe-Ser-Pro	+7	+7	-32	-6	-6	-14
Phe-Arg	+6	+7	0	+2	+7	0

DISCUSSION

With regard to the effect of bradykinin on the central nervous
system, it was reported that the excited state was elicited by the
authentic bradykinin whereas its metabolites might cause a depression
(Iwata et al. 1970).   Previously our group observed that bradykinin
and some fragments containing Ser-Pro, such as Gly-Phe-Ser-Pro,
Phe-Ser-Pro and Ser-Pro prolonged a pentobarbital induced sleeping
time and suggested that a structure of Ser-Pro at the C-terminal
position was required to prolong sleeping time (Okada et al. 1970).

On the other hand, there are many reports for kinin inactivating enzymes in brain.   However, it is not certain which bonds in
bradykinin are cleaved.   Shikimi and Iwata (1970) showed that Arg
and Phe were released from C-terminal of the peptide after incubation
for 24 hr at room temperature using the enzyme purified 32 fold to
the rat whole brain homogenate.   Marks and Pirotta (1971) reported
the appearance of amino acids from bradykinin with time by the enzyme
partially purified from the rat brain supernatant and suggested that
a primary point of cleavage occurred at the Phe-Ser bond.   Furthermore, Camargo et al. (1973) and Oliveira et al. (1976) showed that
there are two kininases in the rabbit cerebral cortex, one cleaved
peptide bond of Phe-Ser(kininase A) and the other released Phe-Arg
from bradykinin (kininase B).   The results obtained here showed
that the pH 5.0 supernatant fraction obtained from 25,000 g supernatant in the rat whole brain contained three different bradykinin
cleaving enzymes.   Namely, these enzymes hydrolyzed a Phe-Ser bond
(F-A), Pro-Gly and Pro-Phe (F-B) and all peptide bonds (F-C).
As shown in Fig. 4, F-A is the same enzyme as kininase A but F-B
is different from kininase B as far as the cleavage of a Pro-Gly
bond is concerned.   F-C is similar to a carboxypeptidase.   As F-B
contained a few F-C under this separation, dansylated amino acids,
Phe and Arg, might be spotted.

```
                    Arg-Pro-Pro-Gly-Phe-Ser-Pro-Phe-Arg
Plasma                                        ↑  ↑
kininase                                      II  I

Rabbit brain                            ↑     ↑
kininase                                A     B

Rat brain
  Fraction A                            ↑
         B                                       ↑  ↑
         C          ↑  ↑  ↑  ↑  ↑  ↑  ↑
```

Fig. 4. Summary of various kininases and their cleaving sites.

Koida and Walter (1976) separated the post—proline cleaving enzyme from the lamb kidny, and showed that this enzyme hydrolyzed post - proline bonds both in bradykinin and its potentiating factor. While this enzyme was not found in the central nervous system as a post-proline cleaving enzyme, F-B seems to be similar to this enzyme. However, the lung angiotensin converting enzyme hydrolyzed bradykinin at the site of Pro-Phe bond (Overturf et al. 1975). But Oliveira et al. (1976) described that brain kininase B hydrolyzed angiotensin I without converting it to angiotensin II. In this point, the determination of the site of hydrolysis in angiotensin has been studied using these enzymes obtained from the rat whole brain.

Arg-Pro-Pro-Gly-Phe, Ser-Pro-Phe-Arg and Gly-Phe-Ser-Pro blocked hydrolysis of bradykinin by F-A. Phe-Arg did not influence this kininase. These results support the hypothesis that the site of hydrolysis is Phe-Ser bond. Similary, F-B was inhibited by Arg-Pro-Pro-Gly-Phe and Ser-Pro-Phe-Arg, but was not influenced by Gly-Phe-Ser-Pro and Phe-Arg. F-B might be concerned in the cleavage of the Pro-X (X: amino acid) in the brain.

Although Ser-Pro-Phe-Arg has potentiated the contraction response by bradykinin of the guinea-pig ileum in vitro (Kameyama et al. 1970), it is interesting to see that this fragment inhibits activities of F-A and F-B in vitro. Furthermore, the results obtained from the observation on the effects of SH reagents, SH blockers and chelator to the brain kininases, did not coincide with other investigators findings, and also they had obtained each different results (Iwata et al. 1969, Camargo and Graeff 1969, Shikimi and Iwata 1970, Camargo et al. 1973, Cicilini et al. 1977). These discrepancies might be due to the different experimental conditions, such as the experimental animals used, the regions of the brain used and the bioassay system. To obtain desirable results, it is necessary to establish the quantitative mircro analyzing system of bradykinin and small peptides using chemical or immunological techniques.

ACKNOWLEDGEMENTS

We wish to express our thanks to Miss M. Okamoto, Miss M. Kami-
mura, Mr. J. Seki and Mr. D. Hazeyama for an assistance in the assay.
We thank Mr. Y. Inoue for helping the preparation of the manuscript.

REFERENCES

Camargo, A.C.M. and F.G. Graeff, 1969, Subcellular distribution and
    properties of the bradykinin inactivation system in rabbit brain
    homogenates, Biochem. Pharmac. 18, 548.
Camargo, A.C.M., R. Shapanka and L.J. Greene, 1973, Preparation,
    assay, and partial characterization of a neutral endopeptidase
    from rabbit brain, Biochemistry 12, 1838.
Cicilini, M.A., H. Caldo., J.D. Berti and A.C.M. Camargo, 1977,
    Rabbit tissue peptidases that hydrolyse the peptide hormone
    bradykinin, Boichem. J. 163, 433.
Da Silva, G.R. and M. Rocha e Silva, 1971, Catatonia induced in the
    rabbit by intracerebral injection of bradykinin and morphine,
    Eur. J. Pharmacol. 15, 180.
Graeff, F.G., I.R. Pela and M. Rocha e Silva, 1969, Behavioural and
    somatic effects of bradykinin injected into the cerebral ventri-
    cles of unanesthetized rabbits, Br. J. Pharmac. 37, 723.
Gray, W.R., Endogroup analysis using dansyl chloride, 1972, in:
    Methods in Enzymology, Vol.25, ed. C.H.W. Hirs (Academic Press,
    New York) p.121.
Iwata, H., T. Shikimi and T. Oka, 1969, Pharmacological signifi-
    cances of peptidase and proteinase in the brain (I), Biochem.
    Pharmac. 18, 119.
Iwata, H., T. Shikimi, M. Iida and H. Miichi, 1970, Pharmacological
    significances of peptidase and proteinase in the brain (IV),
    Japan. J. Pharmacol. 22, 80.
Kameyama, T., K. Sasaki and J. Nabeshima, 1970, Contractile activi-
    ties of synthetic bradykinin fragments on guinea pig ileum,
    YAKUGAKU ZASSHI 90, 1006.
Koida, M. and R. Walter, 1976, Post-proline cleaving enzyme, J.
    Biol. Chem. 251, 7593.
Lowry, O.H., N.J. Rosebrough, A.L. Farr and R.J. Randall, 1951,
    Protein measurement with the Folin phenol reagent, J. Biol. Chem.
    193, 265.
Marks, N. and M. Pirotta, 1971, Breakdown of bradykinin and its ana-
    logs by rat brain neutral proteinase, Brain Res. 33, 565.
Oliveira, E.B., A.R. Martins and A.C.M. Camargo, 1976, Isolation of
    brain endopeptidases: Influence of size and sequence of sub-
    strates structurally related to bradykinin, Biochemistry 15, 1967.
Okada, Y., Y. Tsuchiya, M. Yagyu, S. Kozawa and K. Kariya, 1977,
    Synthesis of bradykinin fragments and their effect on pentobar-
    bital sleeping time in mouse, Neuropharmacology 16, 381.

Overturf, M., S. Wyatt, D. Boaz and A. Fitz, 1975, Angiotensin I
    [Phe^8-His^9] hydrolase and bradykininase from human lung, Life Sci.
    16, 1669.
Shikimi, T. and H. Iwata, 1970, Pharmacological significances of
    peptidase and proteinase in the brain (II), Biochem. Pharmac. 19,
    1399.
Shikimi, T., S. Houki and H. Iwata, 1970, Pharmacological signifi-
    cances of peptidase and proteinase in the brain (III), Japan. J.
    Pharmacol. 20, 169.

Clinical Significance of Kinins

KALLIKREIN SYSTEM DURING TREATMENT OF HEMATOLOGICAL MALIGNANCIES

Yoichi Chiba, Hiroko Ishihara, Yaeko Haneda, Yutaka
Yoshida

1st Department of Internal Med., Hirosaki Univ.,
School of Medicine
5 Zaifucho, Hirosaki, Japan 036

ABSTRACT

Factors of the plasma kallikrein system have been evaluated
following the course of 48 patients with hematological malignancies
which consisted of 15 cases of AML, 6 cases of myeloproliferative
disorders, 14 of lymphoproliferative disorders, 8 of multiple
myeloma and 5 of bone marrow carcinomatoses. Normal range of
spontaneous activity was 11.4 ± 3.0 µM/ml TAMe hydrolyzed, kallikreinogen was 115.8 ± 26.2 µM/ml·h and enzyme inhibitor was $1.02
\pm 0.37$ unit. Lower kallikreinogen level of the range was from
77.2 to 93.1; higher spontaneous activity, 8.4 to 18.0 and lower
enzyme inhibitor activity of 0.46 to 0.92 was seen before treatment.
Kallikreinogen increased up to the range of 95.6 to 120.1 at complete remission and decreased down to 63.1 - 76.5 prior to death.
The causes of the change in these factors were discussed.

INTRODUCTION

Kallikrein-kinin systems have been investigated extensively
as one of autacoids in various fields. However, simple and
practical methods to measure plasma kallikrein in clinical cases
have not been well established and clinical investigations on
plasma kallikrein systems have been scarce. The authors have been
engaged in the study of plasma kallikrein systems in various medical
disorders and found quite a number of patients with hematological
malignancies show definite changes in this system. We have tried
to evaluate here, the changes in plasma kallikrein systems during
the treatment of patients with hematological malignancies to

elucidate pathophysiological roles of kallikrein systems in these diseases.

MATERIALS AND METHODS

Blood samples were taken from patients with hematological malignancies at their various stages, i.e., prior to chemotherapy, under chemotherapy, incomplete remission, complete remission or exacerbation. The patients were those admitted in the author's department or its affiliated hospitals, and their diagnosis were definitely established by a series of hematological examinations prior to treatment.

A total of 48 cases consisting of the following: 15 cases at AML, 6 cases with myeloproliferative disorders including 4 cases with CML and 2 cases with primary myelofibrosis, 14 cases with lymphoproliferative disorders including 6 cases with ALL, 6 cases with malignant lymphoma and one case each of CLL and malignant reticulosis, 8 cases with multiple myeloma and 5 cases with generalized bone marrow metastases, were evaluated.

Treatment schedules in general, were as follows. Remission induction therapy in AML was combination chemotherapy, consisting of Daunorubicin 0.8-1.0 mg/kg, Cytosine arabinoside 1.0-1.5 mg/kg, Prednisolone 0.5-1.0 mg/kg and 6MP 1.0-1.5 mg/kg (DCMP); or, one to two days of Vincristin 0.15=0.35 mg/kg a week in place of 6MP (DCVP). In myeloproliferative disorders, Busulfan 0.04-0.1 mg/kg and/or Carbocon 0.2-0.4 mg/kg were used for induction therapy. In lymphoproliferative disorders, Vincristin, 2 days a week, cyclophosphamide 1.0-3.0 mg/kg daily, 6MP and Prednisolone (VEMP) were used other than radiation therapy in cases of malignant lymphoma or prophytaxis of CNS invasion. In multiple myeloma, Cyclophosphamide or Melphalan 0.04 mg/kg daily or 0.15 mg/kg 5-7 days a month were used. In bone marrow carcinomatosis due to GI tract cancer, Mitomycin C 0.04 mg/kg, f-FU 5-15 mg/kg and Cytosine arabinoside 0.4 mg/kg were given for 5 days in 2 weeks with Urokinase 200 u/kg. Supportive therapy such as transfusion and antibiotics were initiated as needed according to the patient's condition.

Blood was drawn by venipuncture with a plastic syringe and processed by directions originally reported by R.W. Colman. As normal controls, blood samples were obtained from 50 members of healthy, adult subjects.

As a preliminary study, two methods to measure plasma kallikrein systems were used, one of R.W. Colman which used TAMe as the substrate of plasma kallikrein, and the other a synthetic chromogenic substrate of S 2303 (supplied by AB KABI, Sweden).

We used the following procedure (according to a note of preliminary methods from AB KABI) to measure plasma kallikreinogen
with S-2303:

Reagent:
Plasma samples: Citrated plasma is diluted in distilled water
(1+9)
Buffer: Tris hydrochloric buffer 0.05 mol/L, pH=7.8, ionic
strength 0.05
Activator: Cephotest (Nyegaard & Co., Oslo) is diluted in
buffer (1+9)
Substrate: S-2302 is dissolved in distilled water, 2.45 mg/ml
= 4mM.

Procedure:
1.   Tris buffer (prewarmed to 37°C) 1.5 ml
     Diluted plasma (prewarmed to 37°C) 0.1
     Diluted Cephotest (prewarmed to 37°C) 0.7
     Mix well, incubate for 2 minutes.
2.   S-2302, 4mM (incubate for 2 min.) 0.2
     Mix well, incubate for 3 minutes or more.
3.   Stop the chromogenic reaction by acetic acid conc.
4.   Read the absorbance at 405 nm.
Blank: Tris buffer in place of diluted plasma.

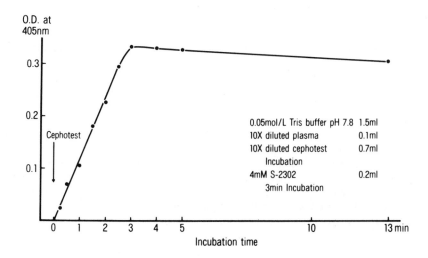

Figure 1.   Kallikrein determination with S-2302. Activation of
            kallikreinogen by Cephotest was evaluated in different
            incubation time. Activation occurred linearly up to
            2.5 minutes.

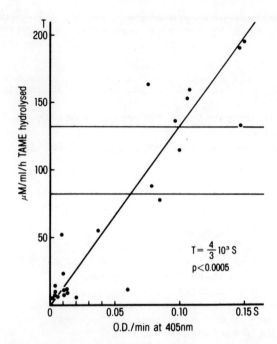

Figure 2.   Kallikrein determination, TAME hydrolysis and S-2302.
Comparison of the kallikrein value determined by TAMe
and by S-2302.

As shown in figure 1, adequate incubation time with Cephotest
was considered to be 2 minutes, as the reaction attained maximal
at 3 minutes. It was confirmed that absorbance at 405 nm. after
incubation with S-2303, under the same temperature, increased
linearly up to 15 minutes.

Twenty plasma samples were evaluated for their plasma kallikreinogen levels by both methods. It was clarified that both
values were quite parallel as shown in figure 2. It was also
evident from figure 1 that the chromogenic method did not show
the inhibitory effect by enzyme inhibitors as sensitive as the
TAMe hydrolysis method. Accordingly, the authors adopted the
TAMe hydrolysis method after R.W. Colman in this study.

RESULTS

Normal ranges of the factors in plasma kallikrein systems
were considered from the value of plasma samples from adult
healthy sugjects as follows. Spontaneous activity was 11.4 ± 3.0

μM/ml·h, kallikreinogen as 115.8 ± 26.2 μM/ml·h and enzyme inhibitor
as 1.02 ± 0.37 units.

Table 1 shows values of spontaneous activity, kallikreinogen
and enzyme inhibitor at various stages of AML at the top column,
and successively downwards, of myeloproliferative disorders,
lymphoproliferative disorders and of multiple myeloma at the
bottom column.

Generally speaking, the values of kallikreinogen were low in
many occasions and highest values were shown at the stage of complete
remission, whereas, the value of spontaneous activity and enzyme
inhibitors showed quite different changes, depending upon the
disorders and stages thereof.

In AML and multiple myeloma, the value of spontaneous activity
showed higher values, and that of enzyme inhibitor were the lowest
at complete remission. In myeloproliferative, and lymphoproliferative disorders, the values of enzyme inhibitors were quite low
prior to treatment and increased to the highest value at incomplete
remission.

Table 1. Kallikrein system during treatment of hematological
malignancies

Disorders (No)	Stage	Prior to therapy	Induction therapy	Incomplete remission	Complete remission
AML (14)	S	13.3	12.3	12.6	16.0*+
	K	81.9*	83.4*	81.1*	95.6*
	I	0.89	0.97	1.04	0.77*
Myeloproliferative disorders (6)	S	15.1*	7.4*+	5.7*+	2.1*+
	K	93.1	88.5	75.6*	111.3
	I	0.46*	0.72	1.53*+	1.13+
Lymphoproliferative disorders (14)	S	10.9	9.7	11.2	11.5
	K	74.4*	95.3*	85.1*	115.9+
	I	0.76*	1.03	1.16+	1.07
Multiple myeloma (7)	S	18.0*	11.5+	34.1*+	33.3*+
	K	73.2*	83.5*	85.5*	120.1+
	I	0.92	1.02	0.53*	0.49*

S: spontaneous activity, K; kallikreinogen, I; enzyme inhibitor *: significantly different from normal value, P<0.01
+: significantly changes after treatment, P<0.02

Spontaneous activity in myeloproliferative disorders were quite high at pretreatment stage, and successively decreased to the lowest value at complete remission.

There were six deaths among these 43 cases of hematological malignancies which included 2 cases of AML, of multiple myeloma, each case of CML and ALL. Four of these had attained complete remission on at least one occasion and the values of kallikrein factors were included into this presentation. The following represents the data after their reexacerbation. The average value of these cases are shown in Table 2. Kallikreinogen and enzyme inhibitor were considerably low, the lowest value was disclosed prior to death, when spontaneous activity showed a significantly higher value.

There were five cases of generalized bone marrow metastases of cancer, origin of which were 3 cases of stomach, one of colon and one case of prostrate. All five died in one to twenty months after treatment. The average value of these cases are shown in Table 3.

Table 2. Kallikrein system in 6 deaths of hematological malignancies

Factor \ Stage	Prior to therapy	Induction therapy	Complication	Exacerbation	Prior to death
S	12.6	7.6*+	9.8	11.2	14.3*
K	77.2*	87.5*	81.8*	88.5	63.1*
I	0.46*	0.92	0.80	0.74	0.37

S: spontaneous activity, K: kallikreinogen, I: enzyme inhibitor
*: significantly different from normal value, $P<0.01$
+: significantly different from pretreatment value, $P<0.02$

Table 3. Kallikrein system in 5 cases of bone marrow carcinomatosis

Factor \ Stage	Prior to therapy	Chemo-therapy	Transient improvement	prior to death
S	8.4	21.8*+	8.5	16.1*+
K	80.6*	122.8	107.0	76.5*
I	0.89	1.19	0.91	1.06

S: spontaneous activity, K: kallikreinogen, I: enzyme inhibitor
*: significantly different from normal value, $P<0.01$
+: significantly different from pretreatment value, $P<0.02$

Kallikreinogen was low prior to treatment and increased to normal levels after treatment. However, marked decreases were noted prior to death where spontaneous activity was quite high in spite of normal values of enzyme inhibitor.

DISCUSSION

Changes in plasma kallikrein systems have been previously reported. Plasma kallikreinogen decreases markedly in liver cirrhosis and moderately in resolving pancreatitis. It has also been noted to increase mildly in patients receiving estrogen and in pregnancy. An increase has also been reported in septic shock and carcinoid flush. Marked decreases of enzyme inhibitor was reported in hereditary angioneurotic edema and pancreatitis also.

It would be quite difficult to explain what significant role the changes of plasma kallikrein systems play in the pathophysiological mechanism(s) of these diseases. Low kallikreinogen level in liver cirrhosis has been explained by the hypothesis that plasma kallikrein is synthetized in the liver. Activation of kallikreinogen was thought to bring about a high level of kallikrein and low kallikreinogen, frequently, but not always associated with low level of enzyme inhibitor which would be combined with kallikrein to form an inactive stochiometric complex.

Although the authors have been engaged in the study of plasma kallikrein systems in various medical diseases and confirmed that kallikreinogen was definitely low in liver cirrhosis, and enzyme inhibitor was low in pancreatitis, cerebrovascular accident, collagen disease and various hematological malignancies as a group; it was not thoroughly evaluated,as this depended upon the stages of various conditions during the treatment of the hematological malignancies. The results of this study however, yielded good evidence of kallikrein system changes during treatment of this disease. The fact that kallikreinogen showed a tendency to increase up to the normal level in remission, presented us with a reasonalble hypothesis, i.e., the derangement of plasma kallikrein system accompanied with the clinical manifestations of hematological malignancies. However, we were unable to determine much about the pathophysiological meaning of the fact that higher levels of kallikrein in AML and multiple myeloma and its low level in myeloproliferative disorders were seen at the remission state. Probably, though the patients' parameters fitted the criteria of complete remission, there may be some equivocal mechanism(s) working on the bone marrow response.

The cause of low level in kallikreinogen and high level of kallikrein before treatment was obscure. Some possibility of hepatic dysfunction might be considered. But, 34 out of 46 cases showed normal or minimal changes in liver profiles. There may be some activation mechanism of kallikreinogen, but it is uncertain whether activation of kallikreinogen played a significant role in the development of hematological malignancies or if it was induced as a result of the diseases. There were a few reports which disclosed that administration of hog pancreatic kallikrein enhanced calcium dependent DNA synthesis of hepatic cell, bone marrow and thymus, but the author could not find any report that evaluated activation of DNA synthesis or cell proliferation by endogenous plasma kallikrein.

Six cases who did not go into complete remission and subsequently died, showed significant lows in kallikreinogen and enzyme inhibitor. Although they increased at induction therapy, the value decreased again at the development of complications, such as sepsis or pneumonia, which may induce an activation of kallikreinogen. Further investigations are needed with an increased number of clinical cases to prove the speculation that low kallikreinogen and enzyme inhibitor is considered to be a poor prognostic sign.

Five cases of generalized bone marrow metastasis showed definite signs of microangiopathic hemolytic states or disseminated intravascular coagulation with fibrinolysis syndrome at their admission. Low kallikreinogen levels could be explained by the activation of kallikreinogen which occurred in some occasions of disseminated intravascular coagulation. High values of kallikrein and low values of kallikreinogen prior to death might be aroused by the derangement of protease systems such as cathepsin, plasmin, trypsin, thrombin, leupeptins, pepstatin, and their inhibitors. Although the authors could not identify specific pathophysiological roles of plasma kallikrein systems in the development of hematological malignancies and its course, definite changes of the system were clearly disclosed. We do emphasize the importance of further investigations on plasma kallikrein systems in clinical cases with keen insight of the basic studies of the system that would open new aspects to the clinical application of kallikrein systems.

REFERENCES

Back, N. et al., 1976. Low molecular weight organic acids as inhibitors of kinin-forming activity of a rodent tumor acid protease and human plasma kallikrein. Pharmacol. Res. Commun. 8: 31.

Chiba, Y. et al., 1976. Clinical study on measurement of human plasma kallikrein system. Jap. J. Clin. Hemat. 19: 214.

Colman, R.W. et al., The human plasma kallikrein-kinin system, 1971. In: Progress in hematology, Vol. VII, eds. C.C. Moore and E.B. Brown (Grune and Stratton, New York) p. 255.

Colman, R.W. et al., Human kallikrein and prekallikrein, 1976. In: Methods in enzymology, Vol. XLV. ed. L. Lorand (Academic Press, New York) p. 303.

Ratnoff, O.D. 1977. In: Haemostasis: Biochemistry, Physiology, and Pathology. eds. D. Ogston and B. Bennett (John Wiley & Sons, London) p. 25.

Rixon, R.H., et al. Kallikrein, kinin and cell proliferation, 1973. In: Kininogenases. eds. G.L. Haberland and J.W. Rohen (F.K. Schattauer Verlag, Stuttgart) p. 131.

POSSIBLE INVOLVEMENT OF KININS AND PROSTAGLANDINS IN THE TRANS-

LATION OF INSULIN ACTION ON GLUCOSE UPTAKE INTO SKELETAL MUSCLE

Gunther Dietze

Matthias Wicklmayr, Ingolf Bottger and Lothar Mayer

Abteilung fur Stoffwechsel und Endokrinologie des
Akademischen Lehrkrankenhauses Munchen-Schwabing,
Kolner Platz 1, 8000 Munchen 40, GFR

INTRODUCTION

Recent evidence suggesting that endogenous liberation of
kinins from kininogen by kininogenases is essential for the well
known increase of glucose uptake occuring during muscle work (1)
and hypoxia (2) and the fact that kinins exhibit a molecular weight
similar to that ascribed to the "Muscle Activity Factor" (3),
points to the possibility that kinins themselves represent the
required mediator. The earlier finding that the factor liberated
during hypoxia accelerated glucose uptake as insulin via enhanced
transport across the cell membrane (4,5) and kinins themselves
exhibited insulin-like activity in normal (6) and diabetic man (7)
implied that kinins might share with insulin its mechanism of
action. Since, furthermore, evidence had been obtained that the
effect of kinins on glucose uptake into muscle was mediated via
synthesis of prostaglandins (8) it was of interest to investigate
whether kinins and prostaglandins are involved in insulin action.
In order to answer this question we studied the action of insulin
on glucose uptake into skeletal muscle tissue of the human forearm (9,19) under conditions where endogenous liberation of kinins
was prevented by infusion of a kallikrein inhibitor (10,23) and
endogenous biosynthesis of prostaglandins was prevented by indomethacin pretreatment (11).

MATERIALS AND METHODS

Nineteen healthy volunteers were recruited from medical
students. All were informed about the aim and the risks of this
study and gave their consent. Physical examination as well as

511

laboratory tests excluded internal diseases. All the subjects
fasted overnight and received no special premedication. The
catheterisation procedure was detailed in (2,8). Arterial and
deep venous blood samples were collected simultaneously at 5 min.
intervals throughout a 15 min. basal period followed by a 30 min.
infusion period for chemical analysis.

Chemical analysis was performed in 6 subjects (group I)
during intrabrachial-arterial infusion of highly purified crystalline bovine insulation (250 µU/kg x min. in 0,2 ml saline/min) for
the whole test period. Another 5 subjects received identical
insulin infusion and simultaneous infusion of the kallikrein
inhibitor (group II) into an antecubital vein of the opposite
forearm for the whole test period (Trasylol^R, Wuppertal, GFR; 500.
000 KIU within 15 min. and then 12.500 KIU per min.). Another
8 subjects (group III) received identical insulin infusion after
the oral pretreatment with indomethacin (AMUNO^R, Sharp and Dohme,
Munich, GFR; 3 daily doses of 100 mg each for 2 days and another
100 mg dose one hour prior to the test). The three groups were
well comparable as to their age, height and weight. Three minutes
after the start of insulin infusion, 1 mg glucose per kg body-
weight per min. was infused into an antecubital vein in group I
and II. Forearm blood flow (FBF) was estimated by venous occlu-
sion plethysmography (12,13) as detailed in (8).

Glucose, free fatty acids (FFA) and β-hydroxybutyrate (β-HOB)
were determined after storage at -20°C overnight, acetoacetate
(AcAc) at least within 6 hours. Blood samples for oxygen (O_2)
analysis were taken in heparinized syringes and analyzed promptly.
Procedure and precision of the tests has been given in (14).
Serum insulin (IRI) was assayed according to a modification (15)
of the Yalow-Berson immunoassay (16), human growth hormone (HGH)
according to (17). Standard statistical methods were employed
using Student's t-test for paired and unpaired samples when
applicable (18). All the mean values are given with the standard
error of the mean (SEM).

RESULTS

Infusion of insulin. The values obtained during baseline
conditions for the arterial concentrations of O_2 (19.9 ± 0.3 ml/
100 ml), glucose (4.52 ± 0.10 mmol/1), FFA (0.743 ± 0.08 mmol/1),
β-HOB (0.11 ± 0.02 mmol/1) and AcAc (0.07 ± 0.01 mmol/1) were well
comparable as to the data from other laboratories (9, 19). This
was also true for the arterial concentration of HGH which was
found to be 7.5 ± 4.1 ng/ml. The concentrations of the substrates
exhibited no significant differences during the infusion of insulin.
Only the FFA showed significant lowering towards the end of the
infusion (0.610 ± 0.08 mmol/1; p < 0.005). FBF, arterial-deep-

Table 1.

FOREARM BLOOD FLOW (FBF), ARTERIAL-DEEPVENOUS CONCENTRATION DIFFERENCES OF OXYGEN AND GLUCOSE DURING THE INTRABRACHIAL-ARTERIAL INFUSION OF INSULIN (A) AND OF INSULIN PLUS THE KALLIKREIN INHIBITOR (B).

| | | BASAL [a] | INSULIN [b] | | | | | |
			5 MIN	10 MIN	15 MIN	20 MIN	25 MIN	30 MIN
FBF [e]	A	2.67 ± 0.43	2.87 ± 0.17	2.60 ± 0.21	2.67 ± 0.31	2.80 ± 0.30	2.90 ± 0.41	2.87 ± 0.32
	B	2.52 ± 0.38	2.58 ± 0.41	2.33 ± 0.26	2.28 ± 0.34	2.50 ± 0.40	2.42 ± 0.42	2.56 ± 0.40
OXYGEN [f]	A	9.6 ± 0.2	9.8 ± 0.6	10.1 ± 1.0	10.1 ± 1.5	10.5 ± 1.5	10.5 ± 1.4	9.8 ± 1.1
	B	9.4 ± 0.6	8.4 ± 0.9	8.3 ± 1.1	8.4 ± 1.1	8.6 ± 1.1	9.7 ± 1.0	9.5 ± 1.0
GLUCOSE [g]	A	0.39 ± 0.03	0.72 + 0.09[c]	1.14 ± 0.19[c]	1.62 ± 0.22[c]	1.84 ± 0.14[c]	1.96 ± 0.10[c]	1.99 ± 0.06[c]
	B	0.35 ± 0.02	0.38 ± 0.05[d]	0.56 ± 0.08[cd]	0.95 ± 0.15[cd]	1.21 ± 0.17[cd]	1.23 ± 0.18[cd]	1.11 ± 0.12[cd]

VALUES ARE INDICATED AS THE MEANS ± SEM OF 6 (A) AND 5 (B) SUBJECTS IN [e] $ml/(100g \times min)$, [f] $ml/100ml$, [g] $mmol/l$

[a] FROM 4 DETERMINATIONS AT 5 MIN INTERVALS AVERAGED FOR EACH SUBJECT

[b] $250 \mu UNITS/(kg \times min)$

[c] SIGNIFICANT DIFFERENCE TO BASAL AT $P < 0.01$ - $P < 0.05$, [d] TO A AT $P < 0.01$

Table 2.

FOREARM BLOOD FLOW (FBF), ARTERIAL-DEEPVENOUS CONCENTRATION DIFFERENCES OF OXYGEN AND GLUCOSE DURING THE INTRABRACHIAL-ARTERIAL INFUSION OF INSULIN (A) AND OF INSULIN AFTER INDOMETHACIN PRETREATMENT (B).

		BASAL[a]	INSULIN[b] 5 MIN	10 MIN	15 MIN	20 MIN	25 MIN	30 MIN
FBF[e]	A	2.67 ± 0.43	2.87 ± 0.17	2.60 ± 0.21	2.67 ± 0.31	2.80 ± 0.30	2.90 ± 0.41	2.87 ± 0.32
	B	2.75 ± 0.32	2.75 ± 0.30	2.75 ± 0.29	2.80 ± 0.30	2.80 ± 0.27	2.88 ± 0.35	2.80 ± 0.31
OXYGEN[f]	A	9.6 ± 0.2	9.8 ± 0.6	10.1 ± 1.0	10.1 ± 1.5	10.5 ± 1.5	10.5 ± 1.4	9.8 ± 1.1
	B	9.2 ± 0.7	9.2 ± 0.8	9.1 ± 0.9	8.8 ± 1.0	8.5 ± 1.0	8.5 ± 1.0	8.5 ± 1.1
GLUCOSE[g]	A	0.39 ± 0.03	0.72 ± 0.09[c]	1.14 ± 0.19[c]	1.62 ± 0.22[c]	1.84 ± 0.14[c]	1.96 ± 0.10[c]	1.99 ± 0.06[c]
	B	0.35 ± 0.05	0.56 ± 0.09[cd]	0.78 ± 0.11[cd]	0.93 ± 0.15[cd]	1.19 ± 0.16[cd]	1.26 ± 0.17[cd]	1.21 ± 0.18[cd]

THE VALUES FOR OXYGEN AND GLUCOSE REPRESENT THE MEAN ± SEM OF 6 (A) AND 8 (B) SUBJECTS IN [f] ml/100ml AND [g] mmol/l FOR FBF OF 6 SUBJECTS IN EACH GROUP IN [e] ml/(100g TISSUE x MIN)

[a] FROM 4 DETERMINATIONS AT 5 MIN INTERVALS AVERAGED FOR EACH SUBJECT

[b] 250 μUNITS/(kg x min)

[c] SIGNIFICANT DIFFERENCE TO BASAL AT P < 0.05, [d] TO A AT P   0.05 - 0.005

venous concentration differences of O_2 and glucose are listed in
Table 1 and 2. This concentration of glucose rose continuously
reaching 5 times the basal value at the end of insulin infusion
($p < 0.005$, paired t-test). While calculated O_2 uptake did not
change, glucose uptake rose correspondingly to the increase of
the arterial-deepvenous difference (Fig. 1 and 2.) The mean
values obtained for the deepvenous insulin concentrations are
indicated in Fig. 1 and 2.

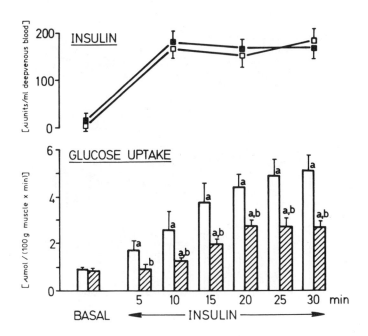

Fig. 1.   Muscle glucose uptake and deepvenous insulin concentra-
          tions during the infusion of insulin and insulin plus the
          kallikrein-inhibitor. The values are indicated as the
          mean ± SEM of 6 (insulin) and 5 (insulin + inhibitor)
          subjects. Empty dots and columns: insulin only.
          a significant to basal at $p < 0.05 - 0.005$
          b significant to insulin at $p < 0.05 - 0.005$

     Infusion of insulin plus the kallikrein inhibitor. As com-
pared to the values obtained for the arterial concentrations of
substrates in the insulin group there were no significant differences during baseline conditions and the infusion of insulin plus
the kallikrein inhibitor. The small but significant lowering of
FFA seen in the insulin group was almost identical (from 0.650 ±

0.08 to 0.507 ± 0.07 mmol/1). FBF and the arterial–deepvenous
concentration differences are indicated in Table 1. During the
infusion of the inhibitor, identical insulin infusion exhibited a
significantly smaller effect on glucose balance throughout the
whole test (p < 0.05 - p < 0.005). Accordingly, calculated uptake
of glucose was significantly smaller (fig. 1) while that of oxygen
was not changed. As shown in fig. 1 deepvenous insulin concentrations did not essentially differ between both groups.

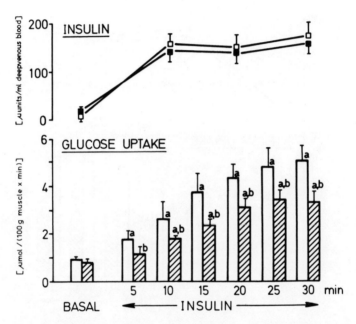

Fig. 2.   Muscle glucose uptake and deepvenous insulin concen-
           trations during the infusion of insulin and insulin
           after indomethacin pretreatment. The values are in-
           dicated as the mean ± SEM of 6 (insulin) and 8 (insulin
           + indomethacin) subjects. Empty dots and columns:
           insulin only.
           a significant to basal at p < 0.05,
           b significant to insulin at p < 0.05.

Infusion of insulin after indomethacin pretreatment. The
arterial concentrations of substrates were also well comparable to
those obtained in the insulin group except that of glucose. After
indomethacin treatment, glucose concentration was significantly
elevated and did not fall during the infusion of insulin, although

no glucose was infused. The arterial concentration of growth
hormone was almost identical to that obtained in the insulin group
(9.6 ± 4.2 ng/ml). Similarly as in the other two groups there was
a small but significant lowering of the concentration of FFA
during insulin infusion (0.848 ± 0.10 to 0.617 ± 0.06; p < 0.05).
FBF, arterial-deepvenous concentration differences of oxygen and
glucose are given in Table 2. After indomethacin pretreatment
the effect of insulin on glucose balance was significantly reduced
throughout the test. Deepvenous (IRI) concentrations exhibited no
significant differences, compared to those in the insulin group
(fig. 2). While oxygen uptake as in the insulin group remained
essentially unchanged, glucose uptake was significantly reduced
after indomethacin pretreatment (fig. 2).

DISCUSSION

Insulin accelerated glucose uptake into skeletal muscle of
the human forearm as described earlier (9,19). As compared to
these data, deepvenous concentration of insulin was in good accord
(19) but the effect of insulin on the arterial-deepvenous glucose
concentration difference was somewhat greater in our experiments.
Accordingly, at variance, infusion of small amounts of glucose was
necessary in order to maintain arterial glucose level, and arterial
FFA declined at the end of the infusion.

The different behaviour of the two groups (infused with the
inhibitor and pretreated with indomethacin) could not be explained
by smaller supply with insulin since mean deepvenous insulin concentrations showed no significant differences (fig. 1 and 2).
Also, the nearly identical values for O_2-uptake, FFA- and ketone-
supply throughout the test provided well comparable metabolic
conditions to the controls. The well known insulin resistance
which occurred after indomethacin pretreatment (20,21) manifested
by elevated glucose concentrations in the presence of normal insulin levels and the reduced action of insulin on glucose uptake
into muscle could not be attributed to an increase of the HGH.

That inhibition of kallikrein by this kallikrein inhibitor
may be responsible for reduction of muscle glucose uptake. has
already been observed in earlier studies (1,2). The specificity
of this effect was confirmed by the finding that administration of
a small amount of kinins during the infusion of the kallikrein
inhibitor was able to normalize the rate of glucose uptake again.
Also, in the present study, the inhibitor could have acted not
only on the kininogenase kallikrein, but in addition on other proteases (22). Since the inhibitor has no effect on glucose uptake
during baseline conditions, it seems to inhibit a protease which
is involved in insulin action. However, since there is no clear
evidence so far that a protease is involved in insulin action (23)
we should like to speculate that diminution of the insulin effect

by the kallikrein inhibitor is a consequence of its inhibitory
action on the activity of the kininogenase kallikrein.

This would for the first time imply that the liberation of
kinins from kininogen is involved in the translation of insulin
action on glucose uptake into skeletal muscle. The consideration
that kinins as the most probable candidates for the muscle activity
factor, increase glucose uptake into muscle as insulin does, via
the acceleration of glucose transport across the plasma membrane
(4,5) gives further support for this notion. Our findings that
physiological doses of exogenous bradykinin introduced into the
brachial artery during muscle rest exerted insulin-like activity
on glucose uptake in normal (6,8) and in diabetic man (7) would
also favour this view. Finally, earlier evidence (24,25) suggesting that the operation of the kallikrein kinin system is dependent
on the presence of small insulin concentrations is also speaking
for a cooperation between both systems.

Since kinins had earlier been shown to translate their metabolic actions via endogenous biosynthesis of prostaglandins it is
not surprising that inhibition of prostaglandin biosynthesis reduced insulin action likewise. This implies that prostaglandins,
besides kinins, also participate in the translation of insulin
action on glucose uptake into skeletal muscle. This view is under-
lined by the findings that prostaglandins as kinins were found to
exhibit insulin-like activity in myocardial (26,27,28) and adipose
tissue (29,30).

Apart from the finding that insulin at pharmacological doses
inhibits one of the kinin degrading enzymes (31), thus possibly
leading to accumulation of these peptides, nothing is known so far
as to whether insulin influences any step of the kallikrein-kinin
cascade. In case of its action on this cascade, from our findings,
one would rather suggest that insulin influences the activity of
kallikrein itself or one of the mechanisms providing activation of
kallikrein from its inactive form (32). That insulin in contrast
to kinins (8) does not accelerate blood flow (Table 1,2), would not
militate against such notion, since insulin exhibits its action
on glucose transport only in insulin sensitive tissues where
appropriate binding is provided to specific receptors (36).

ACKNOWLEDGEMENTS

This work was dedicated to Prof. Dr. E.K. Frey and Prof. Dr.
E. Werle. The authors are indebted to Prof. Fritz, Prof. Kraut,
Prof. Mehnert, Prof. Wieland for valuable discussions and support.
They wish to acknowledge the excellent technical assistance of E.
A. Bauer, A. Bammert, E. Maerker, H. Kirschner and G. Drotleff.
Thanks are also due to Priv. Doz. Dr. R. Landgraf, Dr. T. Ebersmann

and Priv. Doz. Dr. K. v. Werder, for the determination of HGH.
This work was supported by a grant from the Sonderforschungsbereich
51 of the Deutsche Forschungsgemeinschaft.

REFERENCES

1.   Dietze, G. & Wicklmayr, M. (1977) FEBS Lett. 74: 205-208.
2.   Dietze, G., Wicklmayr, M. & Mayer, L. (1977) Hoppe-Seyler's
      Z. Physiol. Chem. 358: 633-638.
3.   Goldstein, M.S. (1966) Fed. Proc. 25: 1-12.
4.   Randle, P.J. & Smith, G.H. (1958) Biochem. J. 70: 490-508.
5.   Morgan, H.E., Randle, P.J. & Regen, D. (1959) Biochem. J.
      73: 573.
6.   Dietze, G. & Wicklmayr, M. (1977) Lin. Wochenschr. 55:
      357-358.
7.   Wicklmayr, M. & Dietze, G. (1977) in Kininogenases (Haberland,
      G.L., Rohen, J.W. & Suzuki, T. eds.) pp. 299-308, F.K.
      Schattauer-Verlag, Stuttgart
8.   Dietze, G., Wicklmayr, M., Mayer, L., Bottger, I. & v.Funcke,
      H.J. (1978) Hoppe-Seyler's Z. Physiol. Chem. 359: 369-378.
9.   Andres, R., Baltzan, M.A., Cadar, G. & Zierler, K.L. (1962)
      J. Clin. Invest. 41: 108-115.
10.   Kraut, H., Frey, E.K., Werle, E. (1930) Z. Physiol. Chem.
      192: 1-12.
11.   Hamberg, M. (1972) Biochem. Biophys. Res. Commun. 49: 720-726.
12.   Gutmann, J., Kachel, V., Brandl, G. (1969) Elektromedizin,
      Sonderh. 87.
13.   Whitney, R.J. (1953) J. Physiol. (Lond.) 121: 1-9.
14.   Dietze, G., Wicklmayr, M., Hepp, K.D., Bogner, W., Mehnert, H.
      Czempiel, H. & Henftling, H.G. (1976) Diabetologia 12: 555-561.
15.   Herbert, V., Kam-Seng Lau, Gottlieb, C.W. & S. Bleicher (1965)
      J. Endocrinol. 25: 1375-1379.
16.   Yalow, R.S. & Berson, S.A. (1960) J. Clin. Invest. 39: 1157-
      1175.
17.   v. Werder, K. (1975) Urban & Schwarzenberg, Munchen
18.   Snedecor, G.W. & Cochran, W.G. (1967) 6th edn., Ames, Iowa
      State University Press
19.   Pozefsky, Th., Felig, P., Tobin, J.D., Soeldner, J.S. &
      Cahill, G.F., Jr. (1969) J. Clin. Invest. 48: 2273-2282.
20.   Syvalahti, E.K.G. (1974) Int. J. Clin. Pharmacol. 10: 111-
      116
21.   Cavagnini, F., Dilandro, A., Invitti, C., Raggi, U., Alessan-
      drini, P., Pinto, M., Girotti, G. & Vigo, P. (1977) Metabo-
      lism 26: 193-200.
22.   Vogel, R. & Zickgraf=Rudel, G. (1970) in Bradykinin, Kalli-
      krein (Erdos, E.G., ed.) pp. 550-578, Handbook of Experimen-
      tal Pharmacology (Eichler, O., Farah, A., Herken, H. &
      Welch, A.D., eds.) Vol. 25, Springer-Verlag, Berlin, New York
23.   Freychet, P., Kalm, R., Roth, J. & Neville, D.M. Jr. (1972)
      J. Biol. Chem. 247: 3953-3957.

24. Gould, M.K. & Chaudry, I.H. (1970) Biochim. Biophys. Acta
    215: 258-263.
25. Berger, M., Haag, S. & Rudermann, V.B. (1975) Biochem. J.
    146: 231-238.
26. Maxwell, G.M. (1967) Brit. J. Pharmac. 31: 162-168.
27. Glaviano, V. & Masters, T. (1968) Circulat. 38: Suppl. VI,
    83-97.
28. Willebrandt, A.F. & Tasseron, S.J.A. (1968) Am. J. Physiol.
    215: 1089-1-95.
29. Bergstrom, S. & Carlson, L.A. (1965) Acta Physiol. Scand.
    63: 195-196.
30. Vaughan, M. (1967) in: Prostaglandins (Bergstrom & Samuelson
    eds.) Proc. 2nd Nobel Symp., p. 139, Almquist and Wiksell,
    Stockholm.
31. Igic, R., Erdos, G.E., Yeh, H.S.J., Sorvells, K. & Nakajima,
    T. (1972) Circ. Res. 31: 11, 51-61.
32. Kraut, H., Frey, E.K. & Werle, E. (1933) Hoppe-Seyler's Z.
    Physiol. Chem. 222: 73-99.
33. Hepp, K.D. (1977) Diabetologia 13: 177-186.

THE INTERACTION OF KALLIKREIN WITH UROKINASE IN PERIPHERAL CIRCULATORY DISORDERS. A MICROCIRCULATORY OBSERVATION

Itaru Ohara

Dept. of Surg. (II), Tohoku University Hospital

Sendai, Japan

INTRODUCTION

In general, peripheral circulatory insufficiency is considered to be greatly influenced by the condition of the main blood vessels. However, clinically there are many cases which show paresthesia, coldness, and color changes of the fingers or toes irrespective of the findings of aretries or veins. The commonly used arteriograms or venograms to outline the blood vessels have limitations to elucidate the microvasculature of the tissue.

The recent knowledge of microcirculation has provided us with some aspects on tissue circulation. In order to understand the characteristic features of peripheral circulatory disorder at the level of vessels which are not appreciated readily by our sensory organs, several techniques, such as radioangiography, photoelectric plethysmography and dye dilution have been helpful in obtaining information regarding the microcirculation in peripheral circulatory disturbance in dogs and patients (1). It was found that the tissue circulation was sluggish and irregular in different parts of the extremities in this situation. Kallikrein showed some effect in changing this phenomena from a slow circulation to a faster one, and was also found to show a similar tendency to change the stagnant tissue circulation to a more easier flowing condition (2).

In this report, kallikrein and urokinase were used successively to see how they influence the microcirculation with each other instead of their independent effect.

MATERIALS AND METHODS

Seven dogs and 19 patients were subjected to the study. Dogs weighing 9 kg-18kg, were used. Following intravenous injection with pentobarbital sodium (30 mg/kg), the dog was held in a supine position. An endotracheal tube was inserted and exposed to room air with a room temperature of 23°C. A reflecting type photo-electric transducer was attached to one of the hindpaws distal to either a patent or occluded femoral artery. 2.5 mg of indocyanine green was injected into the jugular vein. The circulating dye was then monitored by a transducer which was recorded through a dye densitometer. The records were taken for 10 seconds - 5 hours at 5-50 mV, with a paper speed of 1.5 mm per second.

The patients were suffering from various degrees of peripheral circulatory insufficiency, which included paresthesia, coldness, change of skin color and ulcers of the toe or hand. In some patients, intermittent claudication was the only complaint. Clinically, they were diagnosed to have thromboangiitis obliterans, arteriosclerosis obliterans, Raynaud syndrome and lymphedema. The age ranged from 14 years to 75 years, eleven male and eight female. The patient was kept at rest in the supine position for 15-20 min. with the eyes closed. The room temperature was maintained around 23°C with a humidity of 60% in a quiet condition. 2.5-3.8 mg of indocyanine green was injected into one of the veins in the arm and the circulating dye was recorded from the fingers or toes with and without symptoms, using a transducer which was connected with the dye densitometer and recorder.

In both animal and human experiments, a record without drug (control) and with drug, i.e., kallikrein and urokinase were taken. The drugs were used successively in alternative order and the changes of dye pattern were primarily analyzed.

In 5 dogs and human cases, three blood samples were obtained three times, i.e., a) without drug, b) with kallikrein or urokinase and c) with two drugs together, during the measurements of dye study. One volume of 3.9% sodium citrate was added to 9 volume of venous blood and kept in ice water for 2 hours. 0.1 ml of 3.7% calcium chloride was added to one ml of this blood and put in a 275 mm x 3 mm silicone tube. The ends were closed with a connector and rotated for 2 hours in the Chandler's apparatus. Three tests for each blood sample were examined for the clot formation and the fluidity of blood in the tube.

RESULTS

In dog experiments, the dye curve showed a typical pattern. Following injection of dye, the dye was recorded slower and its

concentration gradually increased. The dye became constant after
15-30 minutes. The pattern of the curve showed a faster appearance
of dye and a rapid decline of dye concentration in a given time
when the circulation was not impeded. The degree of changes
depended upon the severity of peripheral resistance which was
caused by a combination of anatomical changes of the blood vessels
and the structure of fluid.

Independent injection of kallikrein or urokinase produced
faster dye dilution than the case without either drug. When
kallikrein was given first and then urokinase was supplemented,
one of the pattern of dye dilution curves appeared similar with
the other (Fig. 1). However, the curve by kallikrein appeared
earlier after urokinase was injected. The same was observed in
human patients. When the dye dilution of a finger was not remarkable at the first recording, kallikrein caused greater initial dye
appearance and faster dye dilution. This tendency was augmented
with urokinase in a shorter time than with kallikrein (Fig. 2).

The effect of kallikrein with urokinase on dye dilution curve
was not only limited to the sites where peripheral circulatory
insufficiency was present, but also similar findings were observed
at the asymptomatic site of measurement. When a patient complains
of circulatory disturbance on the unilateral toe, the toe on the
contralateral side may not be symptomatic. In such a case,
kallikrein and urokinase produced earlier dye dilution on bilateral
toes irrespective of the symptoms (Fig. 3). This dye dilution
continued over 40 minutes once it became stabilized within 5
minutes after the injection was made (Fig. 4). The apparent
difference on the dye dilution curve by kallikrein and urokinase
was not recognized after a single injection of dye was continuously
checked for over 3 minutes.

The change of the order of kallikrein and urokinase caused
earlier drug action of kallikrein than was given prior to urokinase on the dye dilution curve (Fig. 5). The clot formation
and fluidity changed prior to and after the drugs were administered. The clot formation became less and fluidity was increased
in 3 of 5 cases, while in the other 2 it became completely clotted
after the drug was given.

DISCUSSION

The vasodilatory drug action of kallikrein has been considered
to be the primary cause to improve the peripheral blood flow.
It was also found out to accelerate the microcirculation in dogs
and patients with peripheral circulatory disturbance (1).
Recently, plasma kallikrein has been suggested to play a role as
one of the plasminogen activator by way of activating Factor XII

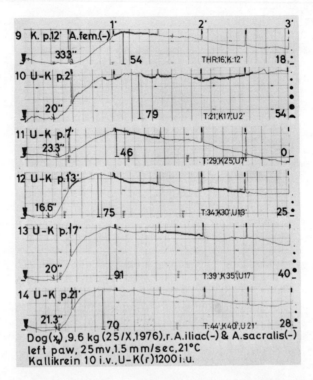

Figure 1.   Dye dilution curves of the canine hindpaw following
            kallikrein and urokinase.   Curve No. 9, 12 minutes
            after kallikrein showed a similar pattern with that
            of No. 11, 7 minutes after urokinase.

which then promotes the conversion of inactive plasma plasminogen
to active form (3).   Urokokinase is known to activate plasminogen
and produce clot lysis in the visible blood vessels from its
product, plasmin.   It was observed that the microscopic findings
of blood vessels in the skin and subcutaneous tissues in amputated
specimen for ischemia was causing stagnation from enhanced viscosity of the blood.   Administration of urokinase accelerated the
dye dilution in those with peripheral circulatory disorder (4).
The dye dilution curves in the dog experiment showed a great
similarity in its pattern except the difference of time when they
were recorded.   Urokinase caused speedier change than that by
kallikrein.   Both drugs showed that the effect of promoting the
dye dilution was augmented with each other.   This finding of dye
dilution did not always correlate well with the results by the
Chandler method.   This method itself may not be adequate to check
the viscosity changes of the blood after these drugs were given.

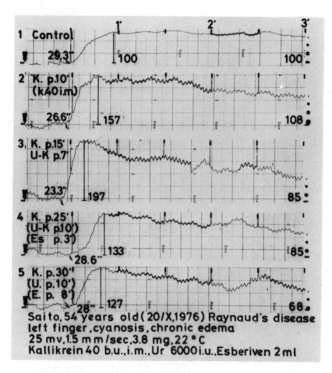

Figure 2.   The effect of kallikrein and urokinase on dye
dilution curve of the finger in a 54 year old
woman.   Curve No. 2 with kallikrein shows
increase of dye concentration with a tendency
of earlier dilution.   Such findings are further
augmented with urokinase (Curve No. 3).

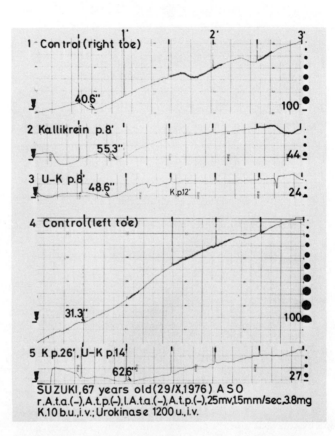

Figure 3. The influence of kallikrein and urokinase on
the dye dilution curves from the right and left
toes in a 67 year old man.
The dye concentrations in both toes are rapidly
diluted, suggesting the general effect of the
drugs.

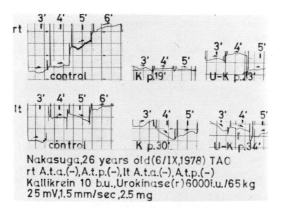

Figure 4. The pattern of dye dilution curves from the right and left toes in a 26 year old man. The control curves show increase of dye with time. Kallikrein (K) and Urokinase (U-K) show a balanced, or decreasing tendency of dye dilution.

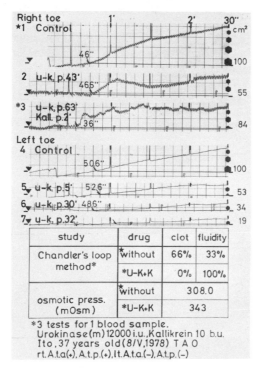

study	drug	clot	fluidity
Chandler's loop method*	*without	66%	33%
	*U-K+K	0%	100%
osmotic press. (mOsm)	*without	308.0	
	*U-K+K	343	

*3 tests for 1 blood sample.
Urokinase(m)12000 i.u.,Kallikrein 10 b.u.
Ito,37 years old(8/V,1978) T A O
rt.A.t.a.(+),A.t.p.(+),lt.A.t.a.(-),A.t.p.(-)

Figure 5. Dye dilution curves of the right and left toes from a 37 year old man and the results after simultaneous blood sampling. Both urokinase and kallikrein accelerated dye dilution curves (No. 2, 3 & 5). Blood sample (*) showed increased fluidity with the Chandler's method.

SUMMARY

Kallikrein and urokinase were used successively in dogs
and patients with peripheral vascular disturbance. It was found
that kallikrein showed similar pattern of peripheral dye solution
curve with that of urokinase. However, its action was slower than
urokinase.

REFERENCES

1. Ohara, I. The effect of kallikrein on body fluid circulation.
    1977. In: Kininogenases (Kallikrein 4), eds. G.L. Haberland,
    J.W.Rohen and T. Suzuki (F.K. Schattauer Verlag. Stuttgart)
    p. 321.
2. Ohara, I. Evaluation of peripheral vascular insufficiency
    by measurements of microcirculation, experimental and
    clinica. 1977. In: Proceedings of the 1st M. E. DeBakey
    International Congress of Cardiovascular Surgery (Athens,
    June 11-15, Greece). p. 507.
3. Haberland, G.L. 1977. In: Kininogenases (Kallikrein 4).
    eds. G.L. Haberland, J.W. Rohen and T.Suzuki (F.K. Schattauer
    Verlag. Stuttgart) p. 1.
4. Ohara, I. 1978. The therapeutic role of urokinase in vas-
    cular surgery. Medical Postgraduates. 16: 79.

KALLIKREIN TREATMENT OF MALE INFERTILITY

H. Sato, F. Mochimaru, T. Kobayashi, R. Iizuka,
S. Kaneko* and C. Moriwaki*

Department of Obstetrics and Gynecology, Keio Univ.
*Science University of Tokyo
35 Shinano-Machi, Shinjuku-ku, Tokyo, Japan

INTRODUCTION

Until recently, any approach for the treatment of male infertility had brought us little satisfactory results, if any. In
1973, Stüttgen showed that kallikrein increased the number of
sperm in patients with oligospermia. Since then, many clinical
studies have been performed successively with promising results
(Schill, 1974). These findings have prompted a similar investigation in oligospermic patients and asthenospermic patients in our
clinic to test the effectiveness of kallikrein on semen parameters.
We have performed artificial insemination with husband's semen for
the treatment of male infertility, but conception rate has not
been improved as we expected.

MATERIALS AND METHODS

100 patients with oligospermia ranging from 4 to 40 million/ml,
with asthenospermia ranging from 5 to 60% motility were selected
for kallikrein treatment. Of these 14 were unsuccessful because
a semen test was not performed, some patients stopped taking kallikrein for unknown reasons, and 4 patients stopped because of pal-
pitation, fatigue, epigastralgia and acute hepatitis. Considering
the side effects of kallikrein three items were checked before
administration, namely, blood pressure, blood sedimentation rate
and urinalysis. Only those patients who passed these check points
were enrolled in the study.

After the sexual abstinence of 4 to 7 days, semen analysis
was performed twice before treatment, as well as after kallikrein

administration. The following parameters were incorporated into the evaluation; the ejaculate volume, sperm count and total sperm motility.

RESULTS

The ejaculate volumes were examined before and during kallikrein treatment with 400 KU daily. The average value immediately before treatment and on the 1st, 2nd and 3rd month after the onset of kallikrein treatment in 24 patients was 2.5 ml, 2.5 ml, 2.7 ml and 2.3 ml respectively. Therefore, during three months of kallikrein treatment, a comparison of the ejaculate volume showed no difference.

Figure 1 shows the changes of sperm count during kallikrein treatment with 200 KU/day orally. Changes are expressed as percent change from the initial number of sperm. The mean value is written in bold strokes. Slight increase was found as a whole. Six patients showed more than 50% improvement of sperm count.

Figure 2 shows the changes with 400 KU/day orally. A significant increase was found in the first month and progressive increases were noted after treatment. Prominent increases were found in some patients, but considerable decreases were observed in others.

Figure 3 shows the changes with 600 KU/day orally. The mean value is increasing gradually, but not up to the treatment of the 400 KU group. It may be caused by the fact that severe oligospermic patients were enrolled in more than 400 KU group.

Figure 4 shows the changes of sperm count in 12 severe oligospermic patients using kallikrein. A significant increase was noted in only 2 patients. To examine if the influence of kallikrein might depend on the initial number of sperm, we arbitrarily formed two subgroups on the basis of their initial values, with below 10 million/ml and 10 to 40 million/ml.

In the former group, initial value was 4.49 mill/ml after the onset of treatment significant increase was not found, but in the latter group, initial value was 20.33 mill/ml, significant increase was found after treatment (Table 1).

Figure 5 shows total sperm motility before and during kallikrein treatment with 400 KU/day orally. Expressing these changes as percent change from the initial motility.

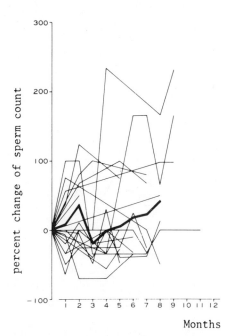

Figure 1. Percent change of sperm count during kallikrein treatment (200 KU daily) in oligospermic patients. (N = 20). The mean value is depicted in bold strokes.

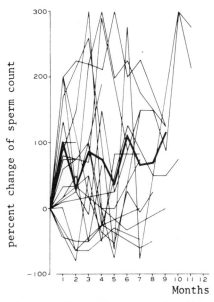

Figure 2. Percent change of sperm count during kallikrein treatment (400 KU daily) in oligospermic patients. (N = 25). The mean value is depicted in bold strokes.

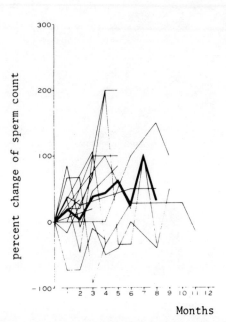

Months

Figure 3.   Percent change of sperm count during kallikrein
            treatment, (600 KU daily) in oligospermic patients.
            (N = 15). The mean value is depicted in bold strokes.

Table 1.   Mean value of sperm count in 36 oligospermic patients
           during kallikrein treatment (400 KU daily).
           Two subgroups were formed on the basis of their initial
           value.

400KU Kallikrein daily Range of sperm count (mill/ml) No. of patients	< 10	10 - 40
	12	22
Time of semen analysis (months)	Mean value	
0	4.49	20.33
+1	5.96	41.02
+2	2.87	27.20
+3	3.50	38.14
+4	5.00	35.66
+5	6.00	28.40
+6	5.83	42.89

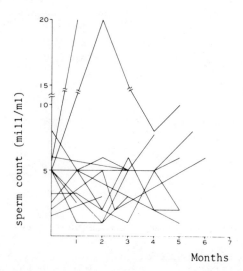

Figure 4.   Sperm Count (mill/ml) during kallikrein treatment
            (400 KU and 600 KU daily) in severe oligospermic
            patients. (N = 12).

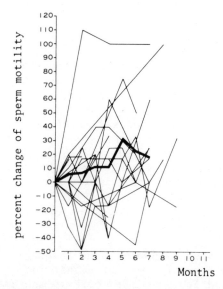

Figure 5.   Percent change of total sperm motility during
            kallikrein treatment (400 KU daily) in asthenospermic
            patients (N = 24). The mean value is depicted in bold
            strokes.

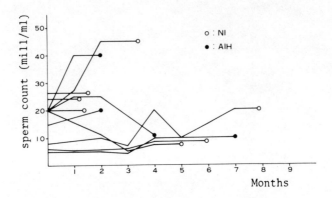

Figure 6. Sperm count (mill/ml) of pregnant cases (N = 11)

       O: Natural insemination
       ●: Artificial insemination with husband's semen

      Increasing tendency during kallikrein treatment was found.
The mean increase rate after the onset of treatment is 5.2%, 5.6%,
11.6%, 11.2% and 31.4% respectively, showing a progressive increase.

      To examine if the influence of kallikrein might depend on the
initial motility, we arbitrarily formed two subgroups on the basis
of their initial value with below 20% and 20 to 60%. In the former
group, there may not always be a tendency to improve the motility,
while in the latter group, about 10% improvement of motility was
found after 3 months (Table 2).

Conceptions

      Figure 6 shows changes of sperm count in pregnant cases.
Changes of total sperm motility was not significant. Eleven cases
of conception were noted from the 1st month to the 8th month.
Seven cases of pregnancy were by natural insemination. Four cases
of pregnancy were by artificial insemination with the husband's
semen. Sperm count was not improved in 8 patients except 3.

Table 2. Mean value of sperm motility in 48 oligospermic patients
during kallikrein treatment (400 KU and 600 KU daily).
Two subgroups were formed on the basis of their initial
value of sperm motility.

400 KU & 600 KU daily Range of sperm motility (%) No. of patients	20 12	20 - 60 36
Time of semen analysis (months)	Mean value(%)	Mean value(%)
0	15.8	50.4
+1	10.0	52.5
+2	12.9	53.8
+3	19.0	62.4
+4	15.0	57.7
+5	10.0	56.9
+6	13.8	60.0

DISCUSSION

It is strongly suggested that kallikrein has an influence on
spermatogenesis in human as indicated by an increase of sperm count
and an improvement of sperm motility. But the mode of actions of
kallikrein on spermatogenesis are not yet known.

Kallikrein-kinin system in the regulation of sperm motility
and spermatogenesis was already suspected by Cushman and
Cheung. We demonstrated high levels of kininase in the
seminal plasma of normospermic patients but low levels of
kininase in the seminal plasma of asthenospermic patients and
oligospermic patients. Kallikrein may have an indirect effect
on the intracellular cyclic AMP levels of sperm (Schill, 1975). On

Table 3   Effective cases and pregnant cases.

dosage	200KU	400KU	600KU
No. of cases	20	40	19
No. of effective cases	6	25	8
rate (%)	30.0	62.5	40.9
No. of Conceptions	2	6	3
rate (%)	10.0	15.0	16.7

the other hand, kallikrein may improve the blood supply of the testis and the accessory male sex glands.

Kallikrein may change vascular permeability in improving the nutritional functions for the sperm. In 200 KU administered group, effective cases were only 6, that is 30%. Two couples became pregnant.

In the 400 KU administered group, effective cases were 25 which is 62.5%. Six couples became pregnant. In 600 KU administered group, effective cases were 8 which is 40.9%. Three couples became pregnant (Table 3).

We administered a kallikrein dose of 50 KU per tablet. The patients in this group must take 12 tablets daily. Some patients found difficulty in taking 12 tablets.

We know both 400 KU daily and 600 KU daily are effective, but which dosage is better needs further research. We believe the effectiveness of treatment should be determined by the rate of conceptions. An improvement of semen parameters was not always accompanied by conceptions in our clinical trials.

REFERENCES

Cushman, D.W., H.S. Cheung, 1971. Concentrations of angiotensin-converting enzyme in tissues of the rat. Biochemi. biophys. Acta, p. 261.

Fritz, H., 1974. The kallikrein-kinin-system in reproduction: Kininogenases 2 (F.K. Schattaure Verlag, Stuttgart, New York) p. 9.

Moriwaki, C., H. Moriya, 1973. Intestinal absorption of pancreatic kallikrein and some aspects of its physiological role: Kininogenases: 1st Symposium (F.K. Schattaure Verlag, Stuttgart, New York) p. 57.

Schill, W.B., 1975. Coffeine- and kallikrein-induced stimulation of human sperm motility. Andrologia, p. 135.

Schill, W.B., 1977. Kallikrein as a therapeutical means in the treatment of male infertility. Kininogenase 4 (F.K. Schattaure Verlag, Stuttgart, New York) p. 251.

Stuttgen, G., 1973. Clinical substantiation of the effect of kallikrein: Kininogenases: 1st Symposium (F.K. Schattaure Verlag, Stuttgart, New York) p. 189.

DETERMINATION OF VARIOUS SEMEN PARAMETERS AND SEX HORMONE LEVELS

IN SUBFERTILE MEN DURING KALLIKREIN THERAPY

W.-B. Schill, A. Krizic and H. Rjosk

Andrology Unit of the Department of Dermatology
and First Department of Obstetrics and Gynecology
University of Munich, D-8000 Munich 2, FRG.

INTRODUCTION

During the last years several groups have shown that hog
pancreatic kallikrein is able to stimulate motility of hypokinetic
spermatozoa (Schill et al., 1974; Leidl et al., 1975; Steiner et
al., 1977; Bratanov et al., 1978). The in vitro studies were
complemented by clinical investigations showing a statistical significant improvement of sperm motility after systemic administration
of kallikrein to asthenozoospermic and oligozoospermic men (Hofmann
et al., 1975; Schill, 1975a, g.; Lunglmayr, 1976; Tauber et al.,
1977; Homonnai et al., 1978; Schirren, 1978). Furthermore, kallikrein treatment of subfertile men with reduced number of spermatozoa led to a significant increase of the total sperm output with
a maximum 2 to 3 months after initiation of the therapy, which
could recently be confirmed by a double blind trial (Schill, 1977).

So far, clinical studies were performed mostly with a medication period of not more than 7 weeks. In the following investigation
subfertile adults with idiopathic oligozoospermia and asthenozoospermia were treated by a daily oral medication of 600 units of
kallikrein over a period of 3 months covering the length of a
spermatogenic cycle of 74 days plus the epididymal passage of
about 1-2 weeks.

MATERIALS AND METHODS

In 54 patients a complete semen analysis with 5 days of sexual
abstinence was performed 1 month and immediately before the clinical

trial, as well as 1,3 and 5 months after beginning of the 3 months'
lasting oral kallikrein administration (3 x 2 tablets of Padutin[R]
100 (Bayropharm, Cologne,FRG)) including quantitative and qualitative sperm motility, sperm count, total sperm output, sperm
morphology, pH, volume, liquefaction time and seminal plasma
fructose levels. The semen analysis was performed according to
Schirren (1971) by the same research technician to avoid inter-
individual variations. Furthermore, in 24 patients, several serum
proteins found in seminal plasma including albumin, transferrin,
immunoglobulins, proteinase inhibitors and acute phase proteins
were determined quantitatively by radial immunodiffusion (Schill
and Schumacher, 1973), in order to evaluate possible effects of
kallikrein treatment on the secretory activity of the accessory
sex glands or the blood-seminal plasma barrier.

     In addition, serum levels of gonadotropins and testosterone
were measured by radioimmunoassay (Rjosk and Schill, 1979) in
order to determine possible hormonal changes during kallikrein
administration, which have been already discussed by Frey, Hartenbach, Igarashi and Werle twenty years ago (Werle, 1975).

                         RESULTS AND DISCUSSION

     Analysis of the semen parameters of 31 men with the semen
criteria of oligozoospermia before, during and after kallikrein
treatment showed no significant changes regarding the ejaculate
volume, the pH, the liquefaction time, the sperm morphology and
the seminal plasma fructose levels.

     Considering the sperm count (Fig. 1), a significant increase
of the number of spermatozoa per ml ejaculate was found already
1 month after start of treatment with a maximum 3 months later.
Two months after withdrawal of the therapy the mean sperm count
decreased, however, was still significantly higher than the
comparable value before therapy. Interestingly, during and after
kallikrein medication the standard deviation increased considerably.
Since the ejaculate volume remained unchanged, the increase of the
sperm density must be due to a real increase of the total number
of spermatozoa per ejaculate, the so-called total sperm output.
In fact, 1 month after initiation of kallikrein treatment, the
mean increase of the total number of spermatozoa was 51% and after
3 months 101%. Two months after withdrawal of therapy, the total
sperm output showed a mean value still 50% above that before
initiation of therapy.

     Regarding the individual response of the 31 oligozoospermic
patients towards the kallikrein treatment, 14 men, corresponding
to 45%, showed an increase of more than 20 million spermatozoa
per ml.

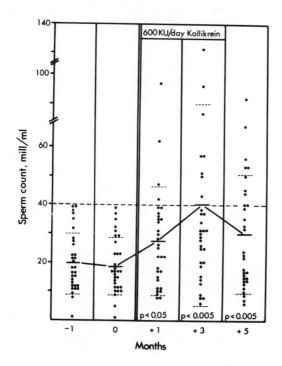

Figure 1. Sperm count (mill/ml) of 31 men with idiopathic
           oligozoospermia (<40 mill/ml) before, during and after
           oral administration of 600 units kallikrein daily
           over a period of 3 months. Mean values and standard
           deviation are plotted. For statistical analysis the
           Student t-test was used.

    Figure 2 shows the mean sperm motility before, during and after
3 months oral administration of daily 600 units kallikrein in the
same patient material. A significant improvement of the quantitative and qualitative sperm motility during the observation period
of 5 months can be observed. The average increase of the total
motility was between 18% and 22% and that of the progressive motility
between 64% and 78%. Interestingly, 2 months after withdrawal of
therapy mean sperm motility was still improved. Regarding the
individual response towards kallikrein therapy, in 58% of the patients
progressive motility was improved, in 19% even considerably.

    From the presented results it can be concluded that kallikrein
therapy with a medication period of 3 months is able to improve the
number of spermatozoa as well as sperm motility in men with
idiopathic oligozoospermia. According to our previous findings ,

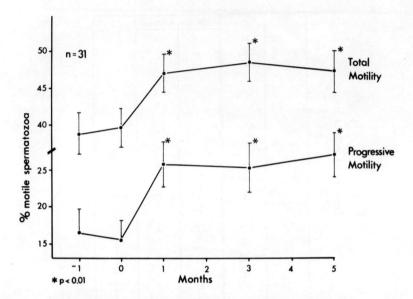

Figure 2.   600KU/day Kallikrein. Mean values (± SEM) of the
             quantitative (total) and qualitative (progressive)
             sperm motility in the same patient material as in
             Fig. 1.

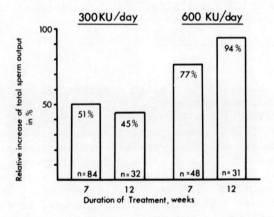

Figure 3.   Efficacy of different regimens of oral kallikrein
             therapy in men with idiopathic oligozoospermia.
             Total sperm output determined 3 months after
             initiation of therapy was used for comparison.

improved semen parameters will also increase the conception chance of infertile couples suffering from a male factor. Conception rate within this study is not known, but will soon be available. Previous studies with a medication period of 7 weeks showed conception rates between 28% and 38% and abortion rates of 7%.

Figure 3 shows a comparison between different regimens of oral kallikrein application in oligozoospermic men from this and previous studies determined by calculating the total number of spermatozoa 3 months after initiation of therapy. It is obvious that the effect of daily 600 units of kallikrein is significantly better than a daily dosage of 300 units. In addition, a medication period of 3 months seems to be more effective than that of 7 weeks.

Results obtained in 23 asthenozoospermic men will be published elsewhere. In summary, kallikrein therapy with a medication period of 3 months improved sperm motility in a greater percentage of asthenozoospermic men, having pronounced long-lasting effects on sperm motility compared to a medication period of 7 weeks.

In contrast to the empirical clinical results in subfertile men, the mode of action of the systemic kallikrein administration on sperm count and sperm motility is at present only poorly understood and still has to be elucidated. From several mode of actions, including enhancement of cell proliferation, stimulation of supply, improvement of sperm maturation during the epididymal passage and a direct effect on sperm motility after entry of the enzyme into the male genital tract secretions, the following actions of kallikrein have to be considered:

1) Improvement of sperm motility via a stimulation of the secretory activity of the accessory sex glands, as has been discussed by Tauber and coworkers (1977) due to a kinin-induced enhancement of blood flow and capillary permeability in the accessory sex glands and,

2) Kallikrein may interfere with the endocrine system by affecting the pituitary-gonadal axis.

Using the split ejaculate technique, Tauber and coworkers (1977) showed significant changes of some serum proteins found in seminal plasma during kallikrein treatment, indicating a possible effect of kallikrein on the accessory sex gland secretions. Thus, enhancement of sperm motility could also be induced via the stimulation of the secretory activity of the accessory sex glands whose components are important factors in triggering and maintaining sperm motility and sperm viability. The work of Tauber prompted us to determine several serum proteins including acute phase proteins in seminal plasma under the influence of kallikrein therapy.

Table 1 shows the results of albumin and transferrin and of the immunoglobulins IgG and IgA.

During kallikrein treatment a small increase of these proteins occurred, however, it could not be statistically confirmed due to greater variations. In contrast, Tauber and coworkers (1977) found a significant increase of albumin, IgG and IgA during kallikrein administration.

Table 2 shows the acute phase proteins CRP and aicd α_1-glyco-protein and the proteinase inhibitors α_1-antitrypsin and $\alpha_{1,X}$-anti-chymotrypsin. As can be seen, only $\alpha_{1,X}$-antichymotrypsin showed a significant increase during and even after withdrawal of kallikrein treatment, confirming the results of Tauber and coworkers (1977). The other three serum proteins were more or less unaffected.

It can be concluded that kallikrein treatment affects at least, to a certain degree, the secretory activity of the male sex glands and the blood-seminal plasma barrier. However, it is still unclear whether changes of the secretory components of the accessory glands are one of the mechanisms stimulating sperm motility and thus needs further investigation.

Finally, the possibility of hormonal changes within the endocrine system of the pituitary-gonadal axis during kallikrein treatment was investigated. Determination of the follicle-stimulating hormone FSH showed certain fluctuations but no significant changes occurred during and after kallikrein therapy.

In contrast, serum levels of the luteinizing hormone LH significantly increased during kallikrein treatment (Fig. 4) with a maximum at the end of the medication period. There were still significantly increased LH values 2 months after withdrawal of therapy.

Parallel to that a significant increase of the serum testosterone levels during kallikrein therapy was found (mean increase: 20%).

Thus, from the presented data it can be tentatively concluded that systemic kallikrein administration is able to induce significant changes of the hormonal balance of the pituitary-gonadal system confirming the observations of Hartenbach (1954) and Igarashi (1962) using crude bioassay methods. Whether these hormonal changes are a specific effect of kallikrein or an unspecific activation of the hypothalamic-pituitary-gonadal axis has to be investigated. At least, the surge of LH levels during kallikrein therapy gives an easy explanation for the observed increase of the spermatogenic function of the human testes via the stimulation of the Leydig cell

TABLE 1. MEAN CONCENTRATION (mg%) OF SEMINAL PLASMA PROTEINS DURING ORAL KALLIKREIN TREATMENT OF SUBFERTILE MEN (N=24)

Seminal plasma protein	Observation period in month			
	Before	During		After Therapy
	0	1	3	5
Albumin	79.79	107.94	96.54	91.46
Transferrin	6.69	7.97	7.05	6.85
Ig A	4.19	3.81	4.31	4.22
Ig G	12.67	12.83	13.17	13.04

TABLE 2. MEAN CONCENTRATION (mg%) OF SEMINAL PLASMA PROTEINS DURING ORAL KALLIKREIN TREATMENT OF SUBFERTILE MEN (n=24)

Seminal plasma protein	Observation period in months			
	Before	During		After Therapy
	0	1	3	5
CRP	2.48	2.46	2.15	2.06
Acid α_1-Glycoprotein	6.58	8.19	6.65	5.65
α_1-Antitrypsin	8.65	8.64	8.49	8.64
$\alpha_{1,x}$-Antichymotrypsin	3.18	3.82^x	4.64^x	4.30^x

^{x}p < 0.005

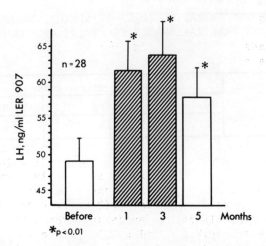

Figure 4.   Determination of luteinizing hormone (LH) levels in
            serum of 28 men with idiopathic oligozoospermia before,
            during and after oral administration of 600 units kalli-
            krein daily over a period of 3 months. Mean values
            (± SEM) thereof are plotted. The dashed lines represent
            mean LH levels during kallikrein therapy.

apparatus leading to increased intratesticular testosterone levels
necessary to maintain and accelerate spermatogenesis. Furthermore,
locally increased testosterone levels may favour epididymal sperm
maturation leading to an improved sperm viability and sperm
motility.

     Lastly, besides the observed increase of the strictly target
cell-orientated sex hormones, the local action of kinins as pharmacological active tissue hormones has to be considered which may be
of additional significance to restore fertility.

ACKNOWLEDGEMENTS

     Financially supported by Deutsche Forschungsgemeinschaft
(Schi 86/5) and Sonderforschungsbereich SFB 51. The technical
assistance of Miss Ilse Meyer is gratefully acknowledged.

SUMMARY

Thirty-one (31) subfertile men with idiopathic iligozoospermia were treated by a daily oral medication of 600 units of pancreatic kallikrein (Padutin$^{(R)}$ 100) over a period of 3 months. Total sperm output increased significantly with a maximum 3 months after initiation of therapy. In addition, quantitative and qualitative sperm motility improved during treatment and was still improved 2 months after withdrawal of therapy. Compared to other regimens, oral administration of 600 units kallikrein for a period of 3 months yielded better results than shorter medication periods or lower dosage.

Quantitative determination of several serum proteins occurring in seminal plasma before, during and after kallikrein therapy showed a significant increase of $\alpha_{1\,x}$-antichymotrypsin. Thus, kallikrein treatment seems to affect, to a certain degree, the secretory activity of the accessory glands or the blood-seminal plasma barrier.

Determination of serum gonadotropins and serum testosterone levels showed a significant increase of LH and testosterone during kallikrein treatment, whereas FSH was unaffected. Thus, systemic kallikrein administration induces significant changes of the pituitary-gonadal axis influencing spermatogenesis and epididymal sperm maturation. However, the local action of kinins as pharmacological active tissue hormones has to be considered too.

REFERENCES

Bratanov, K., B. Somlev, M. Doychevy, A. Tornyov, and V. Efremova, 1978. Effect of kallikrein on bull sperm motility in vitro. Int. J. Fertil. 23: 73-75.

Hartenbach, W., 1954. Über den heutigen Stand der experimentellen und klinischen Untersuchungen der Wirkung und Anwendungsmöglichkeiten von Padutin. Munch. med. Wschr. 96: 429-431.

Hofmann, N., A. Schönberger und H. Gall, 1975. Untersuchungen zur Kallikrein-Behandlung männlicher Fertilitätsstorungen, Z. Hautkr. 50: 1003-1012.

Homonnai, Z.T., M. Shilon und G. Paz, 1978. Evaluation of semen quality following kallikrein treatment. Gynecol. obstet. Invest. 167: in press.

Igarashi, M., S. Sato, H. Kubo and T. Sato, 1962. Über die Wirkung von Kallikrein auf die Funktion des Hypophysen-Gonaden-Systems. Endocr. japon. 9: 81-89.

Leidl, W., R. Prinzen, W.-B. Schill and H. Fritz, 1975. The effect
    of kallikrein in motility and metabolism of spermatozoa in vitro,
    In: Haberland, G.L., J.W. Rohen, C. Schirren and P. Huber (eds.)
    Kininogenases Kallikrein 2, Schattauer, Stuttgart-New York,
    pp. 33-40.
Lunglmayr, G., 1976. Spermienmotilitat unter Kallikrein, Wein.
    lkin. Wschr. 88: 709-711.
Rjosk, H. and W.-B. Schill, 1979. Serum prolactin levels in sub-
    fertile men. Andrologia, in press.
Schill, W.-B., 1975a. Improvement of sperm motility in patients
    with asthenozoospermia by Kallikrein treatment. In. J.
    Fertil. 20: 61-63.
Schill, W.-B., 1975b. Influence of kallikrein on sperm count and
    sperm motility in patients with infertility problems:
    preliminary results during parenteral and oral application
    with special reference to asthenozoospermia and oligozoospermia,
    In: Haberland, G.L., J.W. Rohen, C. Schirren and P. Huber (eds).
    Kininogenases. Kallikrein 2, Schattauer, Stuttgart-New York,
    pp. 129-146.
Schill, W.-B., 1977. Kallikrein as a therapeutical means in the
    treatment of male infertility, In: Haberland, G.L., J.W. Rohen
    and T. Suzuki (eds). Kininogenases. Kallikrein 4, Schattauer,
    Stuttgart-New York, pp. 251-280.
Schill, W.-B. and G.F.B. Schumacher, 1973. Micro radial diffusion in
    gel methods for the quantitative assessment of soluble proteins
    in genital secretions, In: Blandau, R.J. and K. Moghissi (eds)
    The University of Chicago Press, Chicago and London, pp. 173-
    200.
Schill, W.-B., O. Braun-Falco and G.L. Haberland, 1974. The possible
    role of kinins in sperm motility. Int. J. Fertil. 19: 163-167.
Schirren, C., 1971. Praktische Andrologie, Hartmann, Berlin.
Shirren, C., 1978. Kallikrein in der Andrologie, Vol. 6 Fortschritte
    der Andrologie, Grosse, Berlin.
Steiner, R., N. Hofmann, R. Kaufmann and R. Hartmann, 1977. The
    influence of kallikrein on the velocity of human spermatozoa
    measured by Laser-Doppler spectroscopy, In: Haberland, G.L.,
    J.W. Rohen and T. Suzuki (eds), Kininogenases, Kallikrein 4,
    Schattauer, Stuttgart-New York, pp. 229-235.
Tauber, P.F., D. Propping, A. Niesel, E. Kurz and L.J.D. Zaneveld,
    1977. Effect of kallikrein treatment on the composition of
    human split ejaculates, In: Haberland, G.L., J.W. Rohen and
    T. Suzuki (eds), Kininogenases, Kallikrein 4, Schattauer,
    Stuttgart-New York, pp. 237-254.
Werle, E., 1975. Historical remarks on the role of the kallikrein-
    kinin system in reproduction, In: Haberland, G.L., J.W. Rohen,
    C. Schirren and P. Huber (eds), Kininogenases. Kallikrein 4,
    Schattauer, Stuttgart-New York, pp. 5-7.

METABOLIC CHANGES AFTER APPLICATION OF KALLIKREIN IN AN ERGO-
METRICAL TEST

W. Gross, F. Burchhardt

Med. Poliklinik, Universität Würzburg, W. Germany

INTRODUCTION

The pharmacological effect of kallikreins is founded on
enzymatic reactions of kinins from its precursors. Many pharmacological effects were discovered in the last years (Frey, 1968).
Four points of view may be marked: Vasodilatation of the periphery,
exitation of unstrip-muscle, increase of capillar-permeability and
sensitivity to pain.

Furtheron there were several publications of the influence of
kallikrein of transport-mechanisms. At last we were interested to
read, that kallikrein influences the stabilization of ATP in
erythrocytes (Held).

Therefore we asked ourselves how the effect on the whole man
in exercise would be. We thought, that under these conditions
we would get some information about metabolism.

MATERIALS AND METHODS

For this purpose we tested 20 young students. Before exercise we controlled them clinically, further the blood-cells and
made an analysis of potassium, sodium, triglycerides, creatinine,
iron, cholesterol, calcium, phosphate, bilirubin, albumine, protein, uric-acid, blood-urea-N, LDH, glucose, alcal. phosphatase,
GOT, GPT, Gamma-GT, magnesium and electrocardiogram.

During the test we examined ATP, lactate, pyruvate, glucose,
acid-base metabolism and lung-function. During the test the ATP,
pulse and blood-pressure were continuously controlled. The exam-

ination of the lung-function was done for the vital capacity, the
residual volume in % and the residual volume in l., the intra-
thoracal gasvolume, the total capacity, the resistance, the
Tiffenau and peak-flow as well as the middle- expiration-flow.
The ergometric load was done as follows:

1. Before the test we took from an arm vein blood for ATP,
    pyruvate and lactate. For the control of acid-base metabolism
    capillary blood was taken from the ear. The ergometric test
    started with half a watt/kg body-weight and was increased
    per minute for half a watt/kg body-weight. In all, we took
    blood samples five times.
2. In steady state with a pulse of about 120/M,
3. immediately after the maximum,
4. 15 minutes after the maximum and,
5. 30 minutes after the maximum.

ATP, lactate, pyruvate and glucose were tested before and
immediately after the ergometric test. After the first test the
proband received for 7 days, three times 200 KE (biological units
of kallikrein, Padutin[R] 100). On the 7th day (under the treatment
with the drug) the above mentioned test was repeated. The single
data and the significance will be seen on the graphs.

It can be shown, that after the use of Padutin[R] 100, the
average of values of ATP are above the middle value, but there
is no significance on account of the big dispersion. Parallel
herewith lactate showed before the ergometric test a significance
between before and after given kallikrein. After the physical
strain, you can see the difference, but it is no longer statistically significant. Pyruvate showed a significant difference as well
as before and after the application of Padutin[R] 100, and before
and after the ergometric test in the direction of lowering the
values. Of interest is the proportion of the glucose. Before
and after the intake of drugs, we found no significance, and a
little higher value for glucose, but we could see that those
values are within the normal range. After the ergometric test,
we saw before given the drug constant glucose-values and after
the drug, we found a diminishing of the glucose-values. There
was no significance on account of the small difference and the
high dispersion. The acid-base metabolism showed over all the same
proportions. The pH, pCO_2, pO_2, mostly were not significant.
The pCO_2 showed after given the drug throughout a higher level
and the pO_2 a lower level than before. Only after 30 minutes of
rest (point 5) there was a significance. The HCO_3 (standard bicarbonate) was throughout the ergometric test lower, especially
on the maximum. We could not find any significance in these datas.
One could say, that there is a better utilization of O_2.

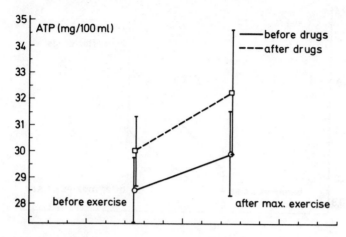

Figure 1. ATP in blood.

a) <u>before exercise</u>

	MW	dispersion	MFM	t
before drugs	28.52	5.64	1.26	0.822
after drugs	30.02	5.95	1.33	n.s.

b) <u>after max. exercise</u>

before drugs	29.92	7.15	1.59	0.814
after drugs	32.25	10.60	2.37	

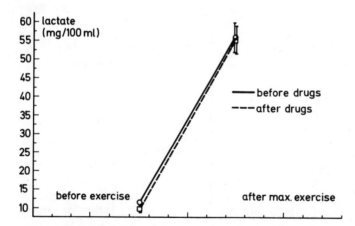

Figure 2. Lactate in blood.

a) <u>before exercise</u>

	MW	dispersion	MFM	t
before drugs	11.49	3.12	0.69	n.s.
after drugs	8.85	3.89	0.87	1.47

b) <u>after max. exercise</u>

before drugs	56.02	17.24	3.85	n.s.
after drugs	55.51	16.22	3.62	0.096

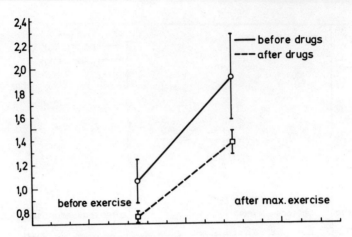

Figure 3.   Pyruvate in blood.

		MW	dispersion	MFM	t
a)	before exercise				
	before drugs	1.05	0.77	0.17	+1.656
	after drugs	0.76	0.2	0.04	
b)	after max. exercise				
	before drugs	1.91	1.53	0.35	1.52
	after drugs	1.37	0.42	0.09	

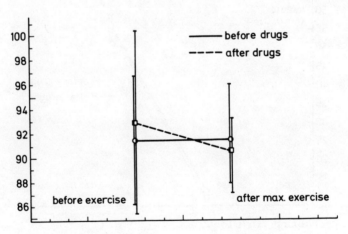

Figure 4.   Glucose in blood

		MW	dispersion	MFM	t
a)	before exercise				
	before drugs	91.47	19.76	5.28	n.s.
	after drugs	92.9	30.86	7.48	
b)	after max. exercise				
	before drugs	91.15	16.48	4.4	
	after drugs	90.59	10.88	2.64	n.s.

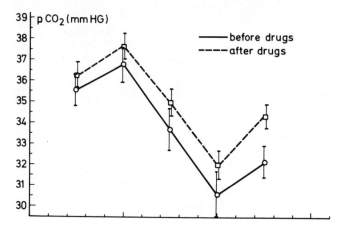

Figure 5.   pCO$_2$

MW	35.37	36.8	33.71	30.61	32.18
bef. d. dispersion	3.4	4.0	4.45	4.83	3.39
MFM	0.76	0.89	0.99	1.1	0.75
MW	36.26	37.63	35.00	32.00	34.34
dispersion	2.8	2.7	2.9	3.0	2.5
MFM	0.63	0.60	0.65	0.68	0.58
significance	n.s.	n.s.	n.s.	n.s.	+
t	0.695	0.767	1.084	1.103	2.278

The static and dynamic volumina of the lung-volumes as well as the capacity of the diffusion showed no significant difference.

While resting, the RQ was in the middle 0.746 and after given kallikrein 0.798 in a significant way. We mean that these values point out a better utilization.

DISCUSSION

Biological systems are mostly open ones. Substrates, quality and quantity of the working enzymes decide the turning over of such a process. We think, that kallikrein/kinin-system is one of the most important systems. Some authors (Haberland et al.) think, that it is a primitive system. Fritz thinks in the same way, but means, that this system is widespread within the organism. There are connections to the prostaglandin-synthesis and to the fibri-nolytic system. In our question the transport-system is important. Caspary, et al. described in their test no influence of the intestinal transport. But they also say, that it may be possible, that the transport rates in vivo changed (p.73). Menk and Haberland

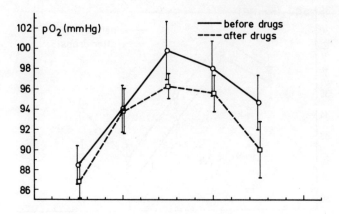

Figure 6. pO_2

	MW	88.4	94.0	99.81	98.04	94.68
bef.d.dispersion		8.3	10.38	12.8	11.81	12.11
	MFM	1.9	2.3	2.8	2.7	2.7
	MW	96.85	93.98	96.29	95.59	90.02
after d.dispersion		7.79	10.03	5.4	7.7	12.15
	MFM	1.7	2.2	1.2	1.81	2.7
significance		n.s.	n.s.	n.s.	n.s.	n.s.
	t	0.63	0.053	1.108	0.743	1.199

measured the transport rates of D-glucose and 3-0-3-methyl-glucose
under the conditions of transepithelial concentrations differences.
Their experiments show in direction that resorption between intra-
and intercellular mechanisms go parallel to the liberation of
kinins. Denhardt and Haberich could demonstrate that kallikrein
leads to an increase of net transport of sodium, resp. the netto
absorption. They think that the increase of this absorption works
on the indirect fluxes from the lumen to the blood. In summary
this would mean that the active-sodium-transport may be direct or
indirect, is activated. The active transport of hexose is not
influenced. Other authors (Johnson and Bades, Marin-Grez) reported an effect on their cell-cultures in the same direction.
Wicklmayr and Dietze discussed an effect between kallikrein and
insulin, but they pointed out that it could not be a real insulin-
effect, more of an insulin-like phenomena. On the other hand, it
may be that kallikrein/kinin increases the influx of glucose to
the muscle. It is our opinion that our experiment goes in the
same direction and shows a better utilization of glucose due to a
higher influx on the one side and on the other hand, a decrease of
pyruvate in blood. Parallel with this, the changes of acid-base

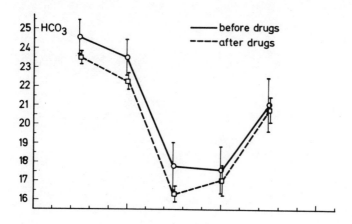

Figure 7.   HCO₃

MW	24.57	23.51	17.80	17.58	21.04
bef.d.dispersion	3.9	4.03	5.41	5.23	6.12
MFM	0.89	0.92	1.24	1.23	1.40
MW	23.51	22.26	16.32	17.04	20.77
after d.dispersion	1.51	1.95	1.84	3.49	2.9
MFM	0.33	0.43	0.41	0.78	0.66
significance	n.s.	n.s.	n.s.	n.s.	n.s.

metabolism takes place without a significant difference. At the end we found a better utilization of the energetic situation. Further we see a change of the RQ in an increase after the kallikrein-influence.

SUMMARY

Kallikrein given in a dose of 3 times 200 KE daily over 7 days caused under our test conditions an increase of ATP in blood and a decrease of lactate and especially of pyruvate. Glucose showed under this condition a higher utilization with a lowering of glucose in blood and an increase of the RQ. The acid-base metabolism follows these tendencies. In other experiments we did not find such effects, so the results must be specific to kallikrein.

PARTICIPATION OF KALLIKREIN, COAGULATION/FIBRINOLYSIS PARAMETERS IN THE DEVELOPMENT OF GLOMERULONEPHRITIS

Kazumichi Nakamura, Mutsuyoshi Kazama, and Takeshi Abe

Department of Medicine, Teikyo University School of Medicine
11-1, Kaga 2-chome, Itabashi-ku, Tokyo 173, Japan

ABSTRACT

Masugi nephritis was induced in dogs in which platelet count, fibrinogen, antithrombin activity, plasma prekallikrein and immediate plasmin inhibitors were coincidentally decreased immediately after the injection of nephrotoxic serum. It was found that the grade of decrease of urinary kallikrein excretion following these immediate reactions were parallel with the grade of renal damages. By the pre-treatment with heparin or the defibrination with snake venom, however, the histological findings of Masugi nephritis showed rather severe damage.

Based on the consumption of coagulation factors, kallikrein, kinin and their inhibitors in the development of this nephritis, it was postulated that inauguration of coagulation and activation of kallikrein contributed to the development of glomerulonephritis. The treatment or prevention of this coagulation process with heparin or snake venom, however, gave untoward effects on the pathological process in this experiment.

INTRODUCTION

As to the pathogenesis of glomerulonephritis in clinical and experimental subjects, immunological phenomena have been regarded as the main cause of tissue damage in kidney. But the fibrin precipitation in kidney was possibly imagined to play an important role in this change to which the activation of Hageman factor and kinin forming system should be closely related. In this paper Masugi nephritis was induced in dogs and the activation of coagulation/fibrinolysis and kallikrein systems were measured and analyzed to elucidate dynamic aspects of this pathologic process.

The possibility of the coagulation process in the pathogenetic participation in human glomerulonephritis has led to a number of trials with anticoagulant drugs in the treatment of patients with this progressive lesion (Kincaid-Smith, P. et al., 1968; Kincaid-Smith et al., 1970; Cade, J.R. et al., 1971; Cade, J.R. et al., 1973). Both anticoagulation with heparin and defibrination with snake venom have been proved to have protective effects on anti-glomerular basement membrane (anti-GBM) nephritis of rabbits (Halpern, B. et al., 1965; Naish, P. et al., 1972). However, the effect of treatments with those drugs have been equivocal in other experimental models and on other species (McGiven, A.R. et al., 1975; Briggs, J.D. et al., 1969). Recent reports failed to show the benefit of heparin administration in animals with anti-GBM nephritis (Bone, J.M. et al., 1975; Border, W.A., et al. 1975). In the present study, we studied the effect of pretreatment with heparin and defibrase on the development of Masugi nephritis.

MATERIALS AND METHODS

Anti-kidney rabbit serum against dog: The antigen was prepared by homogenation of perfused canine kidney with physiological saline for 10 min. New Zealand white rabbits were immunized by intraperitoneal injection of each 3 ml of 20% W/V suspension of this homogenate, twice a week for one month. The harvested anti-serum was adsorbed with an equal volume of canine red blood cell suspension before use.

Induction of Masugi nephritis: Each 1.0 ml/kg of antikidney rabbit serum was injected intravenously to experimental dogs. The urine was collected using metabolic cage.

Assay of kallikrein activity: The activity of tissue and urinary kallikrein was measured with synthetic substrate Pro-Phe-Arg-MCA and plasma prekallikrein was measured with Z-Phe-Arg-MCA after 9 min activation of test plasma with kaolin.

Assay of plasma inhibitor of plasma kallikrein: Plasma inhibitor activity to partially purified bovine plasma kallikrein was measured using synthetic substrate Z-Phe-Arg-MCA.

Immunofluorescence technique for fibrinogen in canine renal tissue: Anti-canine fibrinogen rabbit α-globulin was purified and labelled with FITC in our laboratory.

Defibrination: 0.5 NIH unit of defibrase (snake venom of Bothrops moojeni) was given dogs subcutaneously for defibrination.

RESULTS

Change of coagulation and fibrinolysis in Masugi nephritis.

Immediately after the injection of large doses of rabbit
antiserum into dogs abrupt and marked fluctuation occurred in
coagulation/fibrinolysis system at the first phase: drop of platelet
count, prolongation of prothrombin time (PT) and partial thromboplastin time (A-PTT), decrease of fibrinogen (Fbg), prekallikrein
(PK), plasminogen (PLg), antithrombin (AT) and plasmin inhibitor
activity. These changes however, were recovered within a short
time, except for the platelet count (Fig. 1 & 2). Daily excretion
of urinary kallikrein was gradually decreased within 4 days.

At the second phase the proteinuria suddenly appeared at 5 to
7 days after the injection and the gradual increase of platelet
count, prolongation of A-PTT and increase of fibrinogen were noted
after this phase.

The animal was sacrificed at the sixteenth day of the experiment and renal histology revealed the marked endocapillary and
extracapillary proliferation (crescent formation) in glomeruli
(Fig. 3). The tissue kallikrein activity was high in the cortex
and low in the medulla in intact renal tissue as it was shown at
the left columns in Fig. 4, and these activities were not changed
after Masugi nephritis was induced in the experimental dogs,
although the excretion of urinary kallikrein was apparently decreased.
When the lesser amount of antiserum was injected than in the preceding experiment, the reaction was relatively mild (Fig. 5). The
decrease of platelet count, prolongation of A-PTT, decrease of
fibrinogen and prekallikrein activity were slight, the moderate
decrease of urinary kallikrein and slight proteinuria suggested
mild destruction of renal tissue as they were shown in Fig. 6.

Influence of heparin or snake venom on Masugi nephritis.

After subcutaneous injection of 10,000 u of heparin-Ca into
experimental animals, prolongation of A-PTT and increase of kallikrein inhibitors were observed. Before and after the injection of
nephrotoxin of the same amount as the experiment shown in Fig. 5,
daily doses of 5,000 u of heparin for three days and 2,500 u for
7 days was injected, divided into two parts.

During this period platelet count, PT, A-PTT and concentration
of Fbg realized no significant changes, but the change of urinary
kallikrein content were remarkable; apparent decrease immediately
after injection of nephrotoxin and later obvious increase in its
excretion of urine (Fig. 7).

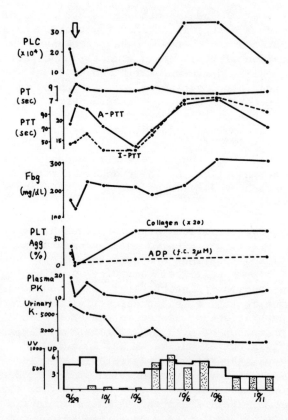

Fig. 1:   Blood Coagulation, Fibrinolysis, Plasma Prekallikrein
and Urinary Kallikrein in Dog with Masugi Nephritis
PLC:Platelet Count, PT:Prothrombin Time, PTT:Partial
Thromboplastin Time, Fbg:Fibrinogen, PLT-Agg:Platelet
Aggregation, PK:Plasma Prekallikrein Activity, Urinary K:
Urinary Kallikrein Activity, UV:Urine Volume(ml/day),
UP:Urinary Protein(g/day).
          Dotted columns show daily amount of urinary protein
and the open arrow shows injection of nephrotoxic serum.
          Plasma prekallikrein was measured with Chromozym PK
and urinary kallikrein was measured with TAME in this
experiment.(See text.)

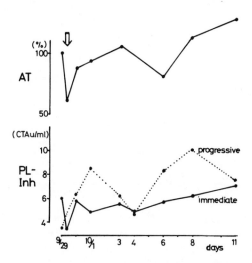

Fig.2:   Plasma Antithrombin and Plasmin Inhibitors Activities
          in Dog with Masugi Nephritis
          AT:Antithrombin Activity, PL-Inh:Plasmin Inhibitor Activ-
          ity. (See text.)

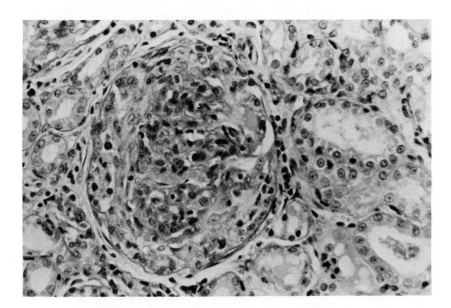

Fig. 3:   Photomicrograph of a Glomerulus from Dog in Experiment
          Shown in Fig. 1 & 2 at Two Weeks after Nephrotoxic Serum
          Injection(PAS Stein).
                  Note extensive proliferative glomerulonephritis
          with crescent formation.

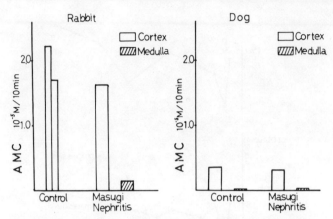

Fig. 4: Tissue Kallikrein Activities in Kidney of Rabbit and Dog
         Open columns for cortical activities and hatched
       ones for medullary activities.
         Kallikrein was measured with Pro-Ph-Arg-MCA.

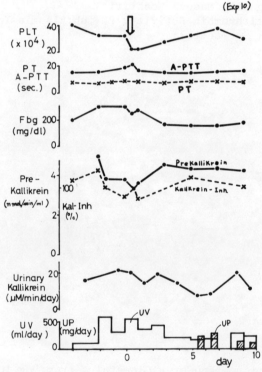

Fig. 5: Blood Coagulation, Fibrinolysis, Plasma Prekallikrein
         and Urinary Kallikrein in Dog with Low Doses of Nephro-
         toxic Serum.
         For legends see those of Fig.1 & 2.

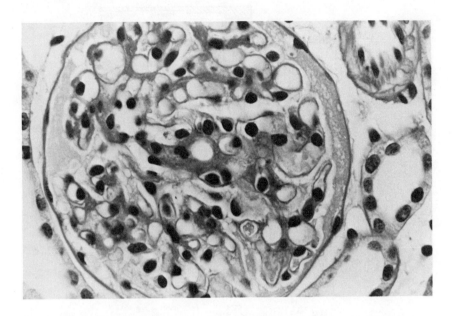

Fig. 6:   Photomicrograph of a Glomerulus from Dog in Experiment
           Shown in Fig. 5 at 14 Days after Nephrotoxic Serum
           Injection.
                Note mild endocapillary and mesangial proliferation.

The histological features in these animals were characterized
by the proliferation of endothelial and mesangial cells in comparison with those of the former experiment shown in Fig. 6 (Fig.
8). This tells us that the injection of heparin invited unrecog-
nizable histological changes.

In order to suppress the deposition of fibrin in kidney
tissue, defibrase (0.5 NIH unit of Batroxobin) was applied to the
dogs. The fibrinogen content in blood was decreased down to 10–100
mg/dl which was continued for 2 or 3 days thereafter, but no
marked changes were noted such as prolongation of PT & A–PTT,
decrease of antithrombin and antikallikrein activity. The rapid
increase of urinary kallikrein at the first stage followed by its
remarkable increase for several days at the second stage, and came
down slowly and gradually (Fig. 9). In these cases the histology
revealed the more marked destruction of glomeruli (Fig. 10) and
the less deposition of fibrin into glomeruli by immunofluorescent
method than those shown in Fig. 3.

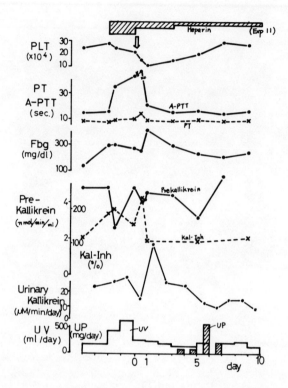

Fig. 7: Blood Coagulation, Fibrinolysis, Plasma Prekallikrein
         and Urinary Kallikrein in Dog with Masugi Nephritis
         Treated with Heparin
             Same amount of nephrotoxic serum was injected as
         the experiment shown in Fig.5.
             For legends see those of Fig. 1 & 2.

DISCUSSION

     The precise role of the coagulation process as a mediator of
vascular and glomerular injury in immune related nephritis remains
to be clarified. In our experiments, the changes of coagulation
and fibrinolysis of Masugi nephritis (Anti GBM nephritis)
summarized as the abrupt drop of platelet count, prolongation of
PT and A-PTT, decrease of fibrinogen, prekallikrein activity and
antithrombin activity as well as plasmin inhibitors. It was postulated that these changes were developed as the result of activation of coagulation system and consumption of its related
factors after the immunological procedure.

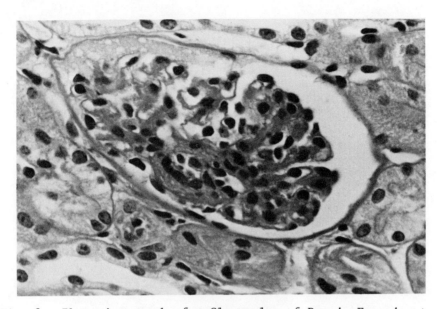

Fig. 8:   Photomicrograph of a Glomerulus of Dog in Experiment
          Shown in Fig. 7 at 14 Days after Nephrotoxic Serum
          Injection.(PAS Stain)
              Note marked endocapillary and mesangial proliferation
          than those   in Fig. 6.

        In these cases the pathogenetic significance of the coagula-
tion system was assumed and interruption or prevention of coagulation might give beneficial influence against the development of
nephritis.   From this point of view anticoagulant and/or platelet
suppressive agents were applied as reported (Michilson, P. and
Verberckmoe, R. 1966).   Kleinerman (1954) and Halpern et al (1965)
insisted that the application of heparin in the rabbit anti-GBM
nephritis showed good therapeutic effects and others reported
that preliminary administration of Warfarin saved the histological
changes as crescent formation and glomerular obliteration before
ànd after nephrotoxin injection (Vassali, P. and McCluskey, R.T.
1964; Vassalli, P. and McClusky, R.T. 1964b; Vassali, P. and Mc
Cluskey, R.T., 1971).   Naish et al. (1972) and Thomson et al.
(1976) also observed the same type of effect by defibrination
with Arvin.   However the anticoagulant therapy was not comprehended
throughly on several aspects.   Bone, et al. (1975) could not show
defensive effect against development of nephritis with heparin
in their experiment, in which proliferation of mesangial cells
and crescent formation might be enhanced and promoted by heparin
administration.   Border, et al. (1975), did observe the same type
of enhancement in histological change.   In our dog experiment
with Masugi nephritis, no effect was realized by heparin therapy.

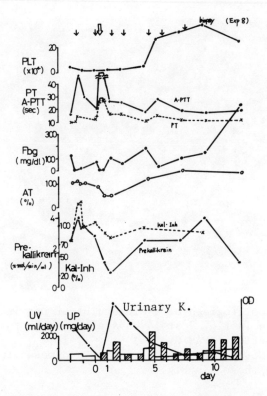

Fig. 9:   Blood Coagulation, Fibrinolysis, Plasma Prekallikrein
          and Urinary Kallikrein in Dog with Masugi Nephritis
          Treated with Defibrase
              Open arrow shows nephrotoxic serum injection and
          solid ones show defibrase injections.
              Urinary kallikrein was measured with TAME and
          indicated by optical density.
              For legends see those of Fig. 1 + 2.

We did observe that defibrination with defibrase in rabbit anti-
GBM nephritis invited intensive renal histological damage (Nakamura, K. 1977), and in the trials defibrination with snake venom
did not show any influence in the development of dog Masugi nephritis, nevertheless, fibrin deposition was only scarce in glomeruli.

          Some other mechanisms of these procedures may be respon-
sible for the development of nephritis. As to the change or
urinary kallikrein in Masugi nephritis, Glasser et al. (1976)

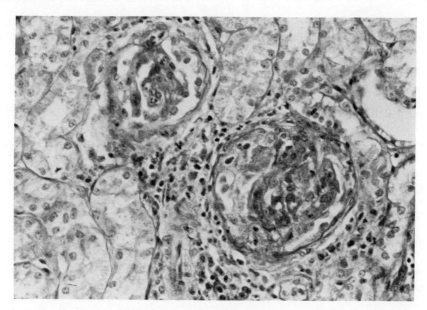

Fig.10: Photomicrograph of Glomerulus of Dog in Experiment Shown
in Fig. 9 at 14 Days After Nephrotoxic Serum Injection.
Note marked extensive glomerulonephritis with
hyalinization and crescent formation.

demonstrated the prompt and significant decrease of urinary kallikrein excretion following the induction of anti-GBM nephritis.
Werle et al. (1968), also found the decrease of urinary kallikrein
excretion in patients undergoing kidney transplant rejection, and
in our experimental nephritis in dogs, marked fluctuation of
urinary kallikrein excretion was observed. These results indicated possible involvement of the kallikrein-kinin system in
the course of parenchymal kidney diseases. The grade of proteinuria was not directly parallel with the fall in urinary kallikrein
excretion, and marked glomerular damages were proved in the cases
with fluctuation and decrease of urinary kallikrein excretion
which were evaluated as a sensitive indication of glomerular
injury in glomerulonephritis.

ACKNOWLEDGEMENTS

The authors express the grateful acknowledgements to Miss C.
Matsuga, C. Tahara, M. Morioka and N. Ohkuni for their laboratory
cooperation.

REFERENCES

Bone, J.M., A.J. Valdes, F.G. Germuth, Jr. and H. Lubowitz, 1975, Heparin therapy in anti-basement membrane nephritis, Kid. Intern. 8, 72.

Border, W.A., C.B. Wilson and F.J. Dixon, 1975, Failure of heparin to affect two types of experimental glomerulonephritis in rabbits, Kid. Intern. 8, 140.

Briggs, J.D., H.C. Kwaan and E.V. Potter, 1969, the role of fibrinogen in renal disease; III. Fibrinolytic and anticoagulant treatment of nephrotoxic serum nephritis in mice, J.Lab. Clin. Med. 74, 715.

Cade, J.R., A.M. DeQuesada, D.L. Shires, D.M. Levin, R.L. Hackett, G.R. Spooner, E.M. Schlein, M.J. Pickering and A. Holcomb, 1971, The effect of long term high dose heparin treatment on the course of chronic proliferative glomerulonephritis, Nephron 8, 67.

Cade, J.R., G.R. Spooner, E. Schlein, M. Pickering, A.M. DeQuesada A. Holcomb, L. Juncos, G. Richard, D. Shires, D. Levin, R. Hackett J. Free, R. Hunt and M. Fregly, 1973, Comparison of azathioprine, prednisone, and heparin alone or combined in treating lupus nephritis, Nephron 10, 37.

Glasser, R.J. and A.F. Michael, 1976, Urinary kallikrein in experimental renal disease, Lab. Invest. 34, 616.

Halpern, B., P. Milliez, G. Lagrue, A. Fray and J.C. Morard, 1965, Protective action of heparin in experimental immune nephritis. Nature, 205, 257.

Kincaid-Smith, P., B.M. Sakerand K.F. Fairley, 1968, Anti-coagulants in irreversible acute renal failure, Lancet 2, 1360.

Kincaid-Smith, P., M.C. Laver, K.F. Fairley and D.C. Mathews, 1970, Dipyridamole and anticoagulants in renal disease due to glomerular and vascular lesions, Med. J. Aust. 1, 145.

Kleinerman, J., 1954, Effect of heparin on experimental nephritis in rabbits, Lab. Invest. 3, 495.

McGiven, A.R., 1967, Blood coagulation and the effect of Warfarin treatment on renal disease in NZB/NZW mice, Br. J. Exp. Pathol, 48, 552.

Michilson, P. and R. Verberckmoe, Treatment of proteinuria with an anti-inflammatory drug, 1966, in: Abstr. II. Int. Cong.

Nephrol. (Washington. D.C.) p. 243.

Naish. P.. G.B. Penn. D.J. Evans and D.K. Peters, 1972, The effect defibrination on nephrotoxic serum nephritis in rabbits, Clin. Sci. 42. 643.

Nakamura, K., 1977, The role of coagulation and fibrinolysis in the development of renal disease, Jap. J. Nephrol. 19, 947.

Thomson, N.M., J. Moran, I.J. Simpson, 1976, Defibrination with ancrod in nephrotoxic nephritis in rabbit, Kid. Intern. 10, 343.

Vassalli, Pl and R.T. McCluskey, 1964-a, The pathogenetic role of fibrin deposition in immunologically induced glomerulonephritis, Ann. N.Y. Acad. Sci. 116, 1052.

Vassalli, P. and R.T. McCluskey, 1964-b, the pathogenetic role of coagulation process in rabbit Masugi nephritis, Am. J. Path. 45, 653.

Vassalli, P. and R.T. McCluskey, The pathogenetic role of the coagulation process in glomerular diseases of immunologic origin, 1971, in: Advances in Nephrology, Vol 1, eds. J. Hamburger, J. Crosnier and M.H. Maxwell (Year Book Medical Publishers, Chicago) p. 47.

Werle, R., R. Busse and A. Schmal, 1968, Über die kallikrein-ausscheidung im Harn des Menschen nach Nierentransplantation, Klin. Wochenschr. 49, 1315.

IMPROVEMENT OF GLUCOSE ASSIMILATION AND PROTEIN DEGRADATION BY BRADYKININ IN MATURITY ONSET DIABETICS AND IN SURGICAL PATIENTS

Matthias Wicklmayr, Gunther Dietze, Bernulf Gunther, Ingolf Bottger, Lothar Mayer and Peter Janetschek

Abteilung fur Stoffwechsel und Endokrinologie des Akademischen Lehrkrankenhauses Munchen-Schwabing, Kolner Platz 1, 8000 Munchen 40, GFR

INTRODUCTION

Impaired glucose assimilation and accelerated protein degradation are concomitant symptoms of insulin deficiency as in diabetes and also of reduced insulin sensitivity as during postoperative stress. Since it is known that kininogen levels are reduced in traumatic stress (1) and that kinin liberation is involved in the peripheral action of insulin (2,3), the influence of kinin infusion on carbohydrate tolerance and urinary nitrogen-excretion was investigated in normal and diabetic subjects and in surgical patients.

MATERIALS AND METHODS

Intravenous glucose tolerance tests (IGTT) (0.33 g glucose/kg body weight) were performed in 10 normal volunteers, in 20 metabolically healthy patients after abdominal surgery, in 10 chemical diabetics and in 10 maturity onset diabetics with and without additional intravenous infusion of bradykinin (BK). IGTT's were carried out first without BK and at least 3 days later with BK in the normals and diabetics after an overnight fast. In the 20 surgical patients the IGTT's were performed at the first and at the second day after operation. In 10 of the patients BK was infused at the first postoperative day (Group A) and in the other 10 patients at the second day (Group B). Glucose was injected into a peripheral vein as a 10% solution within 4 minutes. BK was infused as synthetic bradykinin (Sandoz AG, Nurnberg, GFR) at a dosage of 80 µg per hour, dissolved in 30 ml of physiological saline via infusion pump (Perfusor[R], Braun-Melsungen, GFR).

Samples were taken from venous blood (antecubital) 10 min after
the end of glucose injection for the determination of insulin (4)
and after 5, 15, 20, 25 and 30 min from capillary venous blood for
the determination of glucose (5). Urine volume for the enzymatic
determination of glucose (5) was collected after the injection
of glucose for one hour.

The influence of intravenous infusion of BK (80 µg/h) on fasting blood glucose concentration was studied for a period of 100
min in 9 maturity onset diabetics and in 5 healthy volunteers in
the postabsorptive state in a recumbent position. In another 9
maturity onset diabetics fasting blood glucose was measured under
identical condtions without BK.

In 10 patients after abdominal surgery urinary nitrogen excretion was determined at 12 hour intervals for the 12.-72. postoperative hour. BK was infused intravenously at a dosage of 80
µg/h from the 24.-48. hour. For the whole test period glucose was
infused at a constant rate of 150 g/24 h, water and electrolytes
as necessary. Amino acids have not been applied. The urine was
collected via catheterization of the bladder, which was prepared
for other reasons and not only for the study. Nitrogen concentration was determined according to a modified method of Kjeldahl (6).

The clinical data of all the collectives are listed in Table
1. The protocol for this study was reviewed and approved by the

TABLE 1.   CLINICAL DATA

SUBJECTS	TEST	n	AGE (YEARS)	HEIGHT (cm)	WEIGHT (kg)	BLOOD GLUCOSE (mM)	TRIGLYZERIDES[a] (mM)	CHOLESTEROL[a] (mM)
HEALTHY VOLUNTEERS	IGTT	10	28±2	172±3	71±5	4.38±0.19[a]	1.21±0.08	4.48±0.21
	BLOOD GLUCOSE	5	22±1	175±2	70±3	4.32±0.15[a]	1.27±0.11	4.37±0.28
CHEMICAL DIABETICS	IGTT	10	59±6	168±4	76±5	4.59±0.18[a] 8.06±0.29[b]	1.88±0.15	6.03±0.39
MATURITY ONSET DIABETICS	"	10	70±3	159±2	66±5	12.77±2.9[a]	2.58±0.62	5.85±0.95
	BLOOD GLUCOSE	9	65±5	164±3	69±4	8.61±1.07[a]	2.15±0.20	6.06±0.49
	"	9	69±6	166±4	72±5	12.84±2.6[a]	2.05±0.36	5.90±0.75
SURGICAL PATIENTS	IGTT	10	47±6	174±2	74±3	4.51±0.28[a]	-	-
	"	10	48±5	170±4	73±5	4.53±0.25[a]	-	-
	N-EXCRETION	10	56±9	169±6	65±6	4.47±0.21[a]	-	-

VALUES ARE INDICATED AS THE MEAN ± SEM. [a]AFTER AN OVERNIGHT FAST. [b]2 HOURS AFTER ORAL 100g GLUCOSE

Investigation and Ethical Committee of the Sonderforschungbereich
51 of the Deutsche Forschungsgemeinschaft according to the Code of
Ethics of the World Medical Association (7).

Standard statistical methods were employed (8) using Student's
t-test for paired and unpaired samples when applicable. All the
mean values are given with the sandard error of the mean (SEM).

RESULTS

BK, at the dosage used, did not influence blood pressure or
heart rate.

IGTT (see Figure 1).

BK did not influence the assimilation coefficient in the
normal healthy collective (k-value without BK 2.17 ± 0.21, with
BK 2.46 ± 0.28, p < 0.15).

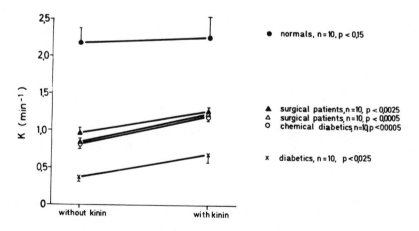

Figure 1.   Influence of bradykinin on intravenous glucose
            tolerance test in healthy volunteers, in surgical
            patients, in chemical and maturity onset diabetics.
            The values are indicated as the means ± SEM. For
            details see "Methods".

However, pathological k-value in chemical diabetics was improved from 0.81 ± 0.03 up to 1.21 ± 0.07 (p <0.0005). Maximal blood glucose concentration 5 min after the injection of the glucose load was not affected (without BK 12.88 ± 0.54 mM, with BK 12.62 ± 0.58 mM). BK did also not increase urinary glucose excretion (without BK 3.89 ± 0.65 mM/h, with BK 3.33 ± 0.68, p <0.1) or peripheral insulin levels (without BK 61.5 ± 5.6 µU/ml, with BK 58.0 ± 5.1).

BK improved assimilation coefficients in maturity onset diabetics from 0.37 ± 0.06 up to 0.69 ± 0.12 (p <0.025). Insulin secretion was not stimulated by BK (without BK 50.6 ± 4.8 µU/ml, with BK 49.9 ± 4.3 µU/ml). Maximal glucose concentrations 5 min after glucose injection were identical in both tests (without BK 13.31 ± 0.71 mM, with BK 13.84 ± 0.69 mM). However, urinary glucose loss was reduced by BK from 17.11 ± 3.80 mMol/h to 13.84 ± 0.69 mM/h (p < 0.005).

Glucose assimilation coefficient was improved in the surgical patients by the additional infusion of BK from 0.96 ± 0.08 to 1.27 ± 0.05 in group A (p < 0.0025) and from 0.85 ± 0.10 to 1.24 ± 0.12 in group B (p <0.005). Both collectives tended to reduce urinary glucose loss under the influence of BK (group A: without BK 3.91 ± 1.02, with BK 2.96 ± 0.75 mMol/h, p < 0.15; group B: without BK 7.52 ± 1.41, with BK 5.26 ± 0.26, p < 0.1). Peripheral insulin concentration did not differ between both days (group A without BK 59.7 ± 3.5 µU/ml, with BK 60.8 ± 7.5; group B without BK 57.7 ± 6.7 µU/ml, with BK 62.1 ± 5.3).

Fasting blood glucose concentration (see Figure 2).

Fasting blood glucose concentration of healthy volunteers was not affected by intravenous infusion of BK (basal value 4.62 ± 0.07 mM, after 100 min BK-infusion 4.59 ± 0.08). However, increased blood glucose levels were continuously reduced by BK in maturity onset diabetics from 12.82 ± 2.60 mM to 11.48 ± 2.47 mM (p < 0.0005). Thereby, peripheral insulin concentrations were not affected by BK (basal value 16.0 ± 2.6 µU/ml, 30 min BK-infusion 14.9 ± 3.2). Another collective of maturity onset diabetics (Table 1) showed no spontaneous change in blood glucose concentration during infusion of identical volume of physiological saline (basal 8.53 ± 1.09 mM, after 100 min 8.51 ± 1.04).

Urinary nitrogen excretion in surgical patients (see Figure 3).

Urinary nitrogen excretion obtained during the 12.-24. postoperative hour was found to be 4.0 ± 0.6 g/12 hr without BK. BK-infusion (24.-48. hour) exhibited no change during the first 12 hours (4.8 ± 0.7 g), however, during the second period (36.-48. hour) a significant decrease occured (2.2 ± 0.2 g, p < 0.01). After the stop of BK-infusion this effect lasted for the following 12 hours

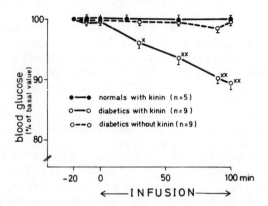

Figure 2. Influence of bradykinin on fasting blood glucose concentration in normals and in maturity onset diabetics at physical rest. For details see "Methods".

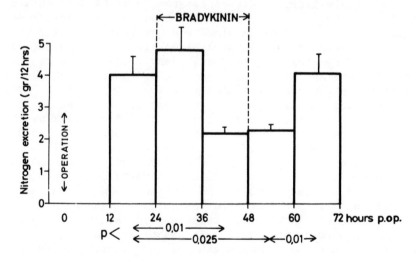

Figure 3. Effect of bradykinin on urinary excretion of nitrogen in surgical patients. For details see "Methods".

(2.3 ± 0.2 g, p < 0.025) and turned once more to increased excretion (4.1 ± 0.6 g, p < 0.01) during the 60.-72. hour interval.

DISCUSSION

In spite of increased insulin levels glucose assimilation is impaired during postoperative stress (9-11). From experiments in animal and man insulin sensitivity of the peripheral tissues, especially of skeletal muscle, was found to be reduced under these circumstances (10,12). One of the reasons discussed was a reduction of muscle glucose uptake due to catecholamine-stimulated glycogenolysis (10,13) or due to inhibition of glycolysis by increased intracellular content of citrate resulting from enhanced uptake of free fatty acids and ketones (14,15). In maturity onset diabetics impairment of peripheral insulin action also was discussed to be one of the events occuring at the beginning of the development of diabetes (14,16). Although all the insulin-antagonizing factors may be partly responsible, the total mechanism of this peripheral insulin resistance is not sufficiently clarified so far.

Recent investigations have shown that kinins have an insulin-like-activity (17,18) and that an insulin resistance may be precipitated by prevention of kinin liberation from kininogen in the resting and working skeletal muscle in man (2,3). Therefore, the present study was performed to investigate whether BK may improve carbohydrate assimilation under circumstances of reduced insulin sensitivity of the tissues. As was expected, pathological k-values of surgical patients and of chemical and manifest diabetics were normalized or improved and elevated blood glucose concentration was lowered by BK-infusion (see Figs. 1 and 2). Since no influence on blood pressure and heart rate was seen and since no change of k-values and glucose concentrations were found in the normal volunteers, an unspecific improvement of glucose tolerance as shown for some vasodilators (19) can be ruled out. BK did not work by changing the glucose pools or by increasing insulin secretion, as could be ascerted by identical blood glucose concentrations shortly after the end of the glucose injection and by identical peripheral insulin levels. In addition, k-values were not improved by BK-induced increased renal glucose loss; on the contrary, glucosuria was lessened slightly in accordance to the quicker disappearance rate of glucose from the blood. From these considerations we may conclude that improvement of k-values in diabetics and surgical patients were due to accelerated glucose assimilation in the peripheral tissues. Since it is known that kininogen levels are reduced in posttraumatic stress (1), one could speculate that disturbances in the kallikrein-kinin-system are the cause of impaired carbohydrate metabolism after surgery. Measurements of the levels of kallikrein, kininogen or kinin in diabetics of maturity onset type are not available so far. However, since BK had no effect on blood glucose concentration and on k-values in healthy volunteers one might suppose that kinin infusion led to substitution of a substance which is less present in the diabetic organism.

Another well known phenomenon occuring under surgical stress is stimulated protein-breakdown (20) which may also be a consequence of the insulin resistance mentioned above. Extremely high doses of insulin and accelerated infusion of substrates (21) are required to inhibit this increased protein-breakdown. It is in line with the improved glucose assimilation observed under BK (see Figs. 1 and 2), that BK was able to reduce urinary N-excretion by 50% (see Fig. 3). That reduced urinary nitrogen excretion was not observed at once during the first 12 hours of BK-infusion and that it persisted for 12 hours after cessation of BK-infusion may be explained by the fact that aminoacid combustion had to be replaced by glucose combustion which may be detected only after a considerable lag phase in urinary nitrogen excretion. Whether there was also a direct inhibitory action of BK on proteolysis cannot be ruled out by the data presented here.

ACKNOWLEDGEMENT

This work was dedicated to Prof. Dr. E.K. Frey and Prof. Dr. E. Werle. The authors are indebted to Prof. Fritz, Prof. Kraut, Prof. Mehnert and Prof. Wieland for valuable discussions and support. They wish to acknowledge the excellent technical assistance of E.A. Bauer, A. Bammert, E. Maerker, H. Kirschner and G. Drotleff. This work was supported by a grant from the Sonderforschungsbereich 51 of the Deutsche Forschungsgemeinschaft.

REFERENCES

1. Hirsch, E.F., Nakajima, T., Oshima, G., Erdos, E.G., and Herman, C.M. 1974. J. Surg. Res. 17: 147.
2. Dietze, G., Wicklmayr, M., Bottger, I., and Mayer, L. 1978. Hoppe-Seyler's Z. Physiol. Chem. 359: 1209-1215.
3. Wicklmayr, M., Dietze, G., Mayer, L., Bottger, I., and Grunst, J. FEBS-Letters, in press.
4. Bergmeyer, H.U., Bernt, E., Schmidt, F., and Stork, H. 1970. D-Blucose. Bestimmung mit Hexokinase und Glucose-6-phosphatdehydrogenase, in Methoden der enzymatischen Analyse, Hrsg. Bergmeyer, H.U., Band II, S. 1163, Weinheim: Verlag Chemie.
5. Herbert, V., Kam-Seng, L., Gottlieb, Ch.W., and Bleicher, S. 1965. J. Endocr. 25: 1375.
6. Parnas, J., and Wagner, R. 1921. Biochem. Ztschr. 125: 253-262.
7. World Medical Association. 1964. Declaration of Helsinki Br. Med. J. ii, 177-180.
8. Snedecor, G.W., and Cochran, W.G. 1967. Statistical Methods, 6th edn. pp. 59-61. Iowa State University Press, Ames. Iowa
9. Ross, H., Johnston, J.D.A., Welborn, F.A., and Wright, A.D. 1966. Lancet I: 563-566.

10. Wright, P.D., Henderson, K., and Johnston, J.D.A. 1974. Br. J. Surg. <u>61</u>: 5.
11. Wright, P.D., and Johnston, J.D.A. 1973. Br. J. Surg. <u>60</u>: 309.
12. Ryan, N.T., George, B.C., Egdahl, D.H. and Egdahl, R.H. 1974. Ann. Surg. <u>180</u>: 402.
13. Wicklmayr, M. and Dietze, G. 1978. Eur. J. Clin. Invest. <u>8</u>: 81–86.
14. Randle, P.J., Hales, C.N., Garland, P.B., and Newsholme, E.A. 1963. Lancet <u>I</u>: 785.
15. Gunther, B., Wicklmayr, M., Dietze, G., Schultis, K., Mehnert, H. and Heberer, G. 1978. Langenbeck's Archiv. Suppl. im Druck
16. Butterfield, W.J.H. and Whichelow, M.J. 1965. Diabetologia <u>1</u>: 43.
17. Dietze, G., and Wicklmayr, M. 1977. Klin. Wschr. <u>55</u>: 357.
18. Wicklmayr, M., and Dietze, G. 1977. Effect of oral kallikrein and intrabrachial-arterial bradykinin on forearm-metabolism in maturity onset diabetics. p. 299–308. <u>In</u>: Kininogenases. Hrsg. G.L. Haberland, J.W. Rohen and T. Suzuki. Stuttgart-New York: F.K. Schattauer-Verlag.
19. Heidreich, H., and Schirop, Th. 1975. Verh. Dt. Ges. Inn. Med. <u>81</u>: Tagung, 315.
20. Cuthbertson, D.P. 1932. Q.J. Med. <u>25</u>: 233–246.
21. Cahill, G.F. Jr., 1971. Diabetes <u>20</u>: 785–799.

AUTOREVERSAL OF BRADYKININ RESPONSE IN THE PERFUSED ISOLATED

CANINE HIND LIMB

Hans J. Wilkens and Nathan Back

Dept. Biochemical Pharmacology, School of Pharmacy

State University of New York, Buffalo New York 14260

Bradykinin lowers the systemic arterial blood pressure in all animal species tested (Haddy, Emerson and others, 1970). This hypotensive effect of bradykinin es the result of a decrease in total peripheral resistance, most probably at the arteriolar level (Baez and Orkin, 1963). However, organ responses are not uniform but display a pattern of selective vasoconstriction and vasodilation (Arcidiacono, Reininger and Sapirstein, 1966). A constriction of larger veins has been observed in rat subcutaneous tissue (Rowley, 1964) and in the rabbit ear (Guth, Bobbin and others, 1966). Also the larger veins in the visceral area appear to be constricted strongly by bradykinin (Tsuru, Ishikawa and Shigei, 1974). Several authors have reported that isolated blood vessels and some vascular beds perfused with artificial fluids respond to bradykinin with constriction (Guth, Cano and Jamarillo, 1963; Moog and Fisher, 1964; Shimamoto, Numano and others, 1966; Wiegershausen, 1966; Northover, 1967). Other have observed a hypertensive response to bradykinin in nephrectomized rats, and in rats with low blood pressure (Croxatto and Belmar, 1961; Croxato, Belmar and others, 1962). Subsequently, it was reported by us that bradykinin elicits pressure increases in the blood-perfused isolated canine hind limb when injected after a large dose of histamine (Back and Wilkens, 1968). This finding was followed by our observation that bradykinin is a potent vasoconstrictor in the isolated canine hind limb when a small amount (3 mg %) of Polyox FRA, a commercially produced high molecular weight ethylene oxide polymer, is added to the circulating blood (Wilkens and Back, 1974). Since neither the vasoconstrictor action in the presence of Polyox FRA, nor the pressor effect following histamine could be abolished by alpha adrenergic blockade, we suggested that bradykinin might act on two types of receptors.

577

We now present the results of three representative experiments showing that successive injections of sufficiently large doses of synthetic bradykinin alone result in autoreversal of its response in the constant flow blood perfused isolated canine hing limb.

METHOD

The limbs were perfused with autologous blood with the aid of a pump-oxygenator circuit as illustrated in Figure 1. With the pump output constant, changes in peripheral resistance were measured as changes in the perfusion pressure recorded onto a polygraph. Various doses of bradykinin were injected into the arterial side of the circuit close to the perfused limb and the elicited reactions recorded.

RESULTS

As shown in Figure 2, doses of bradykinin ranging from .01 to 1 mcg caused dose-dependent decreases in the perfusion pressure. A subsequent 10 mcg dose produced a fall in pressure no greater than the 1 mcg dose, thus indicating a maximum hypotensive response. Three successive 50 mcg doses administered thereafter elicited progressively diminishing hypotensive responses, followed by a rather quick recovery and a considerable pressure overshoot, so as to suggest a biphasic response. Two subsequent 100 mcg doses

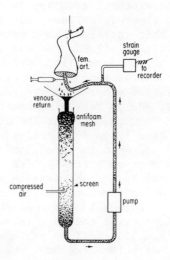

Figure 1.   Pump-oxygenator circuit for perfusion of isolated canine hind limb.

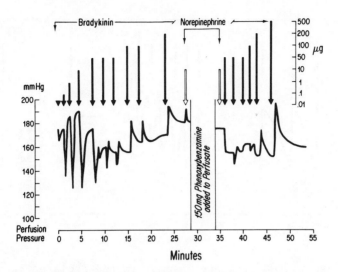

Figure 2.   Perfusion pressure changes in the isolated canine
            hind limb following administration of increasing
            doses of synthetic bradykinin (.01 – 500 µg) before
            and after alpha adrenergic blockade with phenoxyben-
            zamine, 150 mg. Biphasic bradykinin response is
            seen at the 50 µg dose with complete autoreversal
            at the 100 µg doses and higher.

and one 200 mcg dose caused no hypotensive response, but produced
instead significant increases in perfusion pressure. A similar
series of injections administered 13 minutes later, following the
administration of 150 mg phenoxybenzamine and two test doses of
norepinephrine, confirmed the persistence of the reversal phenomenon in the presence of alpha adrenergic blockade. The hypotensive response obtained at the beginning of the second series
of injections indicates that the reversal phenomenon is short
lasting if not maintained by frequent additional doses of bradykinin.

     In a similar experiment, illustrated in Figure 3, two doses
each of 10 and 20 mcg synthetic bradykinin injected at 20 minute
intervals effected maximal decreases in the perfusion pressure,
followed by a slow and continuous recovery. A subsequent 50 mcg
dose also elicited a maximal decrease, but resulted in a biphasic
recovery pattern, consisting of a sharp initial increase in the
perfusion pressure followed by a second decrease and a subsequent
slow return to the pre-injection level over a time period of
approximately 50 minutes. Another 50 mcg dose administered at
this time elicited a similar response, including the biphasic

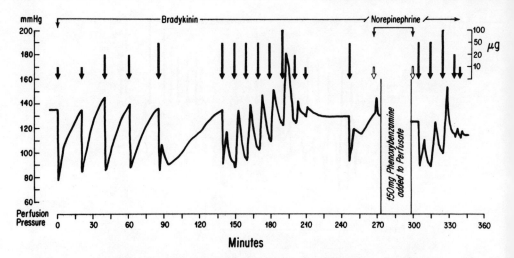

Figure 3. Perfusion pressure changes in the isolated canine hind
           limb following administration of increasing doses of
           synthetic bradykinin (10 - 100 µg) before and after
           alpha adrenergic blockade with phenoxybenzamine, 150 mg.
           Reversal of the hypotensive response can be seen occuring
           when the time interval between bradykinin injection
           was reduced from 20 minutes to 10 minutes. A dose of
           50 µg, given subsequently after a 30 minute interval,
           shows that the normal hypotensive response is restored.

recovery pattern, but four subsequent and more closely spaced doses
of 50 mcg and a 100 mcg dose injected at ten minute intervals
elicited progressive increases in the perfusion pressure well above
the pre-experimental level. Even two subsequent doses of 20 and
10 mcg produced dose related lesser increases. The hypotensive
response to a 50 mcg dose administered 35 minutes later again demonstrated the transience of the reversal phenomenon, whereas its
re-establishment following alpha adrenergic blockade by phenoxybenzamine once more displayed its independence from autonomic
nervous system mechanisms.

    A third hind limb perfusion experiment was designed to test
the premise that even large doses of bradykinin, when administered
during a state of maximal vasodilation produced by other potent
pharmacological agents, should be unable to effect a further decrease
in perfusion pressure, whereas the vasoconstrictor activity occuring
with the development of the autoreversal phenomenon might manifest
itself in the form of perfusion pressure increases. As seen in
Figure 4, a 1 mcg dose of bradykinin injected initially produced
a 32 mm Hg decline in perfusion pressure, followed by recovery.
Methacholine infused subsequently at a rate of .08 mg/min. lowered
the perfusion pressure by 37 mm Hg. Injections at this low pressure

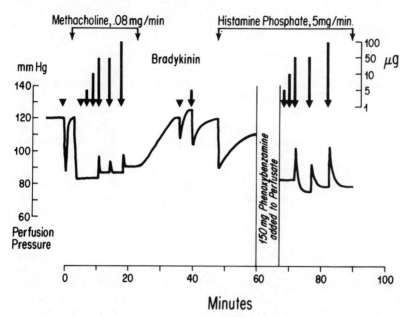

Figure 4.   The autoreversal of bradykinin response in the isolated
            canine hind limb in the presence of maximally hypo-
            tensive doses of methacholine, 0.08 mg/min and
            histamine diphosphate, 5 mg/mkn, respectively. Refer
            to text for further details.

level of 1, 5, and 10 mcg doses of bradykinin were without apparent
effect, whereas two subsequent doses of 50 mcg each, and one 100
mcg dose produced distinct increases in perfusion pressure. When
the methacholine infusion was discountinued, the perfusion pressure
gradually returned to the pre-experimental level, with bradykinin
in doses of 1 and 5 mcg again displaying its usual, if diminished,
hypotensive activity. After inducing once more a state of extreme
vasodilatation with the infusion of histamine phosphate at a rate
of 5 mg/min., and adding 150 mg phenoxybenzamine to the perfusate,
bradykinin in doses of 50 and 100 mcg again caused a rise in the
perfusion pressure.

                          DISCUSSION

     As to the interpretation of these findings, two possibilities
may be considered. The first one centers around the role of
bradykinin as an activator of the prostaglandin (PG) synthetizing
system (Terragno, Lonigro and others, 1972), and its dissimilar

effects in arteries and veins on the relative production of PGE
and of PGF. PGE is a dilator of peripheral resistance vessels in
all animal species tested (Nakano, 1973), whereas PGF has been shown
to exert potent venous and arteriolar constrictor activity in
several species, including the dog (Ducharme, Weeks and Montgomery,
1968; Emerson, Jelkes and others, 1971).

Incubation studies of isolated bovine mesenteric vessels
(Terragno, Crowshaw and others, 1975) have shown the control rates
of PG synthesis to be similar in arteries and veins, and the ratio
of PGE/PGF to be identical in both types of vessels, namely 2:1.
Addition of bradykinin to the incubate resulted in a two- to three-
fold increase in the overall rate of PG synthesis, which was
accounted for by a selective increase of PGE in the arteries (PGE/
PGF ratio 5.7:1), and of PGF in the veins (PGE/PGF ratio 0.3:1).

A possible explanation for the selective release by bradykinin
of PGE from arteries and of PGF from veins has been provided by
studies of Leslie and Levine (1973), and Lee and Levine (1974) on
the enzymic conversion of PGE to PGF by PGE 9-keto-reductase in
mesenteric arteries and veins. The results of these studies led
to the suggestion that activation of this enzyme in veins but not
in arteries might account for these discriminating effects of
bradykinin (Lee and Levine, 1974).

Evidence supporting this view has been obtained by Wong,
Terragno and others (1977), who found that the bradykinin-induced
increase of PGF production in bovine mesenteric veins correlated
with a significant increase in PGE 9-keto-reductase activity,
whereas the increase of PGE production in the arteries was accompanied
by a correspondingly lower activity level of this enzyme. The
further demonstration by these authors that indomethacin treatment
of the mesenteric venous strips abolished the intramural generation
of prostaglandin and prevented the increase in venous tone elicited
by bradykinin, lends support to the suggestion made by McGiff,
Itskovitz and others (1976), that other vessels which constrict in
response to bradykinin may do so as a result of increased synthesis
of PGF or a related substance. Commenting on the possible role of
a PG in mediating the effects of kinin on renal salt and water
excretion, the latter authors have postulated that the capacity
of kinin to activate PGE 9-keto-reductase is determined by the
state of sodium balance. In contrast to the constrictor effect of
bradykinin in veins, which appears to be mediated exclusively by a
PGF compound, the PGE-mediated vasodilatator effect in arteries is
additive to a direct vasodilatator action of bradykinin.

In summary, an explanation of the phenomenon of bradykinin
autoreversal with reference to the prostaglandins needs to consider
the vascular responses to bradykinin as the end result of one or

more of four different actions:
1. direct vasodilator action in most arteries
2. activation of prostaglandin synthetase system
3. activation of PGE 9-keto-reductase
4. preferential production of PGE in arteries and PGF in veins.

As expected, in the perfused isoalted canine hind limb, increasing doses of bradykinin elicited dose-dependent decreases in the
perfusion pressure up to a point at which a maximal hypotensive
response was obtained, suggesting that all available receptors for
the PGE and bradykinin molecules had been saturated. Assuming
furthermore a PGE/PGF ratio of approximately 6:1, similar to that
found in isolated bovine mesenteric arteries (Terragno, Crowshaw
and others, 1975), it would appear that any overt hypotensive
response to bradykinin should mask an antogonistic PGF-mediated
vasoconstrictor component. Considering the PGE/PGF ratio of 6:1,
this vasoconstrictor component would be correspondingly small at
doses of bradykinin up to and including ED 100; i.e., the lowest
dose eliciting a maximal hypotensive response. This dose presumably
produces just enough PGE molecules to saturate all available receptors. With further increasing single or cumulative doses, however,
one should expect the vasoconstrictor effect to become more and more
evident on the assumption that any PGE molecules produced in excess
of the receptor capacity will have no additional effect, whereas
the simultaneous increase in PGF molecules should lead to the
occupation of more and more vasoconstrictor receptors. As a result,
the combined vasodilator actions of PGE and bradykinin itself should
become progressively antagonized and possibly overcome. This view
conceivably could serve as a basis for explaining the changes of
vascular behavior observed in the perfused canine hind limb; namely
the gradually diminishing hypotensive responses at the beginning,
the dose-dependent overt increases in perfusion pressure at the
end, and the transitional biphasic response pattern in between.

Alternatively, these same phenomena could be explained by
postulating the existence of two types of bradykinin receptors, a
high affinity vasodilator (K_1) receptor and a low affinity vasoconstrictor (K_2) receptor. Given such disparate affinities, bradykinin first would occupy all available K_1 receptors and thus exert
a maximal vasodilator action. Thereafter, any molecules offered
in excess of the K_1 saturation limit would be free to interact
with the K_2 receptors and initiate an antagonistic vasoconstrictor
action. As the doses of bradykinin are increased and more and
more K_2 receptors are being occupied, this antagonistic action
would gradually become prominent, expressing itself initially by
progressively diminishing hypotensive responses and thereafter by
visible increases in pressure. A dual receptor interrelationship
closely resembling the above has been described by Ariens, Simonis
and Von Rossum (1964) as a type of noncompetitive auto-antagonism.

While it is not possible without further study to establish the validity of either one of the aforementioned interpretations, it may be stated with some degree of assurance that the findings here reported afford an expanded view of the potential role for kinins under both normal and pathological conditions. In particular, since kinin release occurs in states of underperfusion (Wilkens, Back and others, 1970), it would appear entirely possible that the demonstrated ability of kinin to behave as a potent vasoconstrictor might be displayed in the course of shock, so as to act as an important counter regulatory mechanism. This might be true especially in the presence of histamine which appears to facilitate the development of kinin reversal (Back and Wilkens, 1968). Furthermore, the kinin destroying enzyme carboxypeptidase N is inhibited in a slightly acidic milieu such as may be encountered in underperfused tissues, whereas kinin continues to be liberated rapidly under the same conditions (Edery and Lewis, 1962; Lewis, 1963; Wilkens, Back and others, 1970). Interestingly, in a recent study of the kinin system in patients with acute myocardial infarction, Hashimoto, Hamamoto and others (1974) found that plasma kinin levels were high in the survivors, as opposed to the non-survivors who showed lower levels of kinin. In a subsequent study, (Hashimoto, Wanka and others, 1975) it was shown that the higher kinin levels in the survivors of acute myocardial infarction were due to diminished kinin destroying activity.

SUMMARY

The vascular effects of synthetic bradykinin were studied in perfused isolated canine hind limb preparations. Repeated low doses of bradykinin or high doses administered at sufficiently long time intervals elicited dose-related hypotensive responses. In contrast, administration of bradykinin at short time intervals led first to diminishing hypotensive responses followed by frank increases in perfusion pressure. This autoreversal of bradykinin response tentatively was explained on the basis of known effects of bradykinin on prostaglandin synthesis with specific reference to $PGF_{2\alpha}$.

ACKNOWLEDGEMENTS

This work was supported in part by USPHS grant #HE-11492, National Heart Institute.

REFERENCES

Arcidiacono, F.G. Reininger, E.J. and Sapirstein, L.A. (1967).
    4th European Conference on Microcirculation, p. 29. Basel
    & New York: S. Karger.
Ariens, E.J., Simonis, A.M. and Von Rossum, J.M. (1964). Molecular
    Pharmacology. p. 293. New York & London: Academic Press.
Back, N. and Wilkens, H.J. (1968). Pharmacology of Hormonal Poly-
    peptides and Proteins, Eds. L. Martini, R. Paoletti and N.
    Back. p. 486. New York: Plenum Press.
Baez, S. and Orkin, L.R. (1963). Anesthesiol, 24: 568-579.
Croxatto, H. & Belmar, J. (1961). Nature (London), 192: 879-880.
Croxatto, H., Belmar, J., Pereda, T. and Labarca, E. (1962). Acta
    physiol. lat. amer., 12: 19-21.
Ducharme, D.W., Weeks, J.R., and Montgomery, R.G., (1968). J.
    Pharmacol. Exp. Ther. 160: 1-10.
Edery, H. and Lewis, G.P. (1962). Brit. J. Pharmacol. 19: 299-305.
Emerson, T.E., Jelkes, G.W., Daugherty, R.M. and Hodgman, R.E.
    (1971). Am. J. Physiol., 220: 243-249.
Guth, P.S., Bobbin, R., Cano, G. and Amaro, J. (1966). Hypotensive
    Peptides. Eds. Erdos, E.G., Back, N. and Sicuteri, F. p. 396,
    Berlin, Heidelberg and New York: Springer Verlag
Hashimoto, K., Hamamoto, H., Tijima, N. and Kumura, E. (1974).
    Proc. VII World Congress of Cardiology, Buenos Aires.
Hashimoto, K., Wanka, J., Kohn, R.N., Wilkens, H.J., Steger, R. and
    Back, N. (1976). Kinins: Pharmacodynamics and Biological Roles.
    Eds. Sicuteri, F., Back, N. and Haberland, G.L. p. 245.
    New York: Plenum Press.
Lee, S.C. and Levine, L. (1974). J. Biol. Chem., 249: 1369-1375.
Leslie, C.A. and Levine, L. (1973). Biochem. Biophys. Res. Comm.,
    52: 717-724.
Lewis, G.P. (1963). Ann. N.Y. Acad. Sci., 104: 236-249.
McGiff, J.C., Itskovitz, K.D., Terragno, A. and Wong, P. (1976).
    Fed. Proc., 35: 175-180.
Moog, E. and Fischer, J. (1974). Arch. Exp. Path. Pharmak., 249:
    384-392.
Nakano, J. (1973). Prostaglandins: Pharmacological and Therapeutic
    Advances. Ed. M.F. Cuthbert. p. 41. Heinemann, London.
Northover, B.J. (1967). Brit. J. Pharmacol., 31: 483-493.
Rowley, D.A. (1964). Brit. J. Pathol., 45: 56-67.
Shimamoto, T., Numano, F., Fijita, T., Ishioka, T. and Atsumi, T.
    (1966). Hypotensive Peptides, Eds. Erdos, E.G., Back, N. and
    Sicuteri, F. p. 506. Berlin, Heidelberg and New York: Springer
    Verlag.
Terragno, D.A., Crowshaw, K., Terragno, N.A. and McGiff, J.C.
    (1975). Circ. Res., 36 and 37 (Suppl. I): 76-80.
Terragno, N.A., Lonigro, A.J., Malik, K.U. and McGiff, J.C. (1972).
    Experentia, 28: 437-439.
Tsuru, H., Ishikawa, N. and Shigei, T. (1974). Japn. J. Pharmacol.
    24: 931.

Wiegershausen, B. (1966).   3rd Internat. Congr. Pharmacol., Abstracts,
    p. 186.
Wilkens, H.J., Back, N., Steger, R. and Karn, J. (1970).   Shock:
    Biochemical, Pharmacological, and Clinical Aspects. Eds.
    Bertelli, A. and Back, N. p. 201. New York: Plenum Press.
Wilkens, H.J. and Back, N. (1974). Arch. int. Pharmacodyn., 209:
    305-313.
Wong, P.Y., Terragno, D.A., Terragno, N.A., and McGiff, J.C. (1977).
    Prostaglandins, 13: 1113-1125.

DYNAMICS OF KALLIKREINOGEN UNDER HEMODIALYSIS

T. Shiba, M. Igarashi*, T. Obara**, S. Takeuchi,
T. Asada*, J. Takatsuka, and M. Matsumoto

The 2nd Dept. of Surg., *Dept. of Biochem., and ** Dept.
of Urology, School of Medicine, Toho Univ., Tokyo

ABSTRACT

There are many complications due to hemodialysis, causes of
which seem to lie under disorders of the coagulation system,
fibrinolytic system, and kinin system. Therefore, it is important
to understand the dynamics of these systems during hemodialysis.
Accordingly, kallikreinogen, plasminogen, plasmin inhibitors,
contact factor, antithrombin, and prothrombin were assayed during
the experimental dialysis, experimental ultrafiltration and
clinical hemodialysis.

Plasmin inhibitors decreased remarkably by dialysis. They
then recovered the pre-dialytic values as time went on. Kallikreinogen did not show any definite tendency immediately after
the beginning of dialysis, but two hours later its value rather
increased relative to the pre-dialytic value. It was supposed
that this increase was caused by reactive hyperproduction due to
gradual consumption of kallikreinogen.

Contact factor slightly decreased by dialysis, whereas prothrombin and antithrombin decreased apparently. When hemodialysis is practiced, it is necessary to fully realize that the
coagulation system, fibrinolytic system, and kinin system might
lose their balance.

INTRODUCTION

It has been known that hemodialysis sometimes accompanies
hematuria, retinal bleeding, or increase in capillary permeability.

It is generally accepted that the principal cause of such a hemorrhage diathesis is to be sought in heparin. However, considering
the action mechanism of heparin, it is not reasonable to attribute
the hemorrhage diathesis only to heparin. Apart from this,
correlation between the blood coagulation system and kinin system
has been noted recently. It is natural to suppose that both blood
coagulation system and kinin system are activated by hemodialysis.
However, there has been no report on the systemic determination
of changes in these systems during the hemodialysis.

Thus, experimental and clinical investigations of systemic
dynamics of the coagulation system, fibrinolytic system and kinin
system which have been carried out will be reported here.

MATERIALS AND METHODS

Clinical Cases

Eleven patients with chronic glomerulonephritis, two with
polycystic kidney, one with chronic pyelonephritis, and one with
diabetic nephropathy were subjected to the present experiments.

Apparatuses

Hollow Fiber Dialyzer (b/HFU-1) (Dow Chemical Co.) was used
for the experimental dialysis and ultrafiltration. A twin-coil
hemodialyzer (Kolf type) was used for the clinical hemodialysis.

Dialysate

Kindaly II made by Shimizu Seiyaku was used.

Experimental Dialysis

The experimental dialysis was carried out using the apparatus
as shown in Fig. 1. The sample was 200 mℓ fresh human plasma.
The flow rate of the sample was adjusted between two and three mℓ/
min by Holter pump. The experimental dialysis was made in the
recirculating system and the batch system. Various investigations
were made with the sample before and after dialysis.

Experimental Ultrafiltration

The experimental ultrafiltration was carried out using the
apparatus as shown in Fig. 2. The sample was 10 mℓ fresh human
plasma. Vacuum of 300 mmHg was made and held for five minutes.
Plasma, whole plasmin in the ultrafiltrate, and whole plasmin
inhibitors were assayed before and after ultrafiltration.

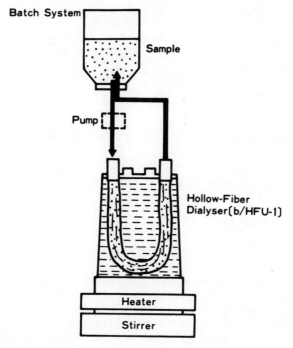

Figure 1.   Experimental Dialysis Apparatus

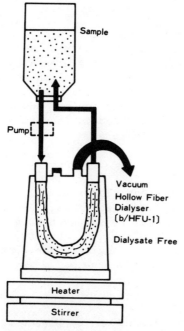

Figure 2.   Experimental Ultrafiltration Apparatus

Clinical Hemodialysis

Clinical hemodialysis was carried out by the system as shown in Fig. 3. Various investigations were made with the samples taken out of the inlet side (A) and the outlet side (V) before and after dialysis.

Plasminogen (Whole Plasmin)

Plasminogen was assayed by the TNP mehtod by Igarashi et al. (1976)(Table 1).

Plasmin Inhibitors (Whole Plasmin Inhibitor)

Plasmin inhibitors were assayed by the TNP method of Igarashi et al. (1976) (Table 2).

Kallikreinogen

Kallikreinogen in plasma was activated by adding dextran sulfate to plasma. Benzen-prolyl-phenyl-arginyl-paranitroaniline-chloride was used as the substrate. Paranitroaniline separated from the substrate by kallikrein was determined by the intensity of the absorption spectral line at 405 nm. Then kallikreinogen was calculated by means of the standard curve (Table 3).

Antithrombin

Blood was taken out of both the inlet and outlet sides and plasma was prepared. By heating the plasma at 53°C fibrinogen was removed from the plasma. Since this plasma contained heparin, heparin was removed by means of the column chromatography using protaminagarose. After adding thrombin of known concentration to this plasma, the fibrinogen solution was added and the clotting times were determined. Antithrombin in plasma was calculated using the standard curve (Table 4).

Contact Factor

Contact factor deficient plasma of 0.1 mℓ was added to 0.1mℓ plasma which had been diluted ten times, then further a reagent for PTT of 0.1 mℓ was added. After incubating this mixture at 37°C for eight minutes, 0.025 M $CaCl_2$ solution of 0.1 mℓ was added and the clotting times were measured. The contact factor was calculated using the standard curve.

Prothrombin

Prothrombin was separated out of plasma after the Masaki method (1968) and assayed by the two-stage method.

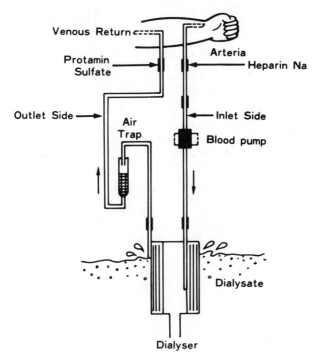

Figure 3. System of Hemodialysis

TABLE 1. ASSAY PROCEDURE OF PLASMINOGEN

1)	SK-activation step	
	Fraction III	0.4 mℓ
	SK (1,000 v/ mℓ)	0.1 mℓ
	Incubated at 38℃ 25 min	
2)	Fibrinogenolysis step	
	The activated solution	0.5 mℓ
	Fibrinogen (2.0%)	1.0 mℓ
	Incubated at 38℃ 10 min	
	TCA (10%)	1.5 mℓ
	Centrifuged at 3,000 rpm for 10 min	
	The supernatant was washed with ether	
3)	Colorimetry	
	The residue	1.0 mℓ
	PBS (0.5 M, pH 7.5)	2.0 mℓ
	TNBS (0.12%)	1.0 mℓ
	Incubated at 38℃ 90 min	
	HCl (17%)	1.0 mℓ
	The color was read at 340 m/u against the control (Zero time activation)	

TABLE 2. ASSAY PROCEDURE OF PLASMIN INHIBITOR

1)	Plasmin preparation step	
	Plasminogen (4 cu/mℓ) or	
	Fraction III	0.3 mℓ
	SK (1.000u/mℓ)	0.1 mℓ
	Incubated at 38℃ 25 min	
2)	Inhibitor binding step	
	The plasmin solution	0.4 mℓ
	Fraction I (inhibitor)	0.1 mℓ
	Incubated at 38℃ 25 min	
3)	Fibrinogenolysis step	
	The above mixtur	0.5 mℓ
	Fibrinogen (2.0%)	1.0 mℓ
	Incubated at 38℃ 10 min	
	TCA (10%)	1.5 mℓ
	Centrifuged at 3,000 rpm for 10 min	
	The Supernatant was washed with ether	
4)	Colorimetry	
	The residue	1.0 mℓ
	PBS (0.5 M, pH 7.5)	2 0 mℓ
	TNBS (0.12%)	1.0 mℓ
	Incubated at 38℃ 90 min	
	HCl (17%)	1.0 mℓ
	The color was read at 340 m/u against the control (Zero time activation)	

TABLE 3. ASSAY METHOD OF KALLIKREINOGEN

Plasma 0.5 mℓ

Dextran sulfate 0.5 mℓ   } 0℃
                                      →
                                   10min ↓

                                   20 μl
                                      ↓

Substrate   37℃
   ≀   } 1.0 mℓ ————→ 10% A₂OH 2.5 mℓ
Buffer   10min
                                      ↓

                                   absorbancy at 405 nm

Dextran sulfate

　　MW: 500,000

　　1.5 mg/H₂O dℓ

Substrate

　: benzen-prolyl-phenyl-arginyl-paranitroaniline-chloride

　: was dissolved by Tris-Imidazol Buffer (pH7.9)

　: 0.37 mM

TABLE 4.   MEASUREMENT OF ANTITHROMBIN IN HEPARINIZED PLASMA

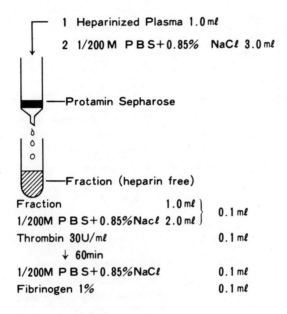

1 Heparinized Plasma 1.0 mℓ

2 1/200 M P B S + 0.85% NaCℓ 3.0 mℓ

—Protamin Sepharose

—Fraction (heparin free)

Fraction	1.0 mℓ	
1/200M P B S+0.85%Nacℓ	2.0 mℓ	0.1 mℓ
Thrombin 30U/mℓ		0.1 mℓ
↓ 60min		
1/200M P B S+0.85%NaCℓ		0.1 mℓ
Fibrinogen 1%		0.1 mℓ

RESULTS

Dynamics of Plasminogen, Plasmin Inhibitors, and Kallikreinogen
under Experimental Dialysis

Plasminogen and plasmin inhibitors in blood and the dialysate
were assayed before dialysis, and two and four hours after starting
dialysis. The amounts of plasminogen were not varied by dialysis.
On the other hand, plasmin inhibitors in blood remarkably lessened
by dialysis. In the dialysate activities of plasmin inhibitors
were not detected in all specimens (Fig. 4).

Kallikreinogen was assayed before dialysis, and at 5, 15, 30,
60, 120, and 180 minutes after starting dialysis. No obvious
change was detected in the amount of kallikreinogen in blood
(Fig. 5).

Dynamics of Plasminogen and Plasmin Inhibitors under Experimental
Ultrafiltration

The sample was 10 mℓ plasma. This plasma reduced to 5 mℓ by
ultrafiltration and 5 mℓ ultrafiltrate was obtained. In plasma
before the ultrafiltration, plasminogen of 3.2 cu/mℓ (total :

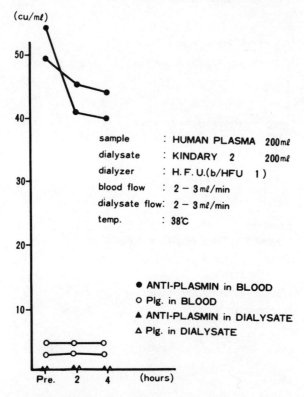

Figure 4.   Dynamics of Plasminogen and Plasmin Inhibitor under
            Experimental Dialysis

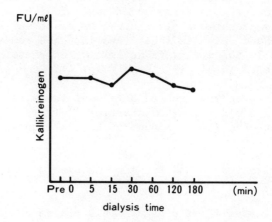

Figure 5.   Dynamics of Kallikreinogen under Experimental Dialysis

32 cu/10 mℓ) and plasmin inhibitors of 62 cu/mℓ (total : 620 cu/10 mℓ) were detected. After the ultrafiltration plasminogen in plasma was 6.0 cu/mℓ (total : 30 cu/5 mℓ) and plasmin inhibitors were 72 cu/mℓ (total : 360 cu/5 mℓ). In the ultrafiltrate, there was no plasminogen, while plasmin inhibitors of 32 cu/mℓ (total : 160 cu/5 mℓ) were detected (Table 5).

Changes in Plasminogen under Hemodialysis

Plasminogen in fifteen cases were assayed twenty times in all. Even pre-dialytic values of plasminogen were a little lower than the normal one. At two and four hours after beginning dialysis plasminogen was assayed with blood taken out of the inlet and outlet sides. The values were nearly equal to the pre-dialytic value (Fig. 6).

Changes in Plasmin Inhibitors under Hemodialysis

Plasmin inhibitors were assayed 20 times with 15 patients. In most of the cases the obtained values were lower than the normal one. The assay of plasmin inhibitors in blood taken out of the inlet and outlet sides at two hours after the beginning of dialysis indicated that all cases had smaller values than the pre-dialytic values. However, the specimens at four hours recovered the pre-dialytic value in most cases. Comparisons were made between the values obtained on the inlet side and the outlet side at two and four hours after beginning dialysis and it was disclosed that there were apparent decreases in plasmin inhibitors in the outlet side specimen at both times (Fig. 7).

TABLE 5. DYNAMICS OF PLASMINOGEN AND PLASMIN INHIBITOR
UNDER ULTRAFILTRATION

	Volume (mℓ)	Inhibitor (Total)	Plasminogen (Total)
		cu/mℓ	cu/mℓ
pre. U.F. Plasma	10	62 (620)	3.2 (32)
post. U.F. Plasma	5	72 (360)	6.0 (30)
Ultrafiltrate	5	32 (160)	0 (0)
Inactivated Inhibitor	100		

b/HFU-1. 38°C.—300 mmHg. 5 min

plasma Flow 2 mℓ/min

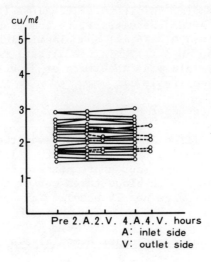

Figure 6. Changes in Plasminogen under Hemodialysis

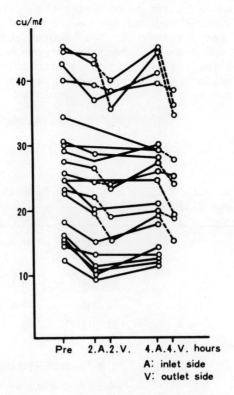

Figure 7. Changes in Plasmin Inhibitor under Hemodialysis

Changes in Kallikreinogen under Hemodialysis

Kallikreinogen was assayed with blood taken out of the inlet and outlet sides at immediately after the dialysis began and two hours afterwards with seven patients. A comparison between the first and second assays disclosed that most cases increased kallikreinogen very slightly in the two hours. A comparison between the values obtained on the inlet and outlet sides did not show any definite trend, although there were quite a few cases which showed a low value on the outlet side relative to the inlet side (Fig. 8).

Changes in Antithrombin under Clinical Hemodialysis

Blood was taken out of the inlet and outlet sides during the dialysis and antithrombin in the specimens were assayed. Seven cases were handled. A comparison between antithrombin in blood from the inlet side and that from the outlet side showed that in all cases the latter was less than the former (Fig. 9).

Changes in Contact Factor under Hemodialysis

Contact factor was assayed with five cases. Blood was taken out of the inlet and outlet sides during the dialysis and the contact factor in the blood was assayed.

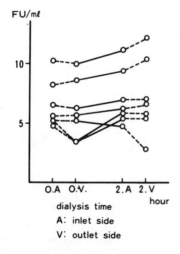

Figure 8. Changes in Kallikreinogen under Hemodialysis

A comparison was made between contact factor values obtained from the inlet and outlet sides. One case out of five showed apparent decrease in the contact factor in the outlet side specimen. A very slight decreasing trend was observed with four other cases (fig. 10).

Changes in Prothrombin under Hemodialysis

Prothrombin was assayed with blood taken out on the inlet and outlet sides during dialysis. Six cases were dealt with. A comparison made between obtained values of prothrombin from inlet side and outlet side disclosed that the latter was less than the former (Fig. 11).

DISCUSSION

Much attention has been attracted in recent years to the activation of the coagulation system and the kinin system by activation of Hagemann factor. This fact implies the possibility that the coagulation system and the kinin system are activated simultaneously by hemodialysis. Many symptoms are observed among complications of hemodialysis which are caused by disorders of the coagulation system, fibrinolytic system, and kinin system. For this reason, it is important to obtain accurate knowledge of the coagulation system, fibrinolytic system and kinin system

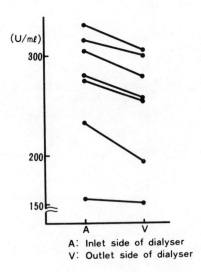

A: Inlet side of dialyser
V: Outlet side of dialyser

Figure 9.   Changes in Antithrombin under Hemodialysis

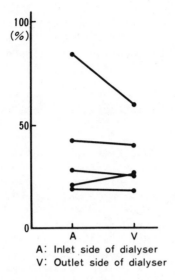

A: Inlet side of dialyser
V: Outlet side of dialyser

Figure 10. Changes in Contact Factor under Hemodialysis

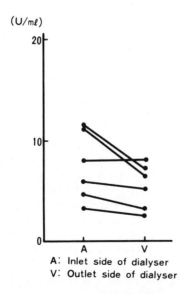

A: Inlet side of dialyser
V: Outlet side of dialyser

Figure 11. Changes in Prothrombin under Hemodialysis

during hemodialysis.

In the present studies, blood was taken during the clinical hemodialysis on the inlet and outlet sides almost simultaneously. Therefore, the difference between the values assayed on both sides is considered to be caused by dialysis. On the other hand, not only dialysis but also reactions of living body have serious effects on the changes in the assayed value on the inlet side or the outlet side with the passage of time. The results of the present assay should be analyzed by taking this fact into consideration.

Plasminogen did not change much by any of the experimental dialysis, ultrafiltration, and hemodialysis. On the other hand, plasmin inhibitors apparently decreased by each of the experimental dialysis, ultrafiltration, and hemodialysis. Also, it was observed that a part of plasmin inhibitors was dialyzed by ultrafiltration. This ultrafiltration method is often applied to patients in order to clinically control body water. It is not necessary to mention that decrease in plasmin inhibitors is caused not solely by dialysis. Adhesion of plasmin inhibitors on the dialysis membrane and inactivation of plasmin inhibitors would also be the causes. Practically no change occurred in kallikreinogen by the experimental dialysis. No consistent trend was observed in the relationship between the values obtained on the inlet side and outlet side during dialysis. The kallikreinogen value two hours after starting hemodialysis was apparently larger, very slightly though, than the value immediately after starting hemodialysis. This increase might be reactive hyperproduction; that is, hemodialysis might induce very gradual consumption of kallikreinogen. The decrease in contact factor due to hemodialysis supports this idea. Moreover, it is said that antithrombin III which is the principal part of antithrombin in terms of both amount and activity is an inhibitor of the coagulation system as well as an inhibitor of the kinin system. Therefore, decrease in antithrombin due to hemodialysis may indicate not only activation of the coagulation system due to hemodialysis but also activation of the kinin system.

It is a fact that hemodialysis causes decrease in plasmin inhibitors, activation of contact factor, and decrease in antithrombin. Decrease in plasmin inhibitors makes activation of the fibrinolytic system easy. As it is already known, it is possible for plasmin to activate the kinin system. Decrease in antithrombin makes activation of the coagulation system easy. There is a possibility that the fibrinolytic system is activated by some reason and further the kinin system is activated.

When hemodialysis is practised, it is necessary to recognize always such pathological physiology.

REFERENCES

Igarashi, M., M. Matsumoto, S. Takeuchi, T. Asada, 1973. Assay
    Method of Fibrinolysis by Affinity Chromatography. J. Med.
    Technol. 17: 713.
Masaki, Y., 1968. Purification of Prothrombin. Seikagaku 40: 890.
Shimada, K., M. Igarashi, T. Asada, 1971. A New Assay Method for
    Heparin - heparin cofactor method. J. Med. Soc. Toho. 18: 939.
Shiba, T., 1976. Influence of Fibrinolytic and Antifibrinolytic
    Factors on Fibrinolysis. J. Jap. Coll. Angiol. 16: 241.
Webster, M.E. and I. Innerfield. Interrelationship of Human Plasma
    Kallikrein and Plasmin in Inflammation. Enzymol. Biol. Clin.
    3: 129.

ALTERED URINARY EXCRETION OF HUMAN KININASE ACTIVITY IN ACUTE

MYOCARDIAL INFARCTION

A. Greco, G. Porcelli, A.G. Rebuzzi, M. Di Jorio,
M. Ranieri and L. Ranalli

Istituto di Patologia Medica and Istituto di Chimica,
Facoltà di Medicina, Università Cattolica S. Cuore, Roma
and Centro Chimica Recettori del C.N.R. Roma, Italy

ABSTRACT

This study concerns the determination of levels of human urinary kininase excretion in acute myocardial infarction (AMI). The results obtained by a biological method show that there is a significant reduction of the enzymatic activity in patients affected by AMI
in comparison with normals (6.4 $\pm$ 0.4 ng of destroyed bradykinin/
min. versus 164.4 $\pm$ 31.4 ng; $P < 0.001$), while urinary kallikrein excretion was close to normal values.

INTRODUCTION

The kallikrein-kinin system seems to have an active role in the
maintenance of blood pressure. A decrease of urinary kallikrein excretion in essential hypertensive patients (Margolius et al., 1971,
Adetuyibi and Mills, 1972; Greco et al. 1974; Abe and Seino, 1975)
has been observed. The kallikrein-kinin system is related to the
presence of kininases. In fact, circulating kinins are very quickly inactivated by kininases (Erdös and Yang, 1970; Vane, 1969).
This study describes the values of human urinary kininase and
kallikrein excretion in acute myocardial infarction (AMI).

MATERIALS AND METHODS

20 normal male subjects (38 ± 2.4 mean ± S.E.) and 19 male patients (40 + 1.5) with a clinical diagnosis of AMI were included in
the study. The patients, hospitalized in the coronary care unit of
Catholic University of Rome, Italy, were carefully monitored for
arrhythmias and changes in cardiac status. All had an AMI within the
preceding 12 hours. The diagnosis was made on the basis of clinical
history, elevation of enzymes (SGOT, SGPT, LDH, CPK) and of diagnostic
electrocardiographic changes. All patients were non-obese, without
known liver diseases and none had diabetes or other endocrinopathies.
None had received diuretics or cortical steroids. A 24-hour urine
collection with controlled cretinine was made in the first period and
the sample was kept in toluene at 4°C for not longer than a week for
testing the enzymes. Eleven of the patients studied were relatively
stable with uncomplicated myocardial infarction. Four patients were
hypotensive, but without other clinical features of circulatory
shock. Four male patients in circulatory shock had a systolic blood
pressure of less than 100 mm Hg. None of the patients mentioned in
this study died. Many of the patients had an indwelling venous catheter in the superior vena cava for the first 4 or 5 days, which was
kept patent by a slow drip of 5% glucose in water. Urinary kallikrein was assayed according to the Porcelli and Marini-Bettōlo
method (1978); the results are expressed in esterase units (E.U.).
Kininase activity in urine was measured according to the Porcelli et
al. method (1978) based on the enzymatic properties of the urinary
kininase which, when incubated with bradykinin, destroys it. The
amount (in ng) of destroyed bradykinin/min. was estimated on isolated
rat uterus. Calculations of statistical significance have been
performed with the Student's t test.

RESULTS

Fig. 1 summarizes our results. The urinary kallikrein mean
level in the normal subjects resulted in 19.6 ± 1.8 E.U./24 hours;
the urinary kallikrein mean level of the infarcted patients resulted
in 18.0 ± 1.7 E.U./24 hours. The urinary kininase activity (mean ±
SE) in the normal subjects was 164.6 ± 31.4 ng of destroyed brady-
kinin/min.; in AMI the urinary kininase activity was 6.4 ± 0.4 ng; P
< 0.001). The analysis of the data did not indicate differences be-
tween the various groups of infarcted patients.

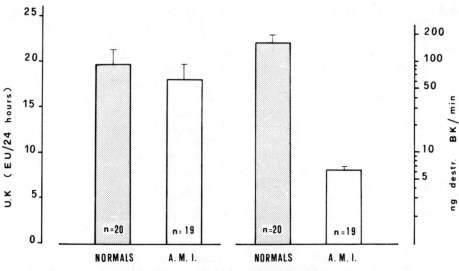

Fig. 1. Kininase in AMI

DISCUSSION

The importance of the kallikrein-kinin system during myocardial ischemia and associated pain was demonstrated (Brunch et al., 1963; Sicuteri et al., 1966; Hashimoto et al., 1974).

Plasma kininases were studied particularly by Hashimoto et al., 1974 and 1975, demonstrating a significantly reduced activity in the AMI survivor patients. In the human urine of a group of AMI patients there was evidence of strong daily oscillations in the amount of kallikrein activity (Del Bianco et al., 1976). In our study we did not observe significant differences in the urinary kallikrein excretion between normal subjects and patients with or without hypotension. Normal urinary kallikrein excretion and low or, in the majority of cases, no urinary kininase activity, can suggest that during AMI the kinins which are formed are not rapidly destroyed.

REFERENCES

Abe K. and Seino M. (1975), Urinary kallikrein excretion and sodium metabolism in hypertention, Life Sci., 16, 817

Adetuyibi A., Mills I.H. (1972), Relationship between urinary kallikrein and renal function, hypertension and excretion of sodium and water in man. Lancet 2, 203

Burch G.E., De Pasquale N.P. (1963), Bradykinin, Amer. Heart J., 65, 116

Del Bianco P.L., Curradi C., De saint Pierre G., Nava G., Sicuteri
    F. (1976) Urinary excretion of kallikrein following myocardial
    infarction, Adv.Exp.Med. and Biol., 70, 329
Erdös E.G.,Yang H.Y.T. (1970) Kininase; in: Hdb of exp.pharmacol.,
    Vol. XXV, Ed. by Erdös E.G., Springer verlag, N.Y. p.289
Greco A., Porcelli G., Croxatto H.R., Fedeli G., Ghirlanda G. (1974)
    Ipertensione arteriosa e callicreina urinaria, Min.Med. 65, 3058
Hashimoto K., Hamamoto H., Tajima N., Kimura E. (1974), Changes in
    Kinin system and hemodynamics in acute myocardial infarction - a
    clinical study - VII World Congress of Cardiology, Buenos Aires
Hashimoto K., Wanka J., Kohn R.N., Wilkens H.J., Steger R., Back N.
    (1976) The vasopeptide kinin system in acute clinical cardiac
    diseases; Adv.Exp.Med.Boil., 70, 245
Margolius H.S., Geller R., Pisano J.J., Sjoerdsma A.(1971), Altered
    urinary kallikrein excretion in human hypertension, Lancet 2,
    1063
Porcelli G., Di Jorio M., Ranieri M., Ranalli L., D'Acquarica L.
    (1978), Method for measurement of human urinary kininase activity
Porcelli G., Marini-Bettòlo G.B. (1978), A simplified method to pre-
    pare human urinary samples for measurement of kallikrein esterase
    activity, V Nat.Congress of Ital. Soc. of Clin.Biochem., Rome,
    October 1978
Sicuteri F., Antonini F.M., Del Bianco P.L., Franchi G.C., Curradi
    c. (1972) pre-kallikrein and kallikrein inhibitor in plasma of
    patients affected by recent myocardial infarction, Adv.Exp.Med.
    Biol., 21, 445
Vane J.R. (1969), the release and fate of vasoactive hormones in
    the circulation, Brit.J.Pharmacol., 35,209